Disaster Medicine · Volume 3
Editors: R. Frey and P. Safar
Sub-Editors: P. Baskett, K. Stosseck, P. Sands, J. Nehnevajsa

D1698006

Cold and Frost Injuries — Rewarming Damages
Biological, Angiological and Clinical Aspects

Hans Killian

In cooperation with T. Graf-Baumann

With 89 Figures

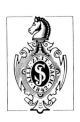

Springer-Verlag
Berlin Heidelberg New York 1981

Prof. Dr. Hans Killian
Riedbergstraße 24
7800 Freiburg/Br.

ISBN 3-540-08991-8 Springer-Verlag Berlin Heidelberg New York
ISBN 0-387-08991-8 Springer-Verlag New York Heidelberg Berlin

Library of Congress Cataloging in Publication Data.
Killian, Hans, 1892–
Cold and frost injuries.
(Disaster medicine; v. 3)
Includes bibliographical references and index.
1.Frostbite. 2.Cold-Physiological effect.
I. Title. II. Series. [DNLM: 1. Frostbite cold–Adverse
effects. 2. Cold climate. W1 DI727 v.3 / WG 530 K48ca]
RC88.5.K54   616.9'88'1   80-26958
ISBN 0-387-08991-8 (U.S.)

Typesetting: SatzStudio Pfeifer, Germering
Printing and binding: K. Triltsch, Würzburg
2127/3321   543210

Contents

Preface

This first manuscript on cold injuries was written in the period 1945–1946 as the result of personal experience gained in the winter months of the years 1941–1943 on the Northern Front in Russia and subsequent experimental work at the "Chirurgische Universitätsklinik" in Breslau (Wroclav) between 1943 and 1945. The intention at the time of writing was to present a summary of our experiences, so that they might serve as a basis for further scientific and clinical work. The manuscript has continually been revised and brought up to date. For purely external reasons publication has been delayed until today.

Our experience of cold preservation and of increased resistance to oxygen deficiency in chilled tissue, acquired during the winter periods of the Second World War in Russia, served as a basis for the development of local *cryanaesthesia* and *hibernation,* which retroactively furthered to a considerable degree our knowledge of cold and frost injuries. See my monograph on the biology and clinical treatment of the cold injury and general loss of temperature, which appeared separately in 1966 and discusses all biological changes. A comprehensive report on cold injuries was written in English in 1952 at the instigation of Captain A. R. Behnke jr. USA (M.C.), (not available commercially).

Even today it must be admitted that the ultimate cause of damage to tissues and cells due to cold is not properly known, and the question, under what conditions cold preserves or necrotises, is not completely cleared, even though cold effects have been used increasingly in cryotherapy in recent years.

The following monograph is concerned with local cold injuries and frostbite in its early stages, not 'however' with later effects and their assessment, which will be the subject of a separate work.

After a period of over 30 years, in which our knowledge has been stagnating and there has been no opportunity for treatment, the experiences of the latest Himalaya expeditions with the use of isovolaemic haemodilution now offer new possibilities to help us to understand cold injuries, and these may also have a favourable effect on treatment.

December 1980   Hans Killian

Introduction

As part of the body's attempt to resist cold with the aim of maintaining thermostability, in other words a positive heat balance, the organism is more ready to sacrifice its extremities than to allow a drop in blood temperature in the body area with its essential organs. Except in the case of an increase in the metabolism due to hormonal influence, and the production of additional heat in the case of danger (especially in the region of the striped muscles) a *centralisation of the circulation* is achieved by a reflex contraction of the peripheral blood vessels and of the small arteries of the limbs, which results in a drop in limb temperature and encourages them to cool down.

The question, whether the human organism possesses qualities which make it more sensitive than other warm-blooded animals with regard to loss of temperature in the whole body and especially in the skin, has been investigated in the last 10–20 years, in particular by English, American, Canadian and French authors (Hiestand 1950; Andjus 1951, Giaja 1952–1954; Smith 1957; Kayser 1933–1959). Some German (e.g. Adler 1920) and Russian authors have also contributed to this research work. The experiments were aimed at comparing the behaviour of a real hibernator with that of other mammals. It was found that the former, as a whole, were considerably more resistant to oxygen deficiency than all other large warm-blooded animals and that their nervous systems, e.g. for respiration, continue to function. Only the newborn warm-blooded animal and the human infant show noticeable resistance to oxygen deficiency in the first 4-6 days after birth. This corresponds to the behaviour of a real hibernator during the winter period (see Eisentraut's diagram in the monograph on loss of temperature). Homeothermal heat regulation only has a limited functional capacity. From a certain critical temperature, which varies according to the animal, onwards there is a sharp drop in the blood and body temperatures. If a negative change in the heat balance occurs, there is an increased danger not only to the life of the particular individual, but especially in that the exposed peripheral tissue may not be preserved. Local cold injuries can occur without the general body temperature being affected to any appreciable degree.

It is, however, normally the case that a critical disproportion between heat emission and input in the exposed areas is the result of a disturbed or defective general resistance to cold (general loss of temperature). The thermostability of a part of the body can only be maintained it the blood-stream is supplied with a sufficient number of thermal units (calories). The loss of heat from a limb is therefore not only dependent on the effect of external cold, i.e. on thermosteresis, but it is also determined by the general circulatory and metabolic state of the body, which undergoes considerable changes during the second to fourth stages of cooling (Fig. 1).

During cooling the extremities are already in danger in Phase II of the cold resistance reactions. The effect of Phase III is unfavourable because it marks the beginning of signs of decompensation in the heat regulation and a negative change in the heat balance as

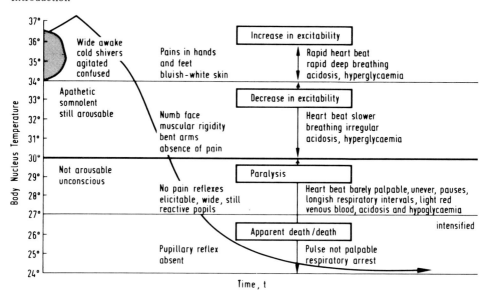

Fig. 1. Phases of general hypothermia according to Grosse-Brockhoff Killian and Souchon. (From Neureuther 1978)

from about 35⁰ C blood temperature (even earlier when the organs are not functioning properly). The danger becomes very acute in Phase IV, due to circulatory failure and arrythmia with the possible development of auricular and ventricular fibrillation. Ventricular fibrillation generally starts at a body temperature of 27° to 28°C and means absolute danger to life. There is also the possibility of the patient collapsing during rewarming (Brendel 1957, 1958, 1961, 1973, 1977), since the warming up phase is never a mirror image of the cooling phase.

Shivering and the centralisation of the circulation associated with it determines the fate of some limbs. The most severe forms of frostbite occur in states of general loss of temperatrue, permanently disturbed heat regulation and of apparent death. Thus it is possible to explain why after cold injuries in the mountains or on polar expeditions additional peripheral frostbite is nearly always observed. It is similar in the case of the wounded or other casualties transported in the cold.

It must be assumed that the physiology of heat balance is wellknown. The essential physiological changes which take place during a general loss of temperature are presented in the following Tables; for all individual factros have an effect on the skin and the limbs (Tables 1 and 2).

The discovery that none of the reactions of physical and chemical resistance to cold occur in isolation but have a mutual influence on each other appears to be of great importance.

We owe the more recent results of the research on the physiological bases of hypothermia mainly to Thauer and Brendel (1932), Messmer (1972, 1975, 1976 a–c, to be published), Messmer and Schmidt-Schönbein (1972), Messmer and Sunder-Plassmann (1973), Messmer et al. (1971, 1972 a, b, 1973, 1975, 1976 a, b) Sunder-Plassmann et al. (1971, 1972 a, b, 1976) etc. New basic information has been obtained from a large

Table 1. Changes in respiration and circulation with loss of body temperature

Blood temperature (°C)	Phase I 37°	Phase II 36° 35° 34° 33°	Phase III 32° 31° 30° 29° 28°	Phase IV (final state) 27° 26°	25° Or	Recovery, rewarming
Whole circulation	Normal	Increased as a reaction to cold	Increasing centralisation of the circulation, spasms of the peripheral arteries due to cold	No circulation in the extremities, heart failure		Gradual recovery
Arterial blood Pressure and Amplitudes	Normal	Increasing by 10 - 20 mm Hg	For a long time high, then dropping with a decrease in the amplitudes	Auricular flutter AV-nodal rhythmn, extension of the conduction time, block type of sinus and AV nodes, i.e. of ventricular and intravenous conduction system — Ventricular fibrillation	Death from ventricular tachycardia and ventricular fibrillation (children and infants more resistant)	Low values, no amplitudes
Heart rate	Normal	An initial slight increase in frequency, then onset of bradycardia		Low		Gradually increasing
Venous pressure	Normal	Slightly increased Slightly increased	Sinking	Low		Gradually increasing
Pulse rate	70	80-90 70 60	40 Becoming irregular and continuing to drop	Total arrythmia		Gradually becoming regular, rate increasing
Cardiac output	Normal	Initial increase, then slight drop	Renewed, constant increase with bradycardia	High, including heart failure		Great drop to below initial value
Minute volume	Normal	Slightly increased	Increased then a sharp drop	Very low, no longer measurable		Increasing moderately
Peripheral resistance	Normal	A slight drop then increasing	Very marked	High, including heart failure		Dropping sharply, then slowly increasing

3

Table 1. continued

Blood temperature (°C)	Phase I 37°	Phase II 36° 35° 34° 33°	Phase III 32° 31° 30° 29° 28°	Phase IV (final state) 27° 26° 25°	Or Recovery, rewarming
Volume of blood flow	Normal	Gradually Increasing	Greatly reduced	Greatly reduced	Very slow increase
A. – v. O_2 difference	Normal	Constantly reduced		Very slight (bright red venous blood)	Sharp increase, increased oxygen requirement
Erythrocyte storage	Normal	More or less unchanged — Increased contraction of spleen	Maximum Spleen contraction	Maximum contraction of the spleen	Gradual increase
Cerebrospinal pressure	Normal	Increasing High	Probably dropping again	Probably very low	Gradually increasing
Oxaemia	Normal	Increased fixing of O_2 to Hbg.	Decreasing dissociation instability of Oxy-Hb.	Release of oxygen to tissue made difficult due to decreased requirement	Phase of relative hypoxaemia, caused by great O_2 requirement
Respiration	16 - 18 min	20-24 min — 14-16 min	Rate dropping below 10 — Irregular, possibly Cheyne-Stokes type	Up to and including respiratory standstill	Spontaneous breathing and increase in rate, possibly above initial value
O_2 – Capacity (Vol %)	Normal	Increasing slightly	Increasing	Relatively high	Compensation
O_2 Saturation	Normal	100 %	98 % - 100 %		Recovery
Total CO_2 (Vol %)	Normal	Decreasing slightly	Increasing drop	Probably unchanged	Compensation
Cell volume in %	Normal	Still normal	Slightly increasing	Relatively high	Compensation
White blood corpuscles	Normal	Still normal	Apparent leucopenia (possible obstruction in the lungs)	Apparent drop in leukocytes	Compensation

Table 1. continued

Blood temperature (°C)	Phase I 37°	Phase II 36° 35° 34° 33°	Phase III 32° 31° 30° 29° 28°	Phase IV (final state) 27° 26° 25°	Or	Recovery, rewarming
Red blood corpuscles	Normal	Initial increase in no. of erythrocytes	Increased release from erythrocyte depots — Then drop No. of erythrocytes	Apparently relatively high value due to loss of plasma caused by lowered resistance		Gradual compensation
Sites of blood production	Normal	Increased activity (reticulocytes, erythroblasts)	Deformation, globular-form, with pseudopodien, fixation on endothel, aggregation	Probably inactive		Increased
Blood platelets	Normal	Still normal	Apparent drop in no. of blood platelets	No longer present		Return
Reflexes	Normal	Slightly increased	Growing increase but not pathological — Slowly becoming sluggish, and the no longer present	Centrally controlled relaxation		Gradual return of muscle tonus and movement
Trembling caused by cold		Trembling	Gradual stiffening of the striped muscles, muscle numbness, great increase in muscular tonus, increasing muscular rigidity	Muscular rigidity		Gradual return
Viscosity of the blood and plasma	Normal	Slightly reduced or normal	Growing increase due to shift of water to tissue	Specific weight of blood also high		Gradually becoming normal
Coagulation factor	Normal	Still normal	Apparently increased activity of the thrombocinase and prothrombin	Apparently high		Probably limited coagulation for some time due to high heparin accumulation

Compiled according to reference data

5

Table 2. Biochemical changes with general loss of temperature (cold accidents)

Blood temperature (°C)	Phase I 37°	Phase II 36° 35° 34° 33°	32°	Phase III 31° 30° 29°	Final Phase or 28° 27° 26° 25°	Rewarming
Glycogen store	Normal	Mobilisation, increased secretion (adrenaline effect)	Increasing requirement and secretion	Subsequent hypoglykaemia	Mostly low values According to length and degree of exhaustion complete depletion of glycogen depots	Gradual recovery
Na^+	Normal	Hardly changed				
Cl^-	Normal		Beginning of a decrease in the blood level			
Cl^{++}	Normal	Hardly changed		Migration to the cells	Possible sequelae of acidosis: high concentration in the cells, depletion in blood and extracellular areas, growing disturbance in the permeability which should only move in one direction possibly preoedemas (in the extremities possibly oedemas)	Gradual compensation of the mostly slight electrolyte imbalance
K^+	Normal	Hardly changed or slightly increasing in the serum				
Ca.	Normal	Gradual drop in Ca level in the extra-cellular areas and in the blood. Increase in the cells. Noticeable increase in the blood plasma with a decrease in the erythrocytes. An initial migration of potassium from the cells, an increase in the potassium level in the blood an in the extracellular areas.				Gradual compensation

Table 2. continued

Blood temperature (°C)	Phase I 37°	Phase II 36° 35° 34° 33°	32°	Phase III 31° 30° 29°	Final Phase or 28° 27° 26° 25°	Rewarming
Hgb	Normal	Unchanged				
Protein plasma	Normal	Unchanged	Moderate decrease	Hypoproteinaemia, possibly albuminuria to the tissue	Low protein values Low oncotic pressure	Slow recovery to normal state
Lactic acid	Normal	Increase in the blood level. Hyperlactacidaemia		decrease: hypolacta-cidaemia	Mostly hypolactaci-daemia with long exposure to cold	Relatively speedy recovery
Pyruvic acid	Normal	Slight initial drop	Similar to lactic acid			Compensation
Inorganic phosphorous	Normal	Unchanged	In general unchanged, occasionally slightly high	No considerable change		Compensation
Plasma bicarbonate	Normal	Unchanged	Mostly unchanged, sometimes slightly low			
Alkali reserve	Normal	Unchanged	Gradually dropping	Respiratoric and metabolic acidosis	Low values	Compensation.
Adrenaline Noradrenaline Cortin	Normal	Increased secretion		Acidosis	Generally low values	Recovery
Thyroxine	Normal	Increase in secretion, activity, and metabolic rate	Growing exhaustion	Greater consumption with longer exposure to cold and exhaustion of reserves	Exhaustion, possible organic changes after longer exposure	Gradual compensation
Water balance	Normal	Hydraemia of the blood (decrease in the viscosity)	Gradual migration from the bloodstream increase in viscosity	Exhaustion in cases of longer exposure	Possible signs of exhaustion and inactivity	Slow recovery
Blood urea level mg %	Normal	Unchanged		In cases of longer exposure preoedemas	Mostly low values	Compensation

Table 2. continued

Blood temperature (°C)	Phase I 37°	Phase II 36° 35° 34° 33°	32°	Phase III 31° 30° 29°	Final Phase or 28° 27° 26° 25°	Rewarming
Rest – N mg %	Normal	Little change	Growing increase	Decreasing values	Generally low values	Gradual compensation
Blood – p^{++}	Normal	Unchanged	Gradually increasing acidosis			Same
Blood liposis and glycerine	Normal	Hardly changed	Gradual increase		Recovery values	Slow compensation
Blood sugar	Normal	Increase	Hyperglycaemic phase sometimes great increase		Acidosis	Compensation
Adrenaline Noradrenaline	Normal	Increased delivery	Periphere Vasoconstriktion	During long cold Exposition diminution Adrenalin and Norandrenalin Reserves and organic changes		Slow recovery
Insulin, Thyroxin	Normal	Increased delivery	Increase of Metabolism	Progressive decrease of metabolisme		Slow compensation
Cortin	Normal	Increased delivery				Compensation

number of animal experiments (warm-blooded animals in deep narcosis) for optimal rewarming and resuscitation, even though this knowledge obtained from animals cannot automatically be applied to human beings after cold injury. One thing, which is certain, is that the organism's resistance to an abnormal loss of heat due to the effects of severe, exogenous cold is a much more complex process than was so far assumed.

A drop in the temperature of the skin as the result of an insufficient blood supply (adrenaline and noradrenaline secretion) lowers the heat gradient to the temperature of the environment and thus reduces the loss of heat by radiation, conduction and convection. If vasoconstriction due to cold becomes too vigorous and lasts too long, it may, of course, lead to ischaemia, intravascular stasis, aggregation of the blood constituents, an increase in the plasma viscosity, failure of the microcirculation and to a blockage of the venous drainage vessels. A disturbance in the permeability of the blood vessels may occur as well as the formation of oedemas, which during the rewarming phase encourages oxygen deficiency and the asphyxiation of the tissues.

In every case the general condition of the heart and circulation remains of decisive importance for the success of the rewarming process.

Brendel et al. discovered that the heart rate follows to about 20°C (in animals) the drop in the nuclear temperature almost in a straight line, below that level, however, (sometimes even earlier) ventricular fibrillation commences. At 10° C the cardiac muscle only contracts occasionally, weakly. This resembles the condition which the author has observed in the final stage of chloroform poisoning. Here the heart reaches maximum dilation and produces only single, worm-like contractions, losing all pumping capacity. The heart should be, however, contracted under the influence of cold. Brendel associates the presence of fibrillation with intracardiac temperature differences (right to left), an assumption which other authors question. The fibrillation also occurs as a result of an increase in the excitability of the spinal reflexes. According to Brendel (1957, 1958, 1961, 1973, 1977) a thermal stimulus of the skin of the back at 20°C blood temperature clearly leads to positive reactions produced by the spine, a temporary increase in the heart rate and in the arterial blood pressure in already paralysed cerebral centres (Fig. 2) This is evidence of a far higher resistance to cold of the spinal reflex centres compared with those of the brain.

The maintainance of spinal reflexes in spite of considerable internal loss of temperature has the effect that, despite reduced cardiac output, the arterial mean pressure still remains relatively high for a long time. It must be considered as the result of a paralysis of the vasomotor centre, caused by cold, with subsequent vasodilatation and the influence of peripheral cold receptors which are still intact, together with vasoconstriction produced by the spine. This relatively high mean arterial blood pressure should not lead to false conclusions about the true state of the circulation, for at the same time the volume of blood flowing is already extremely confined, the strain on the heart due to increased viscosity considerably greater and the cardiac output much lower. There are, accordingly, a number of sources of danger which may affect rewarming, if the latter is carried out incompetently and too hurriedly. Brendel refers to this in particular in his warning about the possibility of a hyperthermic collapse occurring. The effect of intensive, exogenous heat on the skin at about 30°C is to incapacitate the reactions of the peripheral cold receptors, which leads to an acute drop in blood pressure resulting from cerebral paralysis caused by the cold. This can easily lead to a circulatory breakdown and collapse. Conse-

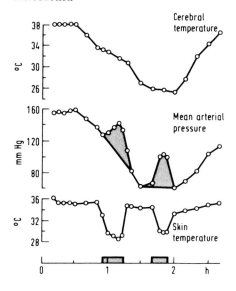

Fig. 2. Influence of a local peripheral cold stimulus (*shaded time interval*) on the reactions of arterial blood pressure during isolated cooling of the brain and normal temperature of the trunk. (From Brendel 1957)

quently there is a sudden, increased reflux of large quantities of cold blood from the extremities to the centre of the body as a result of a decrease in the vascular tone and of dilatation, so that a "rescue collapse" occurs. From the physiological point of view Brendel et al. misgivings concerning rapid rewarming after loss of temperature are justified to a considerable extent, in practice, however, one is mostly obliged to accept the risk of a collapse due to over-heating, as the "rescue collapse" is much more dangerous and has cost many people their lives after a sea rescue.

Another consequence of loss of temperature is an increase in the viscosity of the plasma and of the blood as a whole as a result of its being constricted, an increase in the blood cells (contraction of the spleen), and an increase in the haematocrit, which the heart with its reduced cardiac output, has to cope with. The microcirculation, which is already impaired, thus deteriorates further.

The plasma viscosity already increases considerably in vitro when the temperature falls. In vivo there is an additional increase in the number of red blood corpuscles. The most favourable haematocrit value for the oxygen carrying capacity dependent on it is considered to be 0.3 Maximum values of 0.6–7 may be reached and there is an additional, abnormal loss of water to the outside and to the tissue caused by emigration. According to Krueger and Blumel (1977a, b) the plasma volume decreases by about 11%. Not only is the number of the erythrocytes increased but also their volume due to the cold and their ability to deform is reduced. The growth of the volume of the red cells is the result of a "temperature dependent inhibition of the active cation transport". An impediment or a failure of the so-called sodium pump occurs. The sodium (NaCl) remains in the cells while the potassium migrates to the extracellular areas.

These changes may, of course, be reversed during the rewarming phase, it can, however, happen that after the reopening of the vascular system the blood potassium level rises to such an extent that it causes ventricular fibrillation or at least may help it to develop. In addition, the disturbance of the microcirculation everywhere in the organism may lead to respiratory acidosis due to the metabolic state and to the suppression of breathing, i.e. a drop in the hydrogen ion concentration with its effect on the oxygen dissociation characteristic.

Short-term loss of temperature is tolerable as the experience of numerous cold injuries and heart operations with hibernation have shown. The function of the heart and circulation return to normal after rewarming. This applies in particular to the heart rate, the cardiac output and all changes in the blood. Several measures can be taken to speed up compensation and the risk of ventricular fibrillation can be reduced by rewarming gradually. Whereas in the past only hot baths (39°C) were reccommended to warm the body or in the case of the polytraumatised, hot packs, (warm packs according to Hibler) used, and in Russia in 1941–1942 the author gave warm infusions (5–7% glucose etc.) of hot sweet drinks (41°–43°C), today we have at our disposal a series of other effective methods of rewarming patients, which can even work in cases of unconsciousness and cardiac arrest caused by the cold. Apart from localised short wave therapy (Hirsch et al. 1977; also Leitner and Kronberger 1977), gastric lavages with hot solutions, caned out by Lee et al., as early as 1959, transperitoneal dialysis of the stomach and also artificial respiration with warm damp air (Lloyd et al. 1972; Shanka 1975) were considered to be effective. The lavage of the pericardium with a warm isotonic saline solution or with Ringer's solution seems to be of particular importance in the case of cardiac arrest due to the cold.

What exceptional rescue work can thus be achieved is proved by an impressive incident reported by Höflin (1977) at the congress of alpine rescue physicians in Innsbruck in 1976.

After an avalanche disaster a man of about 40 was found buried about 3 feet under the snow. He was unconscious, unhurt, was breathing spontaneously but weakly and could still move to a certain extent. The rescuer tried to resuscitate him. During the attempt to insert a catheter into his vein the heart came to a standstill. External cardiac massage was the next step and the administration of 10 milliliters of sodium bicarbonate. Mouth to mouth resuscitation and cardiac massage were continued during air transportation shortly after, until arrival at hospital. As the helicopter was equipped with an electrocardiograph it was possible to detect ventricular fibrillation during the flight. An attempt to intubate was at first unsuccessful. After admission to hospital the anaesthetist immediately took over further treatment. He measured a rectal temperature of 22°C. It was therefore not possible to defibrillate (lower threshhold around 26°C). It was decided to perform a thoracotomy and the heart was warmed by lavage of the pericardium with Ringer's solution at 38°–39°C. The heart then began to beat again but during the rewarming process cold blood flowed from the extremities back to the centre of the body, so that once again the heart stopped beating. In all about 30 litres of warm isotonic saline solution were used for pericardial and also gastric lavages. Afterwards heart and lungs began to function normally again. Two days later the patient could be extubated and after 3 weeks discharged fit for work and without any sign of brain damage.

A similar report of Hackl-Haid et al. from 1978. A 51 year old man has a bad fall in the Alps: succedan-fractures on the left side with pneumothorax, multiple contusions and wounds, fracture of the radius left side, second and third degree frostbites in the toes and in the skin of the left arm. He lies in the open air during the night; at first confusion, then unconsciousness. Rescue after 20 h, deep unconscious, dilated pupils without any reflexes. Cold coma, periphery reflexes negativ. Bradycardia. Blood pressure immeasurable. Depression of respiration.

During transport: oxygen inhalation with mask. Massage of the heart and plasma expander infusions. Arriving in the hospital: temperature rectal 24°C, severe acidoses, pH 6,95, PO.2 38 mm Hg, central venous saturation corrected to 88%, Serum potassium 5,9 mol/l. Blood glucose 46 ma/100 ml. Intubation. Rewarming with microwaves (Siretherm, Siemens), beginning in the region of thorax 1°C/h. Off 26°C, first reactions of the patient despite pupils still being large with minimal reflexes.

After 12 h: rewarming stopped because rectal temperature was 37°C. Application of 200 E/h Heparin. Details of pH, p Co2, p 02, 02 saturation, function of the kidneys, treatment of anuria (urea and reatinin), circulation, respiration, coagulation (fibrinogen, thrombocytes), blood glucose, function of the liver see the original communication.

After the primary cold coma, the patient suffered from symptoms of intracranial overpressure caused by oedema of the brain, mid-brain-syndrome and psycho-organic-symptoms which disappeared after 3 weeks.

Report by Neureuther in 1978. A 26 year old woman was caught by wintry weather in the Alps, after a long, hard climbing tour. Bivouac in the open air without any equipment. Discovered after one and a half days. Occasional symptoms of confusion, most of the time unconscious. Irregular respiration, peripheral pulsation negative. At the place of the accident: Hibler packs, transport by acia, cable car, ambulance to the hospital. See Fig. 3: Blood temperature estimated 24°C. Rewarming, after 7 h: 37°C and after 9 h: 38,5°C, off, 30°C conscious, after 2 hours awake, but retrograde amnesia. See the laboratory data of the following 5 days in Fig. 3.

Regular, periodic warming up by temporarily opening the vascular system (Aschoff-Lewis reaction, see Killian 1966, p. 67) rates as the most important means of protecting the extremities during exposure to cold. This heating up phenomenon gradually ceases to function as the tissue temperature drops and may be encouraged by certain medicaments.

The trigeminal region is of particular importance as water, wind and heat reflexes for the circulation are generated from this area of outwardly totally exposed, uncovered skin, which also influences the mechanism of heat production as well as physical heat regulation, in other words, the supply of blood to the limbs. The face is, however, not the only area, from which decisive circulatory and metabolic changes are induced in the interests of heat balance. It is by no means here simpl a question of a centralisation (or decentralisation) of the circulation, but also of changes in the water and electrolytic distribution and in metabolic processes in the area of the skin (skin colour, skin temperature, moistening or dehydration of the skin etc.) It has been known for a long time that the neurovasal and neurohumoral systems, in particular the antagonism between the sympathetic and the parasympathetic nervous systems, play an important part in these changes. During local exposure to cold a disastrous double effect occurs, a directly local and indirectly reflex total change in the circulation, which throttles the blood supply to the endangered limb in an attempt to keep the homeothermally regulated temperature of the interior of the body constant, and thereby inhibits or eliminates the only means of effectively dealing with the cold in the extremities. Local stimuli caused by cold lead in time not only to reflex changes in the whole circulation, the heat balance and the thrombogenesis, but also to functional or even organic changes and to damage to remote

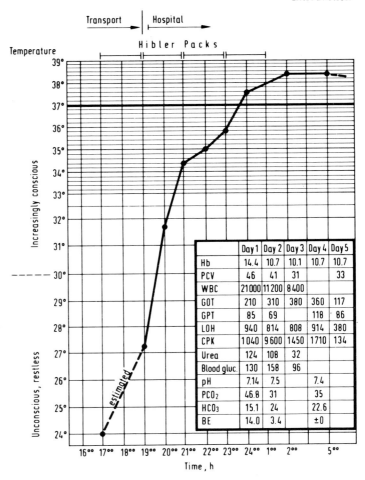

Fig. 3. General hypothermia (rewarming). (From Neureuther 1978)

parts of the body, e.g. to the endocrine glands (Staemmler 1930). The peripheral cooling of larger limbs also has an effect on the whole organism and on the heat balance in as far as the generation of additional heat in the cold muscles is restricted or totally impossible.

Experiments on tissues cultures have shown that the O_2 requirement during the rewarming phase is much greater and that a genuine oxygen deficiency is more likely to occur during the rewarming than during the cooling process (rewarming damage). Apart from this the specific resistance of different organs and tissues to cold as a function of their water and salt content as well as their chemical composition, i.e. their different freezing points, certainly plays an important part. This specific resistance to cold and freezing and the varying freezing points of different tissue substrata have a critical effect on the nature and severity of peripheral forms of frostbite (see the survey in our monograph in the section on the biology of cooling and the data on the specific resistance to cold and the freezing points of lifeless substrata as well as the capacity for survial of living organisms (Killian 1966).

References

Adams RJ, Clemenson CJ (1954) Acta Chir Scand 486
Adams RJ, Falconer B (1951) Acta Chir Scand 101 : 269
Ariev T (1955) Frostbite Defense Coard of Canada
Bezmann FW, Bontke E (1958) Pfenegers Arch 266 : 208
Binhold H (1942) Dtsch Militärarzt 3 : 491
Brendel W (1957) Verh Dtsch Ges Kreislaufforsch 33
Brendel W (1958) Z Gesamte Exp Med 146 : 189
Brendel W (1961) Sportarzt 1 : 372
Brendel W (1973) Aerztl Praxis 39 : 14
Brendel W (1977) V. Internationale Tagung der Bergrettungsärzte. Werk p 19
Campell R (1932) Schweiz Med Wochenschr 62 : 1183
Campell R (1966) VierteljahresSchr Schweiz San Offiz 43 : 20
Couglin F (1973) N Engl J Med I : 326
Davies DM et al. (1967) Lancet 1 : 1036
Davis L, Leuer X (1975) Lancet 2 : 650
Duguid H, Simpson R, Stowers J (1951) Lancet 2 : 1213
Editorial (1972) Lancet 1 : 237
Edward KW (1959) Surg Gynecol Obstet 109 : 743
Ertin MA, Schultz GA, Baxter H (1954) Anesthesiaology 5 : 486
Fay T, Smith GW (1941) Arch Neurol Psych 45 : 215
Fell RJ et al. (1963) Lancet 1 : 392
Fuhrmann FA, Fuhrmann GJ (1957) Medicine 36 : 465
Gerstenbrand F, Lücking CH (1970) Arch psychiatr Nervenkr 213 : 264
Gregorry RG et al. (1972) Lancet 1 : 377
Hackl JM, Haid B (1978) Notfall Med 4 :676
Hegenauer AH, Flynn J, d'Amato H (1951) Am J Physiol 157 : 69
Hirsch WD (1977) Aerztl Praxis 39 : 976
Hirsch WD, Phleps W, Flora S (1977) V. Internationale Tagung der Bergrettungsärzte. Werk p 27
Höflin FG (1977) V. Internatinale Tagung der Bergrettungsärzte. Werk p 25
Höflin FG (1977) Aerztl Praxis 14 : 633
Jesch F, Sunderplassmann L, Pohl U, Messmer K (1975) Chirurg Forum. Springer
Judmaier F (1952) Münch Med Wochenschr 6
Killian H (1952) Zentralbl Chir 77 : 105
Krueger P, Blümel G (1977) Aerztl Praxis 39 : 516
Krueger P, Blümel G (1977) V. Internationale Tagung der Bergrettungsärzte. Werk p 11
Kugelberg J et al. (1967) Scand J Thorac Cardiovasc Surg 1 : 142
Lee JA et al. Synopsis of Anaesthesy. 4th ed
Leitner E, Kronberger E (1977) V. Internationale Tagung der Bergrettungsärzte. Werk p 26
Leitner E, Kronberger E (1977) Aerztl Praxis 29 : 983
Linton Al et al. (1966) Lancet 1 : 24
Loyd E et al. (1972) Scott Med J 17 : 83
Lugger LJ, Phleps (1977) V. Internationale Tagung der Bergrettungsärtze. Werk p 34
MacLean D, Griffith PD, Emslie-Smith D Lancet 2
Meriwether WD, Goodmen RM (1972) Am J Med 53 : 505
Morales P, Carbery W et al. (1957) Am Surg 135 : 488
Mundt ED, Long D, Brown RB (1964) Trauma 4 : 236
Neureuther G (1973) Chirurgie der Gegenwart 4
Neureuther G (1978) Landesarzt Bergwacht. 2 Fallberichte
Neureuther G, Flora G. Kälteschäden. Broschüre der Bayerischen Bergwacht
Neureuther G, Flora G (1978) Kälteschäden. Notfallmedizin 2 : 103
Neureuther G, Ostertag H (1977) V. Internationale Tagung der Bergrettungsärzte. Werk
Schmidt L (1966) Med Welt 20 : 1127
Severinghaus JW (1958) J Appl Physiol 12 :485
Shanka CA (1975) Med J Aust alia 2/9 : 346
Souchon (1974) Seenotrettung. In: Mat Med Nordmark 26
Städler K, Algöwer M et al. (1972) Res Exp Med 158 : 231
Thauer-Brendel (1932) Progress of Surgery 2
Truscott DU, Withmer BF et al. (1973) Arch Surg 106 : 216

Wechselberger F (in Vorbereitung) Referat 3. Internationaler Kongreß über Katastrophen-Medizin Monaco 1979
Westherley-White RCA, Bjöström B (1964) Res 4 : 17
Wickstrom P et al. (1976) Am J Surg 131 : 622
Wynn C (1954) Lancet 2 : 575

Clinical Description of Local Cold Injuries

Internal and External Circumstances Which Encourage Loss of Temperature

Regional Causes

A number of particular exogenous and endogenous factors, which have been partly referred to in the last section play an important part in the cooling of a limb. In addition we would like to draw attention to the following special points:

Actual heat is lost not from the body surface but from the millimeter fine air boundary layer, which constantly surrounds the skin like a fine, protective coat. Within this boundary layer heat transfer only occurs via conduction, not, however, via convection. Only on the outside edge of the air layer is the movement of the air, which causes loss of temperature, effective. The area of the exposed surfaces is critical for the loss of heat, the difference in temperature between skin and air, between skin and inner tissue. the conductivity of the border tissue, especially with regard to *moisture,* wind speed, air pressure and the surface relief. It is wellknown that, when exposed to the cold, man and animals adopt a stooping position to reduce the surface area and prevent loss of heat.

If one takes the above conditions into consideration, it becomes clear that the peripheral areas of the body, especially the limbs, are most acutely exposed to loss of temperature. Although the supply of blood to the facial area, to the nose, the ears, the fingers and to the genitals is particularly good, and the adaptability of the blood vessels in these areas is also relatively good, they often suffer slight cold injuries for lack of cover. The small quantity of tissue is partly responsible for this, e.g. on the fingers and toes.

Another negative factor is the *long distance involved in the blood supply* and heat emission, in addition the relatively *superficial position of some afferent arteries,* as, for example, in the region of the foot, the art. dorsalis pedis and aa. tibialis anterior et posterior, which are most often damaged.

Cold injuries occur for anatomical reasons, especially in areas where the fatty layer is thin and the skin covers tendons and joints or osseous substrata. This includes not only the tips of the fingers, but also the end of the radius, as well as the area of the styloid process, the olecranon and the inner and outer epicondyle. In the legs the kneecap, the head of the fibula, the front ridge of the tibia, the ankle bones and the heel are in more danger than other areas. In the face the tip of the nose, the edges and lobes of the ears, and also the cheeks, cheek bones and the chin are considered to be particularly susceptible.

The water content of the tissue in question also plays an important part, since in the case of a hunger oedema the loss of temperature due to exposure to cold is encouraged as a result of increased heat dissipation from within. In contrast to this, those tissues covered with a thicker fatty layer are well insulated against the cold and suffer less often from frostbite.

Apart from the anatomical causes, unsuitable clothing must, of course, also be considered: tight bandages, tight shoes and puttees, which hinder the blood supply to the extremities and encourage the development of a cold injury. It must be remembered here that leather shoes are inappropriate in cold regions as they offer poor insulation and shrink when wet. (Enderlen 1920 a, b, 1928; Bundschuh 1915; Liebert 1914; Starlinger and Frisch 1944; Killian 1942 a, b)[1]

General Causes

Apart from these regional, anatomical or mechanical predispositions to cold injuries there are a number of constitutional influences which favour the formation of local frostbite or immersion cold injuries. Information on this subject is scarce in literature and its accuracy leaves much to be desired (Schürer, v. Waldheim, 1942, personal communication; v. Brandis, 1943 a, b; Bader and Macht 1948; Sapin-Jaloustre 1956).

Larrey (1817) already knew that certain racial and tribal differences exist with regard to resistance to cold. Monsaignon (1940 a, b) reported in 1940 on the great sensitivity of Arabs and Blacks to the cold in the First World War, compared with Whites. The same was claimed by Black soldiers in American reports from the Second World War.

In general all those who suffer from *vegetative disorders* and easily show signs of over-excitability and *excessive reactions of the blood vessels to the cold* are regarded as being prone to cold injuries. This includes vagotonic as well as sympathicotonic, neurasthenic and lymphatic patients. Excessive reactions to the cold play an important part in the development of local cold injuries. Therefore persons suffering from *digitus mortuus,* Reil's disease, or from *Raynaud's gangrene* or *allergic angiospastic reactions* are considered to be particularly susceptible. The cold cannot cause these diseases, but in can trigger them off or aggravate them. It may also be said in reverse that the presence of a constitutional tendency to Reil's or Raynaud's disease may be the cause of a cold injury and even relatively slight exposure to cold can have serious effects (Table 3).

All those who suffer from an incipient, general blockage of the arteries, combined with a disorder of the lipoidal and cholesteral balance and of the carbohydrate metabolism (diabetes). A local endangiitis caused by cold as the result of preceding frostbite or vascular damage of traumatic and infectious origin, as well as arteriitis nodosa and related conditions also have a negative influence etiologically. Infections of a severe nature and certain infectious diseases must also be included. In this connection we have found that typhoid fever, which affects the arterial vessels, causes gangrene, not only

---

1   On this subject two critical remarks from the book, 'Barbarossa' by Carell: When the Finns saw that the German soldiers were still walking about after the first snow in their army boots with steel nails in the soles, they shook their heads and declared, "The nailed soles of your boots are ideal conductors of the cold, you might just as well go about in your socks or barefoot from the start."
    Schukow explained in the Moscow Officers' Club towards the end of the war that his respect for the German general staff had been shaken when he saw the first German prisoners from the winter battle. Officers and men had all perfectly fitting footwear and, of course, their feet were freezing. In Russia it had been the rule since the eighteenth century to supply the men with larger size shoes for the winter for the purpose of padding them with straw and paper.

Table 3. Diseases which encourage the development of peripheral cold injuries

Endangiitis obliterans	(thrombo-angiitis obliterans, Buerger's disease)
Arterial sclerosis	
Previous cold injuries	(cold endangiitis)
Allergic forms of arteriitis	
(arteriitis nodosa, giant-cell angiitis, vascular sensitisation (Zeeck 1953), erthematosis etc.)	
Traumatic vascular damage	Angiorrhexis Aneurysms with collateral circulation, thrombosis or embolism of the arteries
Arteriitis chronica	After inflammation, general infection, endocarditis lenta
Special infectious disease	with manifest damage to the blood vessels as in typhoid fever, toxoplasmosis
Digitus mortuus (Reil's disease)	
Manifest symmetrical gangrene according to Raynaud	
Chronic diabetes	
Avitaminosis	
Chronic acidosis	

because of vascular occlusion, but because it often leads to additional, severe frostbite due to extremely low blood pressure values and thus a very inadequate supply of blood to the extremities. Often enough genuine gangrene caused by the cold has been confused with typhoid gangrene (Killian 1943).

Larrey (1817) thus mistakenly took typhoid fever to be catarrhal nervous fever caused by the cold. In 1941/42 the author often enough had the opportunity to see highly cyanosed fingers, feet and toes in thyphoid fever, which gave the impression of the beginning of a cold injury necrosis. In most cases, however, the limbs recovered again if the patient pulled through.

It may be said that all general disorders, which lead to a disturbance of thermo-regulation, especially those which belong to the group of *intestinal or anaemic diseases* or concern the *failing of the thyroid gland,* lower the resistance to cold of the exposed regions of the body. The moist state of the skin is of extreme importance in the formation of local frostbite, as it encourages thermosteresis. Constitutional or acquired hyperhidrosis of the hands or feet are among the changes which encourage frostbite (Milian and Jaurison 1941; Bugliari and Canavero 1941a, b; Rosgen and Manier 1942; v. Brandis 1943 a, b; Killian 1942 a, b). A moistening of the top layer of the skin within the normal tendendy to perspire, as occurs during various infectious diseases, e.g. tuber-culosis or as the result of neurohormonal disorders, not only encourages the limbs to lose heat but it also increases the danger of infection, due to maceration. In 1941 Jaurison (Milian and Jaurison 1941) observed in 47 patients with frostbite, in 37 cases signs of tuberculosis.

In the region of the hand, always around the critical borderline temperature of -14° to -15°C, perspiration can cause an immediate freezing onto metals, which, when an attempt is made to remove the skin, results in the epidermis being torn off and the epithelium damaged. The latter may easily become infected.

All those who suffer from depression of circulation are also predisposed to cold injuries. This includes *injuries with an acute loss of blood, states of shock and collapse, irrespective* of their cause (natural disasters, earthquakes). Most of these noxae accompany disorders of thermal regulation, water balance, a reduction of the amount of blood circulating, a sharp drop in the blood supply pressure, as well as a restriction of oscillation, which also particularly affects the peripheral area.

There are references to this in practically all literature relevant to the subject. Every kind of vascular lesion to an artery of a limb presents a particular danger, as it can lead to a deterioration or a stop in the supply of blood to distal areas (Floerken 1915, 1920 a, b; Coenen 1916; Killian 1942 a, b; v. Brandis 1943 a, b; Starlinger 1942, Starlinger and v. Frisch 1944; Paessler 1962). Even without direct arterial damage, however, it often occurs that frostbite only affects the injured and not the healthy limb. This situation can be reconstructed in arterial experiments.

Among the *acute infections* which can cause an extensive disturbance of the heat regulation and of the circulation including profuse loss of water, *gastro-intestinal diseases* play an essential part. It is here not only a question of common *enteritis* but also of dysentery, cholera, typhoid fever and similar diseases.

During the Balkan campaign, as a result of the frequent occurrence of a combination of typhoid fever and cholera with local cold injuries, the assumption was made that gangrene was rather the result of the former diseases than of the effects of cold. One can find particular references to the etiology of this form of illness in the work of Mayer and Kohlschütter (1914). The same has also been pointed out by Wieting (1913), Welcker (1913), Dreyer (1913), Hecht (1915) and Volk and Stiefler (1915). The experience of surgeons during the world wars was also similar. With cases of severe, chronic enteritis and attacks of dysentery and typhoid fever, additional cold injuries very frequently occurred during transport when frost had set in. All states of physical exhaustion, such as *starvation* in association with *loss of weight*, have an unfavourable effect. Acute *hypoproteinaemia, vitamin deficiencies* (A, B and C, perhaps D and E too) and hormonal imbalances, such as a *thyroid insufficiency* (myxoedeama), must also be considered. Disturbances of the tropic hormone of the adenohypophysis, as well as the adrenocortical hormone predispose the patient to cold injuries due to their close relationship to thermogenesis. The poisons which encourage local loss of temperature include all those which relax the muscles. On the subject of hypnotics and narcotics it can be said that in heavier doses they have a disturbing effect on heat regulation and, in fact, lead to a gradual loss of temperature in the body, which is felt most strongly in the limbs.
which is felt most strongly in the limbs.

The consumption of alcohol is of great significance for the cooling down of the whole body, a subject which has been examined elsewhere. Regarding the development of peripheral frostbite, it should not be judged unfavourably, as a moderate amount of alcohol promotes natural defence reactions again, which prevent too great a loss of heat in the limbs. The Aschoff-Lewis reaction can be revived after it has stopped via the administration of small amounts of alcohol. Nicotine with its harmful effect on the whole vascular system, proved by countless statistics, must be seen in contrast to this.

The Role of Nicotine

For a long time a causal relationship has repeatedly been sought between nicotine and the development and deterioration of localised forms of cold endangiitis, real systemic endangiitis obliterans or sclerosis. This was justified as nicotine was considered from the pharmalogical side to be a powerful poison, which initially had a stimulating, then a paralysing effect, not only on the central nervous system but also on the peripheral autonomous ganglia. It appears, however, that individual reactions may vary considerably and habit also seems to play a part. Nicotine has a stimulating effect on some people, a calming effect on others. These effects become most clear after heavy doses. The abuse of nicotine may not only impair the functioning of the heart and circulation, but also produce spasms of the small peripheral arteries and of the coronary vessels.

An increase in the peristalsis and a contraction of the splachnic vessels with increased blood pressure, which seems to be based on a weakening or even a reversal of the depressor reflex may also be observed. According to Straub and Amann (1940) these symptoms should occur before the adrenaline secretion.

Nicotine plays a relatively insignificant part in the general loss of temperature but the reactions of the *peripheral circulation and the blood supply itself are seriously affected even by small quantities of nicotine. The constriction* and drop in the peripheral skin and limb temperatures caused by nicotine favour the development of peripheral frostbite (Maddock et al. 1936; Wright and Moffat 1934; Werle and Multhaupt 1937; Loeser 1944). This vasoconstriction and drop in temperature is most noticeabel in the area of the toes and the fingers. The smoking of just one cigarette leads to a measurable drop in the skin temperature around the fingers.

In 1934 Scherer discovered in connection with the extremities, that the smoking of one cigarette causes the temperature of the finger tip to drop by $2^\circ-7^\circ C$ after $10-40$ min, and that a decrease in the skin temperature of the hand of up to $4.6^\circ C$ and of the foot of up to 3.9° can be observed. The loss of temperature for the rest of the body surface in his experiments was $0.1^\circ-0.3^\circ C$, in one case $0.6^\circ C$. The deeper the smoker had inhaled, the clearer the effect was. These results are in agreement with the experiments of Matthiesen (quoted according to Hochrein). The latter discovered that nicotine in small amounts, as are taken in when one cigarette is smoked, leads to a marked drop in the temperature of the peripheral skin areas, e.g. of the fingers, and a simultaneous drop in the oxygen saturation of the blood and a deterioration in the oxygen utilisation. It would appear, however, that not all areas are affected in the same way by this influence. Matthiesen found the opposite in the region of the ear, namely a rise in temperature and an increase in oxygen saturation. In a series of experiments started by Schulze in 1947 even greater drops in temperature were observed as the effect of nicotine during smoking, namely an average of $3^\circ-4^\circ C$ in the finger area, while the whole body remained below room temperature. The dilatation of the blood vessels caused by exposure to cold counteracted the effect of nicotine. The peripheral vasoconstriction caused by the effects of nicotine is considerable. It leads not only to a slowing of the circulation in some parts but also brings it to a standstill in the capillaries during smoking (Allan et al. 1955). It was quite clear that nicotine or rather the abuse of this poison was to be included among the causes of arterial vascular diseases, especially as the negative effect on arterial sclerosis, endangiitis obliterans, hypertonia or angina pectoris could be explained clinically. This was supported by a series of animal experiments which has apparently succeeded, via the chronic administration of nicotine, in producing vascular changes of the kind observed in arteriosclerosis. Butt and Thieme (quoted according to Hauschild 1956), however, were able to disprove the results of these animal experiments beyond and doubt.

Even though it has been possible to prove with extremely extensive statistics (especially American) the harmful influence of nicotine abuse on vascular diseases, the mode of action remains unclear. In this respect one can support the remarks of Ratschow, who claimed *that nicotine probably interferes in the pathogenetic course of circulatory disturbances but is not itself the cause of arterial vascular diseases.* This nicotine effect apparently occurs via the sympathetic nervous system (secretion of adrenaline). It consists of a disturbance of peripheral vascular regulation with concommitant action of the cathecol amines: adrenaline and noradrenaline. The rise in blood pressure often observed after nicotine consumption may be associated with a secretion of adrenaline during smoking. Such observations were the reason why damage caused by nicotine was ultimately understood to be adrenaline damage due to permanent hypertonia of the peripheral vessels equipped with receptors. Many specialists in internal medicine are convinced of the connection between nicotine abuse and vascular disease, although the pathogenesis is not clear. According to Harkavy (1933) endangiitis or sclerosis occur much more rarely among non-smokers than among heavy smokers.

It is also a fact that a total abstinence from smoking has a positive influence on arterial vascular diseases, and that, if a patient does not totally abstain or starts smoking again, it normally leads to a deterioration in his condition and makes the success of purposeful treatment just about impossible. It has been reported that up to 93% of all patients suffering from endangiitis obliterans are smokers.

Hochrein rejects the causal effect of nicotine on the development of vascular diseases of all kinds but he assumes that nicotine influences the vasa vasorum encourages the development of arterial vascular damage or makes the smoker suseptible to infections, toxis damage to the vascular wall. It is considered to encourage excessive reactions of the autonomous nervous system and possibly cause paradox vascular reflexes. It is also said to encourage a rise in blood pressure and further a disposition to orthostatic failure. As nicotine also restricts the pulmonary circulation the oxygen saturation apparently deteriorates, which mainly affects the heart.

The assumption of a hypersensitivity to nicotine as a cause of the frequent occurrence of vascular diseases and their deterioration had to be rejected for lack of proof. It was, however, possible to establish a lower life expectancy among smokers and according to Sigler (quoted according to Schettler 1959), coronary arteriosclerosis sets in earlier and its progress is more serious in smokers, which Dorn's (quoted according to Ratschow 1963) great veterans' statistic has borne out, with an increase of 63% compared with non-smokers.

Two characteristics of nicotine may be of particular significance here: nicotine apparently inhibits the clearing factor, and according to Marx et al. (1956), the blood flow in the terminal vessels in the retroarteriolar region, which apparently hinders the development of a collateral circulation. It was in no way possible to create genuine vascular damage with nicotine but Hochrein and Schleicher (1959) include this poison among the accumulative effects, which can influence the circulation. Vasoconstriction and arteriolar spasms are particularly noticeable among people with disorders of the autonomous nervous system, who easily perspire, as they suffer from a wetness of the skin of the limbs and their peripheral thermoregulation can be considerably disturbed. This condition favours the development of localised frostbite.

As the result of all these investigations and the experience of the winter of 1941/42 in Russia, the author gave urgent warnings to the sentries on duty not to smoke. Other armies have also, in part, come to the same conclusions. In 1943–44 in a special military hospital for cold injuries in Paris, Paessler (1943) tried to classify the men with heavy nicotine consumption and found that with very few exceptions they were the ones who suffered from frostbite. He attributes particular significance to nicotine abuse in the etiology of arterial circulatory disturbances, especially as he apparently found no vascular diseases among light smokers and non-smokers. We do not assume such an extreme standpoint but consider nicotine to be a supporting factor when a vascular disease is already developing or when exposure to cold and wet occurs. The assumption that nicotine has a negative effect on the blood vessels has been confirmed by the more recent investigations carried out by Forst (1970) and Hess (1970) in Munich, with an electronscanning microscope on large blood vessels, like the aorta and the carotid artery, after smoke inhalation. They found that effects of cold as well as nicotine lead to a change in the relationship between the vascular wall and its contents, which cause the depositing of blood components on the inner surfaces – thrombocyte aggregations, desquamated, endothelial cells and fibrin threads. Perhaps these parallel changes from cold and nicotine have a significant influence. It seems possible that the starting point of obliterating vascular diseases should be sought in these primary reactions.

References

Allan EV, Barker NW, Hines LA (1955) Periphere Durchblutungsstörungen, 2nd edn. Saunders, Philadelphia
Bader ME, Macht NB (1948) J Appl Physiol 1 : 215
Brandis HJ von (1943 a) Vorträge aus der praktischen Chirurgie, vol 27. Encke, Stuttgart
Brandis HJ von (1943 b) Broschüre über Kälteschäden. Encke, Stuttgart
Brendel W (1957) Verh Dtsch Ges Kreislaufforsch 33
Brendel W (1958) Z Gesamte Exp Med 146 : 189
Brendel W (1961) Sportarzt 1 : 372
Brendel W (1973) Aerztl Prax 39 : 14
Brendel W (1977) V. Internationale Tagung der Bergrettungsärzte. Werk p 19
Bugliari G, Canavero G (1941 a) G Med Mil 19
Bugliari G, Canavero G (1941 b) G Med Mil 89 : 505
Bundschuh E (1915) Munch Med Wochenschr 416
Coenen H (1916) Bruns Beitr Klin Chir 103 : 367
Dreyer U (1913) Zentralbl Chir 40 : 1628
Enderlen E (1920 a) Zentralbl Chir 47 : 1051
Enderlen E (1920 b) Die Kälteschäden im Krieg
Enderlen E (1928) Ergeb Chir Orthop 12 : 160
Floerken H (1915) Munch Med Wochenschr 7
Floerken H (1920 a) Zentralbl Chir 47 : 1651
Floerken H (1920 b) Die Kälteschäden im Krieg. Springer, Berlin (Ergebnisse der Chirurgie und Orthopädie)
Forst H (1970) Report. 7. Deutsche Angiologentagung, Berlin
Hauschild F (1956) Lehrbuch der Pharmakologie
Hecht K (1915) Wien Klin Wochenschr 65 : 1487

Hess H (1970) Report. 7. Deutsche Angiologentagung, Berlin
Hirsch WD, Phelbs W, Flora S (1977) V. Internationale Tagung der Bergrettungsärzte. Werk, p 27
Hochrein M, Schleicher J (1959) Herz- und Kreislaufkrankheiten, 2nd edn. Steinkopff, Dresden
Höflin FG (1977) V. Internationale Tagung der Bergrettungsärzte. Werk, p 25
Killian H (1942 a) Zentralbl Chir 1763
Killian H (1942 b) Arbeitstagung beratender Chirurgen, Berlin
Killian H (1943) Zentralbl Chri 70 : 50
Killian H (1966) Der Kälteunfall: Allgemeine Unterkühlung. Dustri
Krueger P, Blümel G (1977 a) Aerztl Prax 39 : 516
Krueger P, Blümel G (1977 b) V. Internationale Tagung der Bergrettungsärzte. Werk, p 11
Larrey JD (1817) Mémoires du chirurgie militaire et de campagne, vol 4. Paris
Lee JA et al. (1959) Synopsis of anaesthesia, 4th edn, chap 27
Leitner E, Kronberger E (1977) Aerztl Prax 29 : 983
Liebert KE (1914) Beitrag zur Kriegsheilkunde. Springer, Berlin
Lloyd E, et al. (1972) Scott Med J 17 : 83
Loeser A (1944) Dtsch Med Wochenschr 71
Maddock W, Malcolm G, Coller RL (1936) Am Heart 12 : 46
Marx H, Schoop W, Zapata C (1956) Z Kreislaufforsch 45 : 658
Mayer AW, Kohlschütter R (1914) Dtsch Z Chir 127 : 518
Milian, Jaurison (1941) Paris Med 2 : 365
Messmer K (1972) Anaesthesiol Wiederbeleb 60 : 149
Messmer K (1975) Surg Clin North Am 55/3 : 659
Messmer K (1976 a) Workshop on pre-operative haemodilution (Lecture), Frankfort 13 Dec 1976. Anaesthesist 25/4 : 123
Messmer K (1976 b) Anaesthesist 25/4 : 185
Messmer K (1976 c) Anesth Analg (Paris) 33/4 : 509
Messmer K (to be published) Lecture held at the "Mittelrheinischer Chirurgenkongreß", Basel 29 Aug 1977
Messmer K, Schmidt-Schönbein H (1972) Review. Internationales Symposium, Rottach-Egern 1971. Microvasc Res 4 : 221
Messmer K, Sunder-Plassmann L (1973) Prog Surg 13 : 208
Messmer K, Sunder-Plassmann L, Klövekorn WP, Holper K (1971) Adv Microcirc 4 : 1
Messmer K, Lewis DM, Sunder-Plassmann L, Klövekorn WP (1972 a) Report. Internationales Symposium, Rottach-Egern 1971. Karger, Basel p 123
Messmer K, Lewis DM, Sunder-Plassmann L, Klövekorn WP, et al. (1972 b) Eur Surg Res 4 : 55
Messmer K, Sunder-Plassmann L, Jesch F (1973) Res Exp Med 159 : 152
Messmer K, Grönandt L, Jesch F et al. (1975) Reprint. Plenum, New York
Messmer K, Klövekorn WP, Pichlmaier H, Sunder-Plassmann L (1976 a) Report. 3rd International Symposium, Rio de Janeiro 1976. Karger, Basel, p 123
Messmer K, Krumme BA Kessler H (1976 b) Microciurculation 2 : 133
Monseignon A (1940 a) Presse Med 48 : 166
Monseignon A (1940 b) Zentralbl Chir 18
Neureuther G (1978) Notfallmedizin 2 : 78
Paessler HW (1943) Zentralbl Chir 44 : 1956
Paessler HW (1962) Referat. Sachverständigentagung, Bonn
Ratschow M (1963) Med Klin 9 : 344
Rosgen MK, Manier (1942) Munch Med Wochenschr 89 : 889
Sapin-Jaloustre J (1956) Enquêtes sur les gélures. Herman, Paris
Scherer E (1934) Z Neurol 150 : 632
Schettler G (1959) Alterssklerose. In: Ratschow M (ed) Angiologie. Thieme, Stuttgart
Schürer F von (1942) Zentralbl Chir 69 : 486, 1797
Schulze W (1942) Klin Wochenschr 646
Shanka CA (1975) Med J Aust 2/9 : 346
Sunder-Plassmann L, Klövekorn WP, Holper K, et al. (1971) Report. 6th European Conference on Micorcirculation, Aalberg 1970. Karger, Basel, p 23
Sunder-Plassmann L, Klövekorn WP, Messmer K (1972 a) Internationales Symposium, Rottach-Egern 1971. Karger, Basel, p 184
Sunder-Plassmann L, Klövekorn WP, Lewis DM, Messmer K (1972 b) Langenbecks Arch Chir (Suppl Forum) 414
Sunder-Plassmann L, Klövekorn WP, Messmer K (1976) Anaesthesist 25/4 : 124
Starlinger F (1942) Zentralbl Chir 69 : 1179

Starlinger F, Frisch OW (1944) Die Erfrierungen. Steinkopff, Berlin
Thauer R, Brendel W (1932) Progress of surgery, vol II. Basel
Volk R, Stiefler G (1915) Wien Klin Wochenschr 28 : 116
Welcker ER (1913) Zentralbl Chir 40 : 1625, 1768
Werle, Multhaupt (1937) Munch Med Wochenschr 84 : 407
Wieting J (1913) Zentralbl Chir 40 : 593
Wright JS, Moffat D (1934) Jama 103 : 318
Zeeck M (1953) N Engl J Med 248 : 764

Terminology and Division Into Groups of Localised Cold Injuries

In 1956, in his "Enquête sur les Gélures", Sapin-Jaloustre referred to the difficulties of defining the different kinds of localised cold injuries, since in French, German, English and American literature varying assertions have been mad. He distinguished between three schools of thought according to authors.

The first, including authors who make a distinction according to the criterion whether or not the tissue was frozen, is represented by Rabout (1939), Shumaker and Lempke (1951), Edholm (1952), Movrey and Farago (1952), and Meryman (1955). The latter tries to distinguish between frost damage and frostbite in that the former is anoxia damage.

A second group of authors differentiates between damage caused by the effects of dry cold to far below 0° C compared with immersion damage, in other words a wet-type of exposure to cold. This group includes a large number of French surgeons, such as Raymond and Parisot (1918), Quenue (1918), Chatelier (1918), Sapin-Jaloustre (1956) who were not familiar with the older reports of German surgeons from the Balkan wars, (Wieting 1913; Meyer 1913; Dreyer 1913; Kohlschütter 1913; Welcker 1913), nor with the reports made by Floerken (1917) on trench foot and Flanders' foot. This classification was often accepted after 1940 in France by Monsaignon (1940 a, b), Ducuing et al. (1940), Paunesco-Podeanu and Tzurai (1940), by the English surgeons Bigelow (1942), Ungley (1949), Heaton and Davis (1952), Higgins et al. (1952), and by American military surgeons (see Whayne and Coats 1958).

A third category of authors rejects this division of cold injuries into groups and considers them to be uniform and independent of their form of origin. According to Sapin-Jaloustre (1956) this group includes Greene (1940), Theiss (1940), further Southworth (1945), Friedmann (1946), Vagliano (1948), Lewis and Moen (1952/1953), and Shumaker (1932).

This standpoint corresponds approximately to that of the second group, although it has been shown that tissues react in a uniform way to the cold noxa and necrosis is always the final link in the chain of reactions. In 1952 Lewis and Moen compared histologically the sequelae of cold effects from minus 15° to minus 30° and typical immersion damage in water at plus 2°C. No difference was to be found. The authors also compared the effects of cold and heat on cases of ischaemia without being able to ascertain histologically a specific change to the injury areas, i.e. to the necrosis. Only one thing is certain, that as a result of the effect of heat all the proteins from the fluid and tissues coagulated, which is not the case after cold damage. This is the main difference between the two kinds of thermal damage. Cold injuries acquired in dry, very windy, air or after exposure at high altitudes to minus 40°C (Hearnly and Buchanat 1952), produced histologically the same tissue damage (Ariev 1939 a,b; Greene 1943; Blair et al. 1951).

The results of this kind of damage were no different from that caused after immersion in water which was minus 15°C, not even when the hindquarters of the experimental animals being used were protected by a rubber cover at temperatures between minus

10° and minus 20° C. According to the report made by Shumaker and Kunkler (1952) who exposed the experimental animals at between minus 10° and minus 20°C for a long time, no histological differences in the sequelae could be found either.

Friedmann's report after the Second World War (1946) on localised frostbite confirmed this finding.

With regard to ischaemia there is a difference, in as far as ischaemic damage occurs much earlier than that caused by cold, which is demonstrated by the increase in the tissue's resistance to oxygen dificiency and the preserving effect of the cold. According to Sapin-Jaloustre (1956) not even frost damage changes essentially the appearance of frostbite, so that it does not seem wise to make a distinction between frostbite with and without freezing of the tissue. Sapin-Jaloustre (1956) quotes in this context the well-known experiments of Smith et al. (1954), on golden hamsters (hibernators), which after exposure to temperatures between minus 15° and minus 38°C in 80 % of the cases apparently survived total freezing easily and without damage. He also refers to the possibility of ice anaesthesia with ethyl chloride, did not seem, however, to be clear about the fact that this is a special form of ultra rapid cooling, which fixes the state of the tissue extremely suddenly without damage occurring as the result of crystallisation or oxygen deficiency. This explains the relatively unscathed state of most tissues after an anesthetic of this kind.

As a result of the similarities in the histological findings on cold injuries, in his critical study Sapin-Jaloustre (1956) came to the conclusion that the terms "gélure" and "froidure" are actually synonymous, but that it is advisable to make a clinical distinction between "gélure", i.e. frost damage, and "froidure", cold injuries. His concluding remark was literally: "Les congélations locales, les pieds gèlés, les gélures d'altitudes, les pieds de trencher, d'abris, d'immersion ne sont que des formes aetiologiques de gélure ou de froidure. C'est du moins étant considéré comme synonyme"

The organism and tissues only have in fact one possible, uniform biological reaction to cold, which ends in necrosis, but we are obliged clinically to make distinctions. Thus the Americans distinguish between six different clinical forms of localised cold injury:
1) Chilblains
2) Shelter leg
3) Immersion foot
4) Trench foot (3 and 4 are more or less identical)
5) Frostbite
6) High altitude cold injury (dry-type)

Inspite of all attempts to clarify the terminology, in our opinion Sapin-Jaloustre (1956) has ignored certain essential points, namely the differences in cold effects, not only according to intensity and speed of development, but also according to duration and degree of penetration. The work of decades on these problems has led to a division of cold injuries into two main groups, which overlap, in which combinations occur and into which the six above-mentioned clinical forms can easily be fitted.

1) *The visible superficial forms of frostbite without any particular degree of penetration* of a localised nature, 1st to 4th degree, with possible loss of tissue from necrosis (the 4th degree corresponds to ice anaesthesia), caused by dry or wet cold action.

2) *Frostbite with depth of penetration and general cooling down,* often of an invisible nature, in which the external layers remain relatively undamaged, the main effect of

the cold being to the inner tissues. It occurs characteristically after repeated *exposure for long periods at around and even above 0° C* and is mainly due to immersion (dampness, wetness, ice, water and cold), because this encourages general loss of temperature and the cooling down of the limbs. It also causes damage to the *muscles, the bone cells and nerves,* especially to their vegetative fibres (partial lesions) as well as direct *vascular damage* (cold endangiitis), as the result of which after months and even years obliterating arterial occlusion of neurovascular origin may occur, which has the appearance of localised endangiitis obliterans.

Such local vascular diseases are not to be confused with systemic arterial occlusion of the multilocular endangiitis or fibrosclerotic type. These forms correspond to Flanders' foot, shelter leg, "pied de trenché", trench foot, immersion foot and immersion hand. They are reproducible but pathologically and physiologically not completely explained.

Clinical Manifestations

According to the exogenous factors and also the endogenous conditions, clinically different forms of cold injury develop, the characteristics of which will be referred to here. Clinically it is possible to distinguish between five group types:
1) Chilblains (caused by mild cold with high humidity and localised moistening of the skin)
a) Perniones
b) Perniosis
2) Erythrocyanosis
3) Shelter leg
4) The common, visible forms of frostbite, 1st – 4th degree (relatively superficial)
a) under normal climatic conditions
b) at high altitudes (effects of dry cold accompanied by hypoxia)
5) Deep-seated cold damage (mostly loss of temperature caused by the effects of wet cold)
a) Immersion foot and hand
b) Trench foot.
   The latter forms of exposure to cold are partly externally invisible and make it difficult to make a prognosis.

Chilblains

Perniones

Perniones (chilblains) are genuine, localised, small forms of frostbite of the skin and subcutaneous area, which occur especially in cold, wet weather.
   French authors considered chilblains to be a form of minor frostbite, others have considered them separately in their monographs on cold injuries.
   In 1946 Paunesco-Podeanu and Tzurai distinguished actual frostbite as *gélures sans engélures* (engélure synonymous with chilblain), gélures, froidures (synonymous with cold injuries), whereas Burton and Edholm (1952, 1955) considered chilblains to be a benign form of actual frostbite. In 1954 Lynn, too, in a careful study of cold damage, made no essential distinction between chilblains and frostbite; it seems to us, nevertheless, advisable to differentiate.
   The main location of simple chilblains of the normal individual are those places which can easily under pressure become ischaemic. They are most likely to form in areas with little padding, on bony protuberances and joints on the extensor sides of the fingers and toes, on the balls of the big and small toes and occasionally even on the knuckles. The thumbs normally remain free from perniones. Seen macroscopically the characteristic

feature of chilblains, which has been investigated by Uschinsky (1893), Hodara (1896 a,b), Rischpler (1900), Marchand (1908), Ricker (1924) and many others, is a nodular swelling the size of a bean or a lentil, which lies in a dark bluish-red field, the edges of which cannot be clearly defined, and in the middle of which a small pit, a tiny point, the source of the bleeding, is sometimes visible. In the middle of this swelling trophic disturbances may be seen and small ulcers with tissue necrosis develop.

Gans's investigations of chilblains (1923, 1925) have shown that an acute widening of the vessels of the corium occurs with a club-shaped swelling of the papillae, pronounced, oedema formation in the lymphatic spaces, a stretching of the epithetial strips and intercellular and intracellular oedema development in the area of the stratum spinosa. Heavy impregnation of the epidermis may occasionally lead to the forming of blisters. The callosity is usually swollen. In the later stages connective tissue proliferation (phorocytosis) in the cutis and desintegration of the elastic fibres occurs.

The small, localised cold injury appears as a painful, reddish swelling, which feels very hot after exposure to cold and is sensitive to pressure. Sometimes excruciating pain is felt or, in the phase of reactive vasodilation with oedemas, a sharp itching. The condition can lead to chronic induration and leave a local disturbance of the circulation. There is a danger of recidivation in following winters. The condition can become chronic. Exogenous factors are mainly responsible for the development of chilblains, i.e. local exposure to cold and wetness combined with mechanical pressure (e.g. from wet shoes). Perniones are not constitutional, anybody can be affected, endogenous influences may, however, occasionally play a part in their development. Young people are normally only affected if the circulation and autonomic nervous system are very instable due to feverish illness with increased sensitivity to cold. Amongst older people those who suffer from a disturbed blood supply, an increase in the neuro-circulatory tonus and excessive reaction to cold are particularly susceptible. A single chilblain normally heals quickly in warm conditions. The unpleasant chronic form takes weeks or moths and is treated like frostbite.

Perniosis

One distinguishes between common perniones and the condition referred to as perniosis, i.e. frostbite disease, which is normally due to constitutional factors. It can be found at any age if endocrine disorders are present, occasionally, too, where chronic infections occur and particularly in the case of disturbed temperature regulation.

Milian mentioned in 1941 that tubercular cases are particularly sensitive to the cold and that their heat regulation is often disturbed by the heavy perspiration. Such patients are most susceptible to chilblains. A steady transition from small, localised cold injuries to perniones and perniosis exists. The frostbite disease is included by some among the angiopathic diseases, Klüken, (quoted according to Ratschow 1959). Kummer (1935, 1938) and Loos (1939, 1953) divided up the different pathological conditions according to the degree of sensitivity to cold (Table 4).

Perniosis causes chronic damage of constitutional nature, which explains the relatively marked development of oedemas and the infiltration, the considerable swelling of the lymphatic spaces and the signs of a capillary paralysis of the cells in the affected

Table 4. Pathological preconditions [a]

Sensitivity to cold	Acute	Chronic	Spreading
Normal	Freezing	Perniones	Localised
Pathological disposition (congenital of acquired)	Cold damage	Perniosis erythrocyanosis cruorum puellarum	Extending to calf area

[a] After Kummer (1935, 1938) and Loos (1939, 1953)

area. The extensor sides of the fingers, of the hand, of the dorsum of the foot, as well as the edges of the big and small toes and of the small finger are mostly affected. In constrast, one never finds chilblains in the hollow areas of the hand or foot. Strict symmetry does not occur either but usually the appearance is similar on both sides. Perniotic changes are seldom observed in the facial area, on the chin, nose, thighs or in the area of the lower leg. Chilblains on the edge of the ear are often the size of hemp seeds, very hard, painful and often hard to distinguish from small, localised cold injuries. According to Klingmüller and Dittrich (1926), the main site of cold action is the follicle. Both authors refer to perniosis follicularis accuminalis sine planus. Later (1926/1929) Dittrich distinguished perniosis follicularis from the infiltrating form with its bullous and ulcerous changes. It usually affects people between the ages of 15 and 35, far more often women than men. As a forefunner of the actual chilblain a kind of acro-asphyxia of the affected area forms with a spastic, atonic condition of the terminal blood vessels. Hands and feet which have undergone such change are cold and damp to the touch. The moistening of the various layers of the skin plays a much more critical role in the clinical picture than has so far been assumed, as it increases the likelihood of the skin cooling down. (See comments in the patho-physiological section.)

Loos observed that in people with perniosis one mostly finds a mottled skin. This condition is characteristic of a change in the autonomous control of heat regulation with an increase in the tonus of the sympathetic nervous system, and provides at the time one of the conditions necessary for the development of actual perniosis. In the changed areas one can find the so-called *iris-diaphragm phenomenon,* as an expression of the increase in tonus of the sympathetic nervous system. In acrocyanotic areas of perniosis it is possible to observe the regression of an anaemic spot created by finger pressure as the spasms of the fine arterial vessels are sustained for a long time and prevent the blood from flowing back quickly. A backward flow from the veins may also occur. In the mottled skin area with its spastic-atonic changes and in goose flesh one finds, as Schneider (1948) points out, the ability of the blood vessels to react to cold stimulus and also to adrenaline and even to suspended histamin. In contrast to this Schulz mentioned in 1943 that the adrenaline reaction changes little after exposure to cold. (cf. our comments concerning the effects of adrenaline in Killian 1966.)

Many dermatologists have concerned themselves with the nature of perniosis and erythrocyanosis but it was not until 1940 that Schneider found evidence to support the fact that it is by no means a type of local cold damage, but that the disease presents essentially a total change in the organism, to be more specific, a disturbance of the thermoregulatory system. As is wellknown, the periphery is exposed to the cold in order to protect the temperature of the centre. This reaction is over-sensitised an pathologically changed in perniosis patients. Schneider used the andrenaline experiment to check the thermoregulatory disturbance of the skin. The effect of a dose of adrenaline in a normally regulating person is to cause a prompt rise in the blood glucose level, a rapid and sharp increase can in fact be observed. In the case of patients with a hereditary tendency to perniosis only weak, protracted changes follow, and hyperglycaemia may not occur at all. By following the blood glucose curves of such patients it was possible to recognise that the vago-insular counter-reaction was not present to compensate for the sympathico-adrenal overbalance (Schneider 1942, 1946). In addition to these investigations the potassium calcium coefficient was determined as this is of decisive significance for the condition of the autonomous system and a predominance of calcium was found in patients with perniosis and erythrocyanosis. The coefficient showed a calcium predomin-ance of 1.6. Parallel experiments on 23 patients who had suffered localised frostbite shortly before showed a coefficient of only 1.49, which was obtained as the potassium was either normal or low, whereas the calcium was more or less increased. This condition corresponds to an increase in the tonus of the sympathetic nervous system, which corres-ponds to the clinical picture of sustained spasms of the arterial vessels after local cold action.

Erythrocyanosis

The *erythrocyanosis cruorum puellarum* is marked by a bluish-red discoloration of the skin and a swelling of the lower leg in young females, most of whom suffer form dyorarism. This is a particularly striking example of the *influence of the endocrine genital glands.* Besides the externally visible discoloration, a follicular hyperkeratosis and a pasty infil-tration can also be observed in the affected area. The same triad in the outward appearan-ce is to be found in frostbite and, with differences in degree, also in acute frostbite (1st and 2nd degree).

In 1929 Perutz described an erythematous swelling on the inside of the knee in young girls and women with a tendency to ulcerous desintegration, after exposure to cold, a clinical picture which in our opinion also fits into the group of constitutional damage caused by a prevalent oversensitivity to cold.

Shelter Leg

This mild form of wet-type cold damage is referred to in the observations of American surgeons after the landing in Leyte (Philippines). The damage is predominantly of exo-genous origin. Men were affected who had to remain relatively still at night in damp conditions with a mild degree of cold. The same damage was observed in 1940 in people who had sought refuge in the tunnels of the London Underground during the night air raids (Whayne and Coats 1958). A heavy swelling similar to that found in trench foot and immersion foot without externally visible signs of cold injury (i.e. without formation of blisters and necrosis) is characteristic of this condition. Persons of all ages and both sexes were affected. Shelter leg was particualarly frequently found in fat women who had spent a long time in a sitting position in air raid shelters. Shelter leg is not dependent on the presence of varicosis or a damaged heart. As causal factors besides coldness and wet the motionless bent kneejoint and the reduced blood supply to the major politeal artery must be considered. The same also applies to people who were exposed to cold and wetness for a long time and had to sit motionless with dangling legs. The absense of any sort of pathological disposition to this kind of injury has been referred to in the literature. The effect of heaviness is apparently felt by part of the circulation. The fact that the marked tissue oedema encourages the tissue to cool down must be taken into consideration here.

A change in position generally led to an improvement and return to normal in a short time. On the other hand it sometimes led not only to oedemas but also to thromboses and in one case described by Simpson even to a pulmonary embolism.

In Germany the disease acquired the name "Schuppenbein" (Schuppen = scales, bein = leg, = scaley leg [approximately]) because after cold damage with oedemas a marked scaling off of the skin takes place. The condition of this cold damage is related to the acrocyanosis in young girls in puberty but is not identical.

Frostbite, 1st — 4th Degree

Under Normal Climatic Conditions

Frostbite under normal air pressure conditions used to be divided into three groups according to the degree of severity. Then, during the second world war, we experienced the state of total freezing of tissue and have termed this the 4th, the worst degree of localised frostbite, which mostly ends in total loss of tissue or limb. Mild frostbite normally remains fairly superficial. It can occur in damp, cold conditions at relatively low temperatures over or just under $0°$ C, or in dry cold with heavy frost. This shows the influence of the climatic conditions of wind and humidity. The time of exposure also plays an important part and this inspite of a certain effect of preservation which cooling exerts on tissue. Uncovered, exposed areas are most likely to be affected. The amount of tissue exposed is sometimes also of significance. Smaller limbs cool quickly as the quantity of heat is not so great, large limbs more slowly as their heat input via the arterial blood supply is considerably greater and cold spasms of the main arteries do not lead to ischaemia due to a blockage.

With common frostbite the etiological emphasis is on the *exogenous* factors and not as Ratschow assumed on endogenous influences. Anybody can be affected by a cold injury. The natural resistance to cold of the tissue and the general state of the health play a decisive part.

The surrounding contact area is of great significance for effective thermosteresis within a certain period of time, in particular humidity (icy water), cold mud and contact with metal. The clinical description of mild frostbite and its pathological physiology will be discussed in the following chapters.

At High Altitude (The Effects of Dry Cold Accompanied by Hypoxia)

High-altitude cold injury is considered as a special form of local frostbite. It is marked by the fact that in addition to the above-mentioned exogenous factors there is also a reduction of the oxygen partial pressure. It is clear that this form of frostbite due to *dry cold* and wind is mostly observed in flight personnel and occasionally on arctic expeditions or in high mountains (See Herlinghofen's report on his experience in the Himalayas). An inadequate outfit, the loss of gloves or a protective face mask etc. are often to blame for the injury (Davis et al. 1943). These forms have been regarded separately from common frostbite, the pathological substrate is, however, in no way different from the common forms of frostbite. As one very often finds temperatures as low as minus 40° C to minus 50° C and even lower at high altitudes the cold damage normally occurs rapidly and it takes only a few minutes or seconds for the tissue to freeze completely. The consequences are as to be expected.

If a cold spasm (shivering) coincides with an exogenous drop in the oxygen partial pressure, endothelial damage to the small arteries and veins or venous capillaries may occur (Whayne and Coats 1958). The relaxing of the ischaemic state after cold injury at high altitude apparently takes place particularly slowly. In the terminal blood vessels, especially in the veins, stases and thromboses then form. In dry-type cold injuries, which set in very rapidly, the otherwise normal, initial symptoms like pain and a clamminess and numbness of the limbs is often not experienced. Functio laesa, total anaesthesia and ischaemia set in at once, as does a hardening of the tissue, which as a result of freezing, normally leads to primary necrosis.

Deepseated Cold Injury (Loss of Temperature Due to Wet-type Cold Damage)

In The group of deep-seated cold injuries the delayed damage is of major significance. In the literature a distinction has been made, it is true, between immersion foot and trench foot, because of the external conditions, but clinically as well as patho-phsiologically no sharp division can be made. In both cases the damage is generally caused by long exposure to relatively mild coldness in a damp environment or in water.

The loss of heat from the limb is so acute that the inner tissue is also damaged. The frigostability and sensitivity of the different tissue substrata, for which scales have been set up, is here of great significance. Ungley already suspected that immersion cold injuries were primarily neurovascular disorders of an inflammatory nature, a view which the author has held for a long time and which has been proved correct by Thorban's (1962) experiments.

The term immersion foot was coined after sea disasters. This form of cold injury was observed when the rescued had to sit for a long time without moving in icy cold and wind, sometimes exhausted and in wet clothes and cramped positions in the rescue boats. Often they stood or hung with their legs in icy water for hours. Another factor was the *depressive effect on the circulation of sea sickness.*

Dunning recently reported (1964) on a 15-year-old patient who had hidden in a rescue boat at only −4° C. Both of his feet froze, both feet becam gangrenous and had to be amputated.

Trench foot differs from immersion foot only in that different external conditions cause it. The term was invented during the First World War in the muddy fields of Flanders. Here, too, two damaging factors are concerned, exposure of long duration and cold action caused by the cold mud which need not necessarily be frozen. As a rule in the development of trench foot the air temperature does not exceed 0° to $+ 10^{\circ}$ C, the ground temperature is around 0° C. The immobility of the limbs in these forced positions and the mechanical restriction of the blood supply to the extremities may also be partly to blame.

Only under these conditions can deeper penetration of the cold and disturbances of the cell metabolism of large limb areas occur, so that the inner arterial walls of an extremity also suffer damage in the form of a serous inflammation. Corresponding to trench foot there is also trench hand but it fairly seldom occurs. Fère deBoye (1917) quoted 30 cases of "main de trenchée".

The predominant symptom in the case of immersion foot and also of trench foot, even during the early stages of development (in the state of numbness of limb and relative functio laesa), is the growing cold oedema, which can later develop into a marked oedema due to disturbances in the permeability and loss of plasma in the tissue. If the inner temperature of a limb drops below the marginal temperature of minus 30° C, the tissue may freeze, which is more or less identical to 4th degree frostbite according to our experience and always leads to the total loss of the limb. (Details on the symptomatology of deep-seated cold injuries, see p. 81.)

Comments on Deepseated Cold Injuries at Temperatures Around and Above 0° C and on Ultra Rapid Cooling

In general experience has shown that it is not only the absolute degree of cold which is decisive in the development of a cold injury, that there is no absolute threshold temperature, but that the duration of exposure plays an almost more important part. In animal experiments it was easiest to produce changes in tissue if a mild degree of cold was applied.

For a long time it was believed that frostbite could only occur at outside temperatures under 0° C and frostbite was understood to be result of a *freezing* of the cells and tissue at different depths. This view had to be abandoned as wrong because it was discovered in time that even at temperatures over 0° C with high air humidity, wind and wetness but without the possibility of freezing more severe cold injuries with gangrene could occur. Temperatures over 0° C preclude a destruction of tissue by ice crystals. There must, therefore, be other biological causes for the necrosis. There is plenty of evidence available in the literature of cold damage including even gangrene at over 0° C outside temperature, although it must be mentioned with the reservation that the outside temperature can differ considerably from the ground temperatures and that one never knows exactly which subnormal temperatures the tissue has actually reached. If, on the other hand, marshland, for example, or mud or icy water are not frozen, a limb which is immersed in them cannot have reached, or ever reach, a temperature under 0° C, in other words, can never freeze, especially as the freezing point of animal tissue is generally around -3° C.

According to Melchior (1914), Delorme was the first to have observed cold injuries to the limbs in the Crimean war (1854–1855) at outside temperatures over 0° C. During the Franco–Prussian war (1870–1871) cases of genuine 1st to 3rd degree frostbite and cases of cold gangrene occured in November and March, in other words during the inter-seasonal period, at outside temperatures of 6.1°-7.9° C Wieting (1913), Dreyer (1913), Welcker (1913), Liebert (1914), Koehler (1913) and Lauenstein (1913) reported on frostbite due to wetness and loss of temperature in the Balkan wars at temperatures of over 0° C. The same thing repeated itself during the First World War, especially before Verdun and in the muddy fields of Flanders. At that time the terms trench foot, Flander's foot and pied te trenche were invented, which we today classify under the name *cold immersion damage,* which owes its development to the physical fact that the conductivity of water is twenty times greater than that of dry air, so that the loss of heat of a limb is abnormally great.

Hecht observed frostbite at plus 6° C, and even at 8° C. In 1915, at Przemysl, Volk and Stiefler experienced frostbite at plus 4° C and Floercken (1915), who has reported on this in detail, diagnosed cold gangrene in 1914 at 12° C. This is a rather dubious case, as the patient had suffered a bullet wound in the aa. tibialis anterior et posterior, which can in isolated cases itself cause an area to become gangrenous. In 1936 Osterland in his textbook of military hygiene found it necessary to refer to gangrene due to wetness as a special form of frostbite, whereas Dreyer (1913) and Wieting (1913), coined the term "cold-paralytic gangrene", which is misleading since the state of the arteries does not correspond to paralysis.

During the Second World War, especially during the inter-seasonal period, surgeons at the front diagnosed cases of wet-type gangrene. Unfortunately German surgeons did not concern themselves more closely with this special form nor did they make a note of them in their reports. This is the only explanation available for the fact that no detailed reports on immersion damage or trench foot exist. This is also why in Toppe's (1949) report on his experiences the false claim was made that in the Second World War on the German side trench food did not occur.

The distribution code for cold immersion damage and actual frostbite, defined according to degrees, is shown in Fig. 32.

In the autumn of 1940 Friedrich and Kroh observed cold and wet damage and in the autumn and April of the winters 1941, 1942 and 1943 the author observed them in Russia. On the other hand, American naval physicians, in particular, reported on immersion foot during the Second World War. We quote here the data provided by Harris and Maltby (1944), as well as White and Scoville (1945), whose experiences derive from fleet operations around Iceland and the Aleutians. They described forms of cold and wet immersion damage, particularly in young people who had sat for days without moving in rescue boats, with their feet in icy water. Their reports are reminiscent of the data provided after the battle of Monastir by Budisavlevic (quoted according to Sonnenburg and Tschmarke 1915), who referred to wet-type gangrene, which developed after soldiers had been standing in icy water for 4 days.

In the Second World War Webster et al. (1942) observed the development of immersion foot with loss of sensation and gangrene after 8 days among shipwrecked persons in the Gulf stream at temperatures of 15.6° C and higher. Old, i.e. subnormal temperatures, alone could never have produced this effect. According to Lewis, in a damp environment the skin already loses considerable heat as from around 16º C.

From the Korean war, too, similar reports exist, for example from Blair et al. (1951) and de Bakey (1951), who at the conference on cold injuries in 1951, reported on immersion foot, whereby de Bakey particularly stressed the danger of the *thawing periods,* which our experience confirms. Orr and Fainer, too, in 1952, reported on cases of trench foot in Korea.

As the prognosis of the cases varies so much, and delayed damage to the vascular system after immersion foot (invisible frostbite) in our experience becomes apparent almost exclusively after a long period, often after years, a clinical separation is justified.

In contrast to the experience of the effects of mild coldness over a longer period, it was discovered that a *short, intensive cooling of the tissue,* including *freezing,* does no harm worth speaking of, otherwise it would be hardly possible to use ice anaesthesia. Here we are concerned with the principle of ultra rapid cooling which fixes the tissue in an amorphous state, and prevents the crystallisation of the cell water and free water in the tissue. This suddenly stops at the same time the complete tissue metabolism and all the fermentation processes, so that the oxygen requirement of the tissue is reduced to nil. The tissue metabolism already reaches a standstill at plus 6° C, belowe this temperature the preserving effect of cold can be observed. Ultra rapid cooling, however, also has its limits.

Cold preservation often has a clinical influence. In 1941–1942, for example, we observed that in ischaemia produced by Esmarch's rubber bandage (exsanguination) the tissue survived much better after hours in the cold than in the warm (Killian 1942 a,b). In 1942 v. Schürer published approximate values for the recovery capacity of cold limbs with signs of ischaemia:

4–6 h	almost regular recovery capacity
6–8 h	frequently still capable of recovery, particularly after additional periarterial sympathectomy within 24 h
8–12 h	only in exceptional cases capable of recovery

This data, which he provided from experiments carried out in 1942, is very much outdated. Schaar et al. (1944) have since investigated the survival time of ligated rate tails with and without cooling. In a cold state the tissue survived 4 days without gangrene, whereas, otherwise, in only a few hours a state of necrosis had been reached.

It is very clear from several publications by Allen (1939, 1945) that after a tourniquet has been put on a limb and it had been cooled to plus 5° to 8° C, it can be preserved without damage from approximately 4 h to over 54 h. As is well and known, Allen (1939, 1945) and other American surgeons, such as Blalock and Mason (1941), Blalock and Duncan (1942), Coulter (1944), as well as Bruneau and Heinbecker (1944), have made this technique applicable to accident surgery.

References

Allen FM (1939) Am J Surg 45 : 495
Allen FM (1945) J Int Coll Surg 8 : 439
Ariev TV (1939 a) Vestn Khir 57 : 527
Ariev TV (1939 b) Sov Krad Zhur 43 : 391
Bigelow GW (1942) Can Med Assoc J 47 : 529
Blair JR, Dimitroff, Hingdey (1951) Fed Proc 10 : 15
Blalock A, Duncan GW (1942) Surg Gynecol Obstet 75 : 401
Blalock A, Mason MF (1941) Arch Surg 40 : 1054
Bruneau J, Heinbecker P (1944) Am J Surg 120 : 716
Burton AC, Edholm OG (1955) Monograph, Physiological Society, No 2. Arnold, London
Davis L, Scarff JE, Rogers N, Dickinson M (1943) Surg Gynecol Obstet 77 : 561
de Bakey ME (1951) Vasc Surg 64
Dreyer U (1913) Zentralbl Chir 40 : 1628
Ducuing J, Harcourt J, Folch H, Bofold J (1940) J Chir (Paris) 55 : 385
Dunning WMD (1964) Surgery 51 : 883
Edholm OG (1952) Practitioner 168 : 583
Floerken H (1915) Munch Med Wochenschr 7
Floerken H (1917) Bruns Beitr Klin Chir 106 : 4
Friedmann NB (1946) Am J Clin Pathol 634
Gans (1923) Handbuch der Haut- und Geschlechtskrankheiten 3 : 4
Gans (1925) Geschichte der Hautkrankheiten. In: Handbuch der Haut- und Geschlechtskrankheiten, vol 1. Springer, Berlin
Greene R (1940) Zentralbl Chir 695
Greene R (1943) J Pathol Bacteriol 55 : 259
Harris, Maltby (1944) Lecture. American Academy of Neurological Surgery
Heaton LD, Davis RM (1952) J Ky Med Assoc 50 : 206
Hecht K (1915) Wien Klin Wochenschr 65 : 1487
Higgins AR, et al. (1952) US Armed Forces Med J 3 : 369
Hodara H (1896 a) Munch Med Wochenschr 14 : 341
Hodara H (1896 b) Z Dermatol 22 : 445
Killian H (1942 a) Zentralbl Chir 1763
Killian H (1942 b) Arbeitstagung beratender Chirurgen, Berlin
Killian H (1966) Der Kälteunfall: Allgemeine Unterkühlung. Dustri, Deisenhofen
Koehler H (1913) Zentralbl Chir 35 : 1362
Kummer (1935) Geschlechtskrankheiten 2
Kummer (1938) Endokrinologie 20 : 326
Lauenstein (1913) Zentralbl Chir 951
Lewis RB, Moen PW (1952) J Med Sci 224 : 529
Lewis RB, Moen PW (1953) Surg Gynecol Obstet 97 : 59
Liebert KE (1914) Beitrag zur Kriegsheilkunde. Springer, Berlin
Loos HO (1939) Dermatol Wochenschr 1017
Loos HO (1953) Munch Med Wochenschr 90 : 155
Marchand F (1908) Handbuch der allgemeinen Pathologie, vol 1
Melchior E (1914) Berl Klin Wochenschr 48
Milian (1941) Paris Med 2 : 365
Monseignon A (1940 a) Presse Med 48 : 166
Monseignon A (1940 b) Zentralbl Chir 18
Movrey FH, Farago PJ (1952) Mil Surg 110 : 249
Orr KD, Fainer DC (1952) US Armed Forces Med J 3 : 95
Osterland (1936) Lehrbuch der militärischen Hygiene. Springer, Berlin
Paunesco-Podeanu A, Tzurai I (1946) Kälteschäden, Masson, Paris
Perutz (1929) Dermatol Wochenschr 88 : 709
Rabout R (1939) Presse Med 47 : 1683
Ratschow M (1959) Angiologie. Thieme, Stuttgart
Raymond V, Parisot J (1918) J Chir (Paris) 14 : 329
Ricker G (1924) Pathologie als Naturwissenschaft. Springer, Berlin
Rischpler A (1900) Beitr Pathol Anat 28 : 541
Sapin-Jaloustre J (1956) Enquêtes sur les gélures. Herman, Paris

Schaar, Jones, Lehan (1944) Surg Clin North Am 1326
Schneider E (1940) Zentralbl Hautkrankh 66 : 11
Schneider E (1942) Med Klin 1 : 389
Schneider E (1946) Arch Dermatol 4 : 186
Schneider M (1953) Langenbecks Arch Klin Chir 276 : 5
Schürer F von (1942) Zentralbl Chir 69 : 486, 1797
Schulze W (1943) Arch Dermatol 184 : 61
Shumaker HB, Kunkler AW (1952) Surg Gynecol Obstet 94 : 475
Shumaker HB, Lempke RE (1951) Surgery 30 : 873
Smith AU, Lovelock JE, Parker AS (1954) Nature 173 : 1136
Sonnenburg E, Tschmarke P (1915) Neue deutsche Chirurgie. Encke, Stuttgart
Southworth JL (1945) N Engl J Med 233 : 673
Theiss F (1940) Zentralbl Chir 102 : 424
Thorban W (1962) Bruns Beitr Klin Chir 207 : 87
Toppe (1949) Experience report for the Americans, World War II
Ungley CC (1949) Adv Surg 1 : 269
Uschinsky N (1893) Beitr Pathol Anat 12 : 115
Vagliano M (1948) Erfrierungen. Masson, Paris
Volk R, Stiefler G (1915) Wien Klin Wochenschr 28 : 116
Webster DR, Woolhouse FH, Johnston JL (1942) J Bone Joint Surg 24 : 785
Welcker ER (1913) Zentralbl Chir 40 : 1625, 1768
Whayne TF, Coats (1958) Cold injuries groundtype. USA General Surgeon of the Army, Washington
    DC
White JC, Scoville WB (1945) N Engl J Med 232 : 415
Wieting J (1913) Zentralbl Chir 40 : 593

Historical and Statistical Data on Frostbite

In peace time cold injuries relatively seldom occur and then only in isolated cases. We experience them most frequently in accidents in high mountains or during arctic expeditions, winter sports, at sea and on high-altitude flights. It must on the whole be admitted that our statistics on cold injuries of all different kinds are not very reliable, as many cases of mild frostbite (without treatment in hospital, sick quarters or military hospital), even cases of white death, have not been registered.

A whole series of reports on peace time cases do exist, but they tend to disappear among the reports on the mass disasters, which occurred during the two world wars. Nevertheless here are a few examples:

Around 1858 Braschnewsky (quoted according to Sonnenburg and Tschmarke 1915) reported on 800 cases which occurred near Maikop in the Caucasian mountains. In his dissertation from Petersburg, Hübener (1871) compiled a list of 340 cases of civilian cold injury from 54 clinics and assessed the total annual number at about 700 cold accidents of all kinds, including the most severe forms and deaths from freezing. According to Krjukow (1914), there was an average of 500-700 deaths from freezing each year in Russia. In 1880 Fremmert compiled a list of 494 cases of partial freezing (92.3% men and only 7.7% women), 40% of which were in a drunken state. Over a period of 20 years not more than 38 cold injuries were observed and treated in the surgical university hospital in Zürich (six of which were sport accidents).

By contrast, in the period between 1938 and 1940 Loos (1941) was nevertheless able to register 70 cases of different kinds of frost damage in the Innsbruck area. Seven of them had taken place during winter sports. In 1939 a disaster occurred on the top of the Schauinsland near Freiburg due to the fact that some British school children had got caught in a heavy snow storm and lost their way. Eleven school children died from the "white death" according to the reports of von Brandis in his brochure on frostbite (1943b). In the winter of 1940 a group of 26 men from a Swiss military detachment suffered considerable frostbite, especially to their hands. In 1941 Debrunner put this information together in the form of a monograph as the observations appeared to be of particular significance. He gave an exact description of the area of frostbite and the degree of each case, from which it could be seen that the skin across the knuckles is very sensitive to the cold, due to its tautness, and can be affected in isolated spots by frostbite (see Fig. 4 and 10a–c).

In 1940 Davis reported on frostbite among the members of the Tibet expedition of 1903/4 among Europeans and some local carriers. Dry cold was seldom the cause of the trouble. The combination of dampness and cold was the main cause of the damage. Amongst the more recent statistical data with information on the treatment of frostbite in peace time I would like to mention the work of Theiss et al. (1951) with 30 cases, Edwards and Leeper (1952) with 71 cases, Sarkisov (1952) with 180 cases of amputation, Lapras (1957, 1959) with 40 cases and Zaretzky (1959) with 64 cases.

Table 5

Wars	Data on cold injuries	Sources
3rd-4th centuries Greek armies in Armenia	Anabasis narrated by Xenophon: Greek armies suffered heavy losses in Armenia due to cold	Grattan (1922) v. Brandis (1943 a, b)
1700–1709 Russian campaign of Charles XIIth of Sweden	Charles XIIth's army suffered heavy losses during winter campaign in Russia due to cold	v. Brandis (1943 a, b)
1803 Napoleon's Russian campaign	Heavy losses in Napoleon's great army in Russia and Poland due to the cold	Larrey (1817)
1854 Crimean War	Approximately 2 % of all losses were due to the cold of 300,000 Frenchman 5,290 cases of cold injury, of which 1,178 were severe. English troops: 2,398 cases (total) with 178 deaths - many cases of immersion foot Of 50,000 Englishmen 1,924 cases of cold injuriy, 437 severe. At Sebastopol: 2,800 cases of cold injury, 900 of which were severe, some fatal Pirogow: of 116,000 wounded 2,632 cold injury cases	Sonnenburg and Tschmarke (1915) Holmes et. al (1915) Hays and Coats (1955) Pirogow (1864) Floerken
1862 American Civil War	Heavy losses due to cold on both sides, 15,273 cold injuries, of which 1,075 serious, 6 deaths and 166 amputations	Whayne and de Bakey (1958) Hays and Coats (1958)
1870–71 Franco-Prussian war	1,014 cold injuries, 6 fatal	Sanitary Officer's report (1880)
1877-78 Russian-Turkish war	Of 300,000 men in Bulgaria 5,403 cold injuries	Pirogow (1864) Sanitary Officer's report (1878)
1905 Russian-Japanese war	Both armies suffered heavy losses due to cold injuries (assessed at about 10,000) 1,200-1,500 amputations (67 % feet, 28 % hands)	Mac Pherson (1908) Whayne and de Bakey (1958)
1912–13 Balkan wars	Many cold injuries, even at temperatures over 0º C. wet-type cold gangrene, immersion foot, 2,000 cold injuries on the Serbian side.	Meyer and Kohlschütter (1914), Welcker (1913) Wieting (1913) Dreyer (1913) v. Budisavlevic (quoted according to Sonnenburg and Tschmarke 1915)

Table 5. continued

Wars	Data on cold injuries	Sources
1914-1918 1st World War	800 cold injuries quoted in Lemberg (Zuckerkandl), of 5,374 losses 434 cold injuries (East Front, 1915 according to Witteck) On the Russian Front: 8 % of all losses were cold injuries. In one night 10,000 cold injuries According to Tuffier: 79,465 cases of "pied de trenché" = 3.02 % of total losses At Verdun 3000 cold injuries (about 30,000 per year in all) Many cases of immersion foot (Floerken) according to Mignon 120,000 total losses due to cold (1914−18) English losses due to cold injury in all 115,367 in all theatres of war. High percentages of trench foot. At the Dardanelles of 14,584 losses 6,602 cold injuries, mostly immersion foot (from cold mud). At Gallipoli (1915) 15,900 cold injuries, in Serbia 998. In the Italian army: In the Alps in all 300,000 losses due to cold (according to Castellaneta)	Floerken (1915) Zuckerkandl (1916) Pranter (1915) Witteck (1914) Friedrich (1919) Tuffier (1918) Mignon (1918) Floerken (1920 a, b) English Sanitary Officer's Report (1931) Greene (1941) Castellaneta (1940)
1937 Spanish Civil War	Of 12,000 men at Ferstell in the Sierra Palomea 4.16 % cold injuries, (only 10 to the hands), 5 deaths	Jimeno-Vidal (1942) Lopez-Muniz (1941, personal communication) Ducuing et al. (1940)
1940-1941 Albanian-Italian Greek war	Of 400,000 Greek soldiers 28,000 cold injuries apparently occurred.	Katsar, Agnatis (1977)
1939-1945 2nd World War	incomplete data According to Mikat 252,664 cold injuries, over 90 % of them 2nd and 3rd degree by the end of 1942. 8,578,624 total losses of which 26.7 % from diseases, 3 % cold injuries (data excludes those treated in sick quarters) Upper extremities: 2,050 = 7.9 % Lower extremities: 230,557 = 91.4 % In the 16th army 19,694 alone in winter battle 1941/42, of which only 17 deaths U.S.A. (Navy and Air Force): 60,000 cold injuries. Many occurred in Iceland and the Aleutians. In Alsace in 1939/40: 10,000 cold injuries among French troops	Mikat (1951) Killian (1966) Webster et al. (1942) Schumaker et al. (1947) Lesser (1945) Harris and Maltby (1944)

Table 5. continued

Wars	Data on cold injuries	Sources
1950/52 Korea	5,629 cold injuries among American troops (many cases of immersion foot) 9.9 % of total losses with 10 % extensive loss of tissue Of 10,172 prisoners of war 720 cold injuries	Blair (1951) Orr and Fainer (1952) de Bakey (1951)

The reports on winter campaigns are, however, of far greater significance. A short summary is given in Table 5.

Frostbite occurs on a large scale in peace time particularly after natural disasters, e.g. earthquakes during cold periods, as was recently experienced in Turkey. There physicians not only had to cope in frost and snow with the injuries and state of shock of the casualties but also with cold injuries to the limbs and this caused further difficulties.

Classification of Cold Injuries

The years 1941–42 provide the most important statistical data. According to my own observations there were 18, 694 cases of cold damage in the 16th Army Division in the Northern Sector of Russia between 12.12.1941 and 31.8.1942. 393 early amputations were necessary. Seventeen patients died, mainly from septic complications, two of them being cases of tetanus. The distribution according to degrees of injury shows the following picture:

1st Degree: 4, 243 (26 %)
2nd Degree: 12, 993 (66 %)
3rd Degree: 1, 458 (8 %)

The 4th degree cold injury had not yet been distinguished by us at that point in time. No single case of immersion cold injury is cited in the statistics; these cases unfortunately got lost in the multitude and were not separately tabulated. In the Anglo-American medical reports of the Second World War, on the other hand, deep cold injuries (immersion foot, immersion hand, trenchfoot) are listed separately from ordinary cases of cold damage, whereby the former type almost always predominates (see Fig. 32). In another analysis of 25,781 cases of cold damage during the same time-span there were 15,404 1st degree, 8,998 2nd degree and 1,119 3rd degree injuries.

In all large-scale catastrophes it has been found that the lower extremities are much more frequently affected than the upper ones. In our data the distribution was as follows: 93.5 % damage to the extremities, 5 % facial region and 1.5 % other parts of the body. By way of comparison Koehler (1913) reports 90 % (extremities): 10 % (other parts), of which 6 % are 1st degree, 88 % 2nd degree and 6 % 3rd degree injuries.

Partsch (1943), on the other hand, found 77 % damage to the legs and 23 % to the upper extremities and other parts of the body. All together 55 % were bilateral. Reports by Witteck (1915) and Kirschner (1917) do not differ to any notable extent.

Cold damage to all four limbs is relatively rare. In 900 cases of cold injury from various military hospitals Frey (1942) found 826 cases of damage to the lower extremities, of which 262 were unilateral and 564 bilateral. There were 55 cases of combined cold damage (feet and hands).

The entire statistical evidence shows clearly that unusually localised forms of cold injury make up only 1 % - 2 % of the total data. In peace time males are three to four times more often affected than females. Cases of cold injury in children are rare.

Forms of Local Frostbite and Areas Likely to Be Affected

In the head region the scalp is at risk, though really only when it comes into contact with metal. At the front we saw cases of 3rd degree frost damage to the scalp due to the skin being in contact with a steel-helmet. In general these cases only occurred at temperatures of less than $-15°C$.

Cold damage to the *face* often arose through pressure points. Even the pressure of a wet veil on the bridge of the nose, the tip of the nose and the cheeks or a ribbon round the chin in females is sufficient to cause cutaneous frost damage (acrocyanosis). Women and girls with double-chins are particularly at risk. The fact that the ear-lobes and especially the rim of the ear are susceptible to damage through cold is understandable if we take the wet and air-flow into account (Fig. 4). That is why this type of cold injury occurs especially in lorry drivers, sailors, mountaineers and airmen. Cold damage to the cheeks and cheekbones is much rarer.

Moreover we are acquainted with cases of cold damage to the *lips* and, very rarely, to the *tongue* (Fig. 5). The partaking of ice and snow sometimes plays a part in cold injuries to the mucous membranes of the mouth, apart from the considerable cooling down of the lips, which are always moist, in cold and wind.

We have never encountered cold damage in the region of the *neck*. On the other hand cases have been reported of cold damage with deep tissue necroses in the region of the *trunk* and *abdomen* through the misuse of ice-packs, e.g. Williams (1923).

There have been numerous reports of cold damage to the male *genitalia* and also to the perineum. Such cases occur particularly in lorry drivers, skiers and mountaineers, especially when trousers and underclothing are not sufficiently well fitting and are easily penetrated by icy wind. Often people exposed to the cold have been unable to fasten their clothing again properly due to numbness in their fingers, and this has resulted in severe frost injuries to the penis (especially the glans region), and also to the testicles, perineum and anus. In some of these cases frostbite was the result of wetting. Men suffering from cystitis due to cold were mainly involved here. In 1950 Guerasimenko described a case of total gangrene of the scrotum and penis due to 3rd degree frostbite in a man who had fallen into water at $-30°C$ and was not able to be rescued until 3 days later. Genital frost injuries have been observed by Riehl (1915), Boehler (1917), Floerken (1920 a, b), Partsch (1943), Starlinger and Frisch (1944), Killian (1943), (Fig. 6). [Furthermore we have seen cases of men, who sat in armouredtanks for longish periods of time in icy weather conditions (escort infantry) with isolated frostbite necroses in the area of both sciatic bones and at the perineum.]

In the *upper extremities* hands, fingers and elbows are at risk. Frostbite rarely occurs in other parts, unless cold damage occurs to the fore-arm as a whole. In the area of the hands particularly the fingers, and of those the distal phalanges, the middlephalanx, finger-tips and also the area of the nail are at risk. Of the fingers the first and the fifth are particularly sensitive to cold, although there are considerable individual differences.

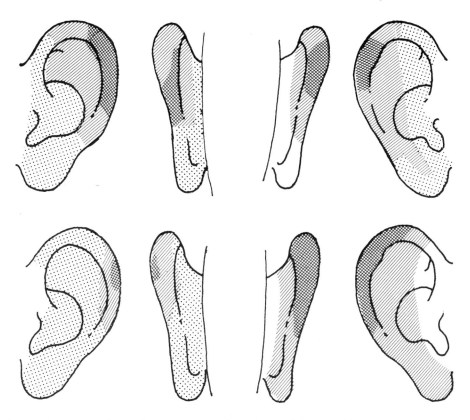

Fig.4. Damage to ears, severity of damage corresponds to degree of shading. (Observation by Debrunner, accident during manoeuvre of the Swiss Army)

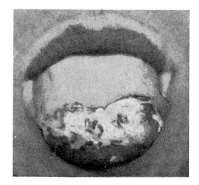

Fig. 5. Second degree frostbite of the lip and tongue. (Observation by Loos 1941)

Sometimes only the thumb is affected by cold damage und becomes necrotic to the basal joint. At other times only the fifth finger or each finger on its own is affected by cold damage and becomes necrotic to the basal joint, sometimes only the thumb remains intact. The couses of this phenomenon are not really clear but it may have something to do with peculiarities of dietary conditions (Figs. 7–12).

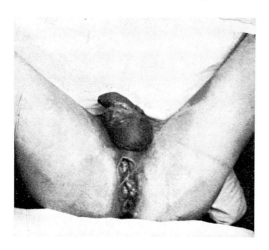

Fig. 6. Frostbite of the perineal region and area of the anus. (From a case by Partsch 1943)

In the case of cold injuries to the metacarpus the main point is whether or not the superficial or deep arcus volaris is occluded. If this is the case then the first segment including the thumb will not be preserved but becomes necrotic. If the entire hand including the main arteries is damaged by cold, then the area of cold injury generally extends to the end joints of the bones of the fore-arm, since the small wrist bones are supplied by fine retrograde branches from the arcus profundus (Figs. 8 and 9). This is known as „glove frostbite", because it extends as far as that part of the limb covered by a glove. Parts of the wrist are also particularly at risk, namely those areas where there is an accumulation of tendons without muscular covering, i.e. where the insulating warming muscular coat and the fatty tissue are minimal or non-existant and those areas over which the skin is taut. That is, for example, the region of the styloid process - the ulna. According to Debrunner (1941), who recorded schematically quite a large number of cases of cold damage to the hand, the degree of risk to the fingers increases from the second to the fifth, and the distal phalanges are particularly sensitive (Figs. 10a-c). According to Debrunner (1941) the thumb is fairly resistant to cold due to its better blood supply and greater bulk. One can see clearly from his diagrams, that zones of particular sensitivity are to be found over the joints.

In the *lower extremities* two areas are known to be particularly susceptible to cold damage. These are the frontal region of the knee joint and the area of the foot. At the knee joint the area over the knee cap is at risk, and this is most frequently so when the trousers are wet through and taut over the bent knee joint. Deep frost necroses are a possibility at this spot. Necroses over the head of the fibula appear relatively seldom (Figs. 11 and 12).

In the area of the toes the first, second and fifth toes are particularly at risk. The first toe on its own or all the toes except the big toe may be frozen. Furthermore the zone of cold injury may extend into the metatarsus and reach well beyond the ankle joints, cases of which are unfortunately by no means rare.

My diagrams show not only the *typical lines of frost injury* but also zones which are particularly susceptible to cold damage e.g. the area over the ankles, the outside edges of the feet, the balls of the small toes, the balls of the big toes and the dorsal side of the toe joints (Fig. 13).

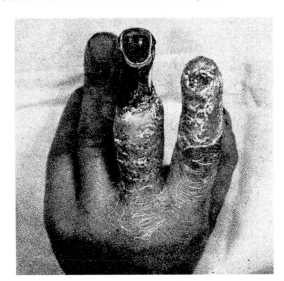

Fig. 7. Frostbite of the 2nd and 3rd fingers with mummification of the distal phalanx and parts of the second phalanx of the 3rd finger; damage to the other fingers. (From the collection of Sponholz, according to Starlinger 1944)

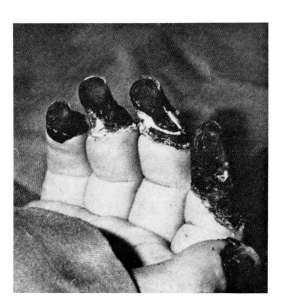

Fig. 8. Mummification of the fingers. (From Riedler and Floser 1970)

In the small toe one generally finds that the frost damage extends as far as the basal joint. In the big toe, however, 3rd degree frostbite is often found, which only affects the outer surface or the tip of the toe, or the first toe is frozen to the basal joint (Fig. 13). In these cases of total necrosis of the first toe the metatarsal bone is very frequently damaged as well, and during amputation cannot be preserved. Isolated frostbite at the tips of the toes is usually associated with pressure from the shoe. The shoe does not have to be too small; shrinking of the leather due to thorough wetness is enough (Figs. 14 and 15).

47

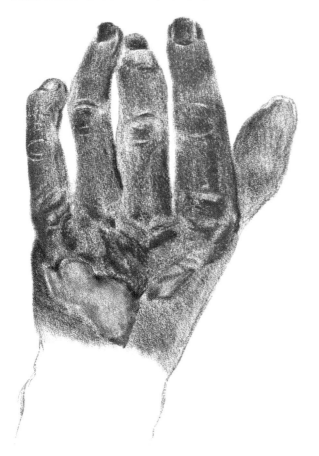

Fig. 9. Frostbite and dry tissue necrosis of the four long fingers of the left hand. Incipient demarcation of the gangrenous tissue. Characteristically, the thumb often remains intact. (From Schweizer Militärzeitung Nr. 1, 1944, according to Zofinger)

Apart from the typical frostbite zones at the level of Lisfranc's joint and Chopart's joint, the frost damage to the outer edges of the foot with complete preservation of the sole of the foot, we are familiar with the notorious *sandal-necrosis*, which mainly occurs through standing with bare feet on ice or on the metal deck of ships. When the necrosis mummifies and becomes hard the entire sole of the foot can then be peeled of (Figs. 16-18).

Not only are cases of isolated frost damage to the ankles, an area, which in itself is poorly nourished, extremely unpleasant, but also the necroses of the heels due to the profound effects of cold. In this condition the bone und insertion of the Achilles tendon are often affected. Chronic ulcerative processes, which extend deep into the balls of the heel, are the result (Figs. 19 and 20).

In cases of the most severe cold injury with damage to the arteries of the lower leg, the whole foot up to above the ankle is lost, sometimes even to about the middle of the lower leg. In general cold injuries do not extend any higher than this, even in the case of acute gangrene due to cold and wet and immersion (early injuries). Only in unusual cir-

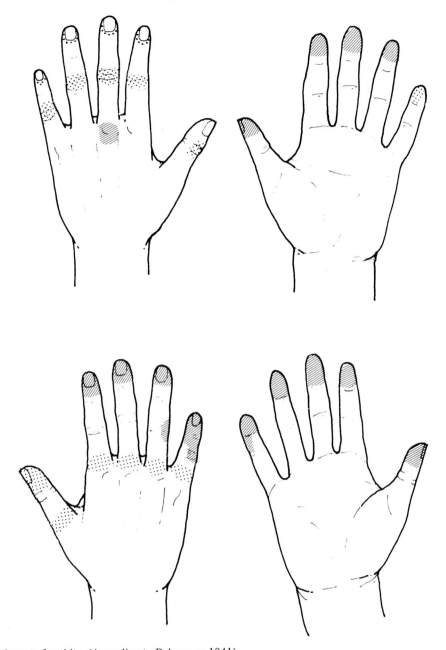

Fig. 10a. Schemata frostbite. (According to Debrunner 1941)

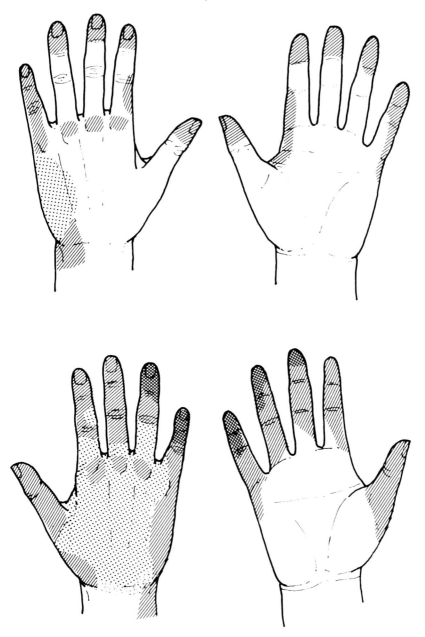

Fig. 10b. Schemata frostbite. (According to Debrunner 1941)

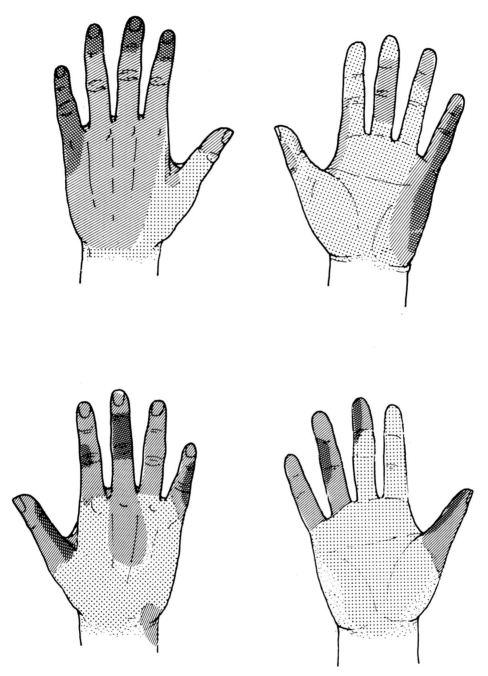

Fig. 10c. Schemata frostbite. (According to Debrunner 1941)

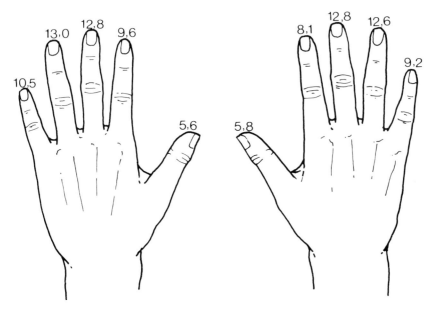

Fig. 11. Distribution (%) of frost-injuries to the hands. (From Guerasmenko 1950; Sapin Jalustre 1956)

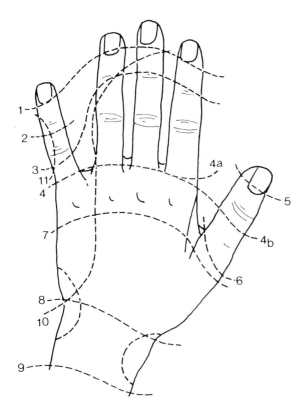

Fig. 12. Typical border lines of frost injury on the hand. *1* Frostbite of the finger tips 2 to 5. *2* Loss of the distal phalanx of 5 alone. *3* Frostbite of the distal phalanges 2 to 4 and of both distal joints 5. *4* Frostbite of the fingers down to the base of the metacarpophalangeal joint 2 to 5 alone (4a or 4b) including the distal phalanx of 1. *5* Frostbite of the thumb only. *6* Loss of the entire thumb. *7* Total finger loss including the distal metacarpal capitulum. *8* Loss down to the level of the wrist. *9* Total loss of hand including wrist.

52

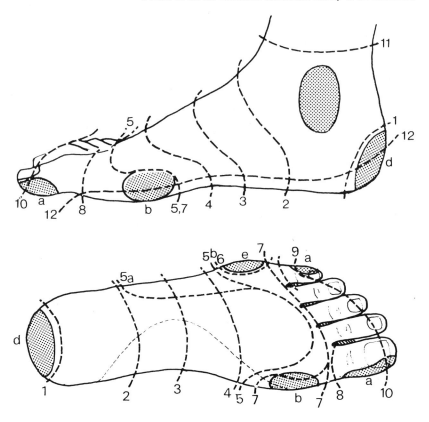

Fig. 13. Typical lines of frost-injuries on foot and toes. *1* Isolated frostbite of the heel area, with deep necrosis *2* Frostbite of the entire foot, without the ankle and heel area *3* Cold-injurie till the Chpart-joint *4* Cold-injurie of the entire forefoot including the balls of 5th and 1st toe. (*5a* with outgord of foot) *6* Isolated frostbite of the outbord of the little toe-ball *7* Cold-injuries of all toes till the basl-joints (*7a* with ball of the 1st toe, *7b* without the ball of the 1st toe) *8* Total necrosis of the 1st toe *9* Total necrosis of the 5th toe *10* Frostbite of all tiptoes *11* Total necrosis of the foot inclusive the ankle *12* Isolated necrosis of the entire sole (Sandalen-Nekrose) *a* Isolated frostbite of the outboard of the 1st toe *b* Isolated frostbite of the outbord ball of the 1st toe *c* Isolated frostbite of the inside of the ankle *d* Isolated necrosis of the heel, often with deep necrosis of the calvaneus *e* Isolated necrosis of the outbord of the ball of the 5th toe

cumstances does the loss of a whole leg up to the thigh occur, e.g. due to freezing under a very wet, icy transportation plaster (my own observation).

Bonomi, who particularly studied frost damage to the foot, has specified typical zones of frost damage according to the architecture of the arteries. He distinguishes three zones:
1) The zona phalangea (digital arteries), which extends to Lisfranc's joint.
2) The zona metatarsalia (interosseal arteries), which extends to Chopart's joint.
3) The zona tarsea, extending to the ankle.

One could undertake a similar division for the hand as well. Apart from these typical boundary lines at the extremities certain types of frost damage have been described and named on the basis of practical experience according to etiology and localisation.

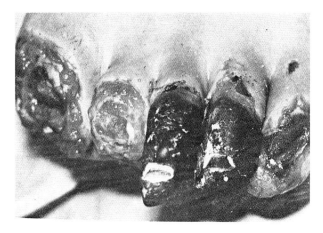

Fig. 14. Mummification of the toes. (From Spiegelberger et al. 1976)

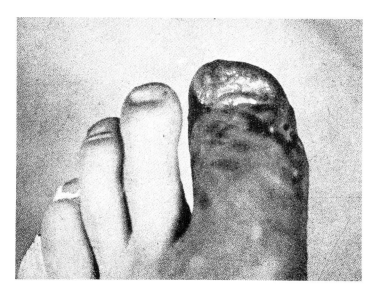

Fig. 15. Isolated 2nd degree frostbite of the large toe including outer edge and ball of the toe and parts of the metatarsal bone 1. (From the Sponholz collection according to Starlinger 1944)

A typical form of frostbite to the hand in riders due to pressure of the reins is known, an isolated frostbite of the 2nd. finger in marksmen due to contact with the metal of the trigger-guard, a typical frost injury of the under-side of the fore-arm or the elbow due to leaning on metal and a typical frost injury in the bearers of metal equipment. Furthermore we are acquainted with a characteristic type of frostbite to the forefoot in lorry drivers due to contact with the metal accelerator pedal and one of the heel due to prolonged supporting of the foot on icy-cold metal-plate, and also the typical frostbite of the feet in riders through contact with the stirrup.

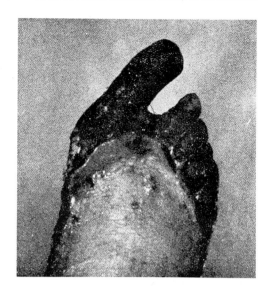

Fig. 16. Total necrosis of the entire forefoot including all the toes and edges of the foot in typical frostbite delineation. (From the Sponholz collection according to Starlinger 1944)

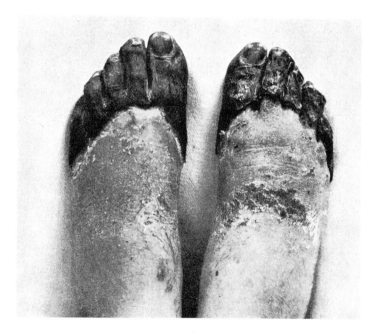

Fig. 17. Frostbite after development of demarcation. (25-year-old nurse, Engadin. Collection E. Ruppanner)

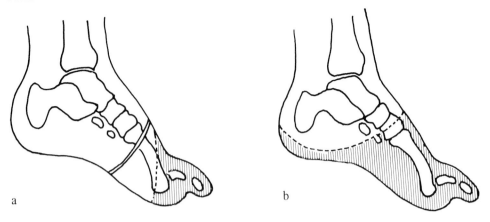

a   b

Fig. 18. *a* Shaded area gangrenous. Dotted line demarcation zone. Double line point of amputation. b Outline of a sagittal section. Shaded area gangrenous. Dotted line demarcation zone, which axtends to the sole and heel. (According to Sharp; Radasewski 1947)

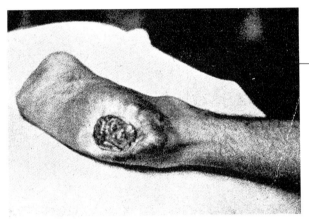

Fig. 19. Typical local 3rd degree frostbite of the heel with deep necrosis down to the level of the bone. (From a case of Frey 1942)

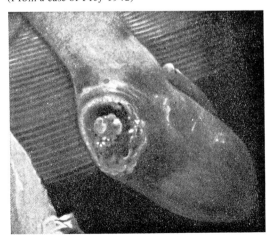

Fig. 20. Severe frostbite of the heel area with bone necrosis

Symptomatology of Localised Cold Injuries

Since every type of localised cold injury offers a changing picture in its total progress over days, weeks and months, it is useful to distinguish at least four developmental phases, as has been suggested by Russian, American and French authors (Guerasimenko 1950; Ungley 1949; White and Scoville 1945):

Phase I.   Acutal cooling process
Phase II.   Rewarming
Phase III. Reactive hyperaemia and development of manifest frostbite forms according to degrees.
Phase IV.   Reparative phase up to the point of recovery with or without permanent damage.

    During the first phase, that is to say, during the stage of cooling down of a limb or other part of the body, it is impossible to know what damage the cold has afflicted, i.e. what degree of local frostbite will develop, since the phase of rewarming is of the utmost importance for the survival of cells and tissue. From the practical clinical point of view this means that it is impossible to make an exact prognosis concerning the fate of the exposed region. This is also true in the case of freezing of the tissue, since, as we know, ultra rapid freezing is sometimes tolerated. Furthermore one can never assess the internal effects of cold on the basis of external signs. This only becomes evident on examination of the consequences.

Phase I[1] of Common Forms of Frostbite Classified According to Degrees

The localised action of cold on the skin of a limb leads in a reflex manner to an immediate contraction of the erector pili muscles. Areas with hard skin, the volar sides of the hands and feet as well as hairless parts of the body (face and neck), remain free from the phenomenon.

    On the other hand goose flesh develops rapidly on the dorsal sides of the extremities and varies in intensity according to the distribution and density of the original pelage. The symptom does not remain confined only to the point affected by the cold but rather irradiates, and the entire surface of the body may be seized by shivering and shuddering. Conciding with the development of goose flesh the flow of blood to the affected limb is reduced and water begins to vanish form the skin, it becomes dry and its ability to conduct warmth is thereby reduced. A progressive shrivelling of the skin takes place; it becomes wrinkled, flaccid and creased as its elasticity is lost. The skin may become taut

---

1   Guerasimenko (1950) and Ariev (1950 a, b) termed these events the pre-reactional or latent phase.

over bony parts and joints on the other hand and develop a smooth, even shiny appearance.

Any reduction in blood flow through a limb is connected with a loss of tissue fluid; dehydration occurs, the course of which can be followed on the plethysmogram (Wilkins et al. 1942; Mullinos and Shulman 1939; Burton and Taylor 1946; Behnke 1950, 1952). A brief increase in blood supply, which has nothing to do with the Aschoff-Lewis Reaction. Hunting symptom, may precede this event (initial rise in the plethysmogram).

The phenomenon has been subject to various interpretations. Probably this peripheral capillary reaction is an attempt to effectively counteract the cooling of the skin through an increase in the circulation and temperature. To some extent this has been proved by Behnke (1950).

If the action of cold continues for any length of time, a reverse shift of water occurs: cold oedemas of the tissue develop, so that a progressive increase in volume becomes evident (second rise in the plethysmogram). The drying-up of the skin is also related to a lowering in sweat secretion. It would appear that the second layer of the cutaneous capillary nets, which enclose the sweat glands, ceases to supplied with blood to any notable extent. Superficial arteriovenous connections remain open, the blood flows via short-circuits (Fig. 21).

Particular significance is attached to this dessication of the skin, especially of the horny layer, since it generates a considerable decrease in thermal conductivity and improves insulation (Rein 1943).

The presence of a bright red or lobster-red skin, which gradually becomes bluish red, is a typical initial reaction to cold. At the same time the skin is cold and remains so. This reddening of the skin with prolonged exposure to cold, especially after the hands have beeing in contact with snow, with standing in icy water or with the action of frost on the face is known to every layman. The condition is reversible and in no way represents a genuine 1st degree cold injury-frostbite erythema.

The development of a bluish redness signifies a dilatation of the veins and venous plexus of the skin, which is reversible, since it does not yet cause damage in the sense of an irreparable paralysis of the plexus-manifested as a permanent acrocyanosis, which appears very unattractive in the facial region, on the nose and cheeks and is related to unpleasant sensations in the hands and feet, particularly when it is warm.

We do not always find an initial reddening of the skin due to cold, but really only in the presence of a good circulation and adequate blood supply to the periphery. The anaemic or sickly person always looks pale and sometimes really marasmic in the cold and in this case we seldom find that lobster-like bright redness of the skin, such as develops from standing in icy cold water.

The bright redness is due to a particular state of the circulation. The reaction is due not only to a narrowing of the terminal arterial pathways with increased velocity of blood flow, but also to a decreased utilisation of the available oxygen in the cold tissue with regional arterialisation of venous blood. For more details see the section on the pathologic physiology of localised cold effects.

Even during the development of this bright redness a burning cold pain is experienced, especially in areas of abundant sensory supply, e.g. the fingers (Sapin-Jaloustre 1956; Vagliano 1948), which soon fades however, since paraesthesias develop and the affected region or limb becomes numb through anaesthesia. This is particularly the case with rapid

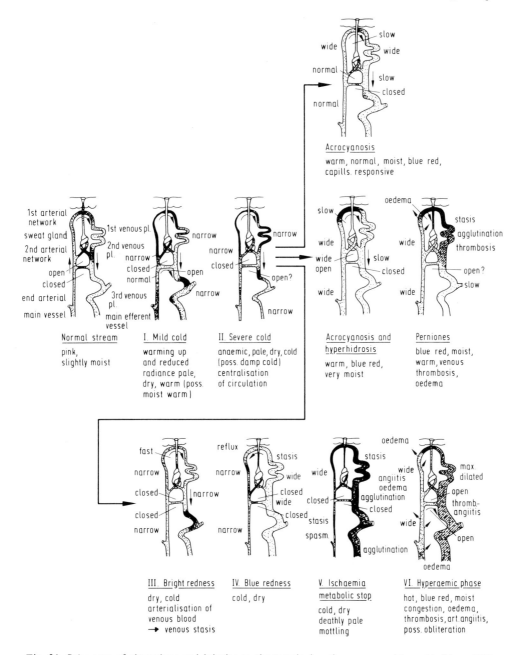

Fig. 21. Schemata of alterations and injuries to the terminal pathways coused by cold. (From Killian 1959)

cooling. In the case where an overall cooling-down occurs at the same time the initial warning cold pain is often missing, unfortunately. This is why the development of frost-bite is often not noticed by the affected person. The cold anaesthesia prevents cold pain, which only reappears, albeit in a vehement manner, during the thawing out phase.

Progressive cooling is more likely to be noticed in the highly sensitive region of the fingers than in the face and in the feet. Affected persons do in fact mention that the areas or limbs have become cold but that they did not notice frostbite (Larrey 1817; Killian 1942 a, b, 1943; Starlinger 1942; Vagliano 1948; Guerasimenko 1950; Allan et al. 1955; Sapin-Jaloustre 1956). Many people only become aware of the state of frostbite when they return to warmer surroundings, the typical intense thawing-out pains appear and the limbs gradually lose their stiffness.

Loss of sensitivity in a limb generally occurs prior to its total loss of serviceability. This is particularly so in the case of the lower extremities, for we were repeatedly able to observe that men with frozen feet still continue walking due to the fact that the calf-muscles still remain capable of functioning even after damage and loss of feeling to the toes and feet. Movement becomes slow however due to loss of the normal rolling action of the foot. On occasion we have even seen men with fully developed 3rd degree frost-bite still able to walk. Similar observations were already reported by Larrey (1817) and Legouest (1855) in the Crimean War (1854/55). (Hence the resistance of many casualties, who do not want to believe the doctor's words, to the necessary amputation.)

The phases of bright redness and bluish redness do not yet signify any particular danger. This only arises when spasms occur in the arterioles and small or middle-sized arteries and the affected zone suddenly develops a *waxy paleness due to ischaemia.* This later merges into a bluish-grey discoloration or mottling. The appearance of this ischaemia through a maximal cold spasm in the small afferent arterial vessels is a sign of acute danger. The bloodless regions now become icy cold. If no help is available they rapidly cool down to the temperature of the surroundings, and as a result can also be-come frozen. Whilst waxy, death-like paleness of a limb signifies ischaemia it does not necessarily have to become necrotic yet, because the cold itself increases resistance to lack of oxygen and has a preservatory effect. It usually starts unexpectedly after the dis-appearance of bright redness at the points of the most extreme loss of warmth, especially therefore at the ends of the limbs, the finger tips, the ends of the toes, the tip of the nose, the rims of the ear, earlobes and the glans and extends upwards in the limbs according to the length and intensity of the action of the cold.

In the case of sharp frost, metal contact and rapid deep-freezing the phase of bright redness may be omitted and a fatal paleness immediately appear, which has on many an occasion led to early necrosis. Davis et al. observed such cases in pilots in 1943 (rapid cooling in dry cold). On thawing out the damaged area does not warm up from within, because the circulation breaks down. Within a few days dessication due to water evapor-ation and mummification, which is easily recognisable from the black colour, occur. In these cases neither oedemas nor blister-formations develop, but only dry necrosis with shrivelling.

In 1953 Lewis and Moen simulated this form of rapid cooling experimentally and described it as coagulation necrosis. It can only occur when cold penetrates the tissue sufficiently deeply and damages the vessels since ultrae-rapid cooling and superficial freezing can be coped with by the tissue if it does not last too long.

Now, if exposure to cold is more prolonged, i.e. many hours or days, then the icy cold limb swells with oedema and bluish spots (mottling) appear, although blisters only rarely occur. The tissues become hard and the solidification process progresses in a central direction. (Shumaker and Lempke 1951.) Not only does circulation of the blood cease but also of the lymphatic stream. We have never seen brittleness of the limbs, which has sometimes been considered to occur in freezing and icing up. It is not supposed to appear until -80° C.

The limbs, especially the fingers may become very hard, however, and lose their elasticity through solidification of the subcutaneous fatty tissue, whilst at the same time their rough, dry surface feels like cardboard. In that sensational case described by Laufmann in 1951 of a Black woman, who was found with rectal temperature of -18° C, the limbs were as hard as glass and the pulse in the axillary and femoral arteries was completely absent. Loss of limbs also occurred afterwards.

The area first affected by cold tends to suffer the greatest degree of frost damage and later requires the longest time to recover. In the case of the cooling down of a limb that alteration in the musculature takes place, which we usually describe clinically as numbness, with an evident loss of motility and strength. Due to a disturbance of deep sensibility patients lose their sense of feeling for the positioning of limbs and joints. Motion and grasp become uncertain, cumbersome and awkward. Thereafter various limbs increasingly develop a rather bent, clutching attitude. The phenomena are based on changes in muscle protein, nerves, nerve conduction and also on swelling processes in the area of the tendons and joint-capsules, which Fox (1961) particularly called to attention recently.

During the first phase of actual cooling no further change occurs, the state of the tissue becomes fixed according to the duration of exposure, a preservatory effect takes place. Only in the border regions, with tissue metabolism still preserved at a temperature of over 6° C and with insufficient blood circulation, may a hypoxaemic state just possibly occur, which is not tolerated for any length of time.

Phase II: Rewarming and Thawing Out

The main feature of this phase is the inflow of warm blood into the areas damaged by cold or rather into the network of the obstructed or injured vessels and the transition into the picture of an inflammation with all its cardinal signs: rubor, calor, dolor, tumour.

The more quickly the action of cold occurs, the sooner a fixation of tissue with metabolic inertia can take place and consequently conservation without notable damage. The slower, the more intensively and the longer cold operates, however, the more intense is the cooling down of the deeper tissue and the sooner do the arteries, arterioles and terminal arterial ducts reach a stage of maximal spastic contraction, which can only be relieved with difficulty. Blood particles and fibrin threads become attached to the inner surfaces of the arteries as Hess was recently able to show with the electron microscope.

The capillary flow, the microcirculation, becomes reduced or breaks down completely and the blood in the dilated, paralysed veins silts up (sludge phenomenon)[1]. Accumula-

---

1   This can best be seen at the perionychium and especially at the conjunctival vessels. A distinction is made between red and white sludge.

tions of thrombocytes develop and ultimately, after engorgement by erythrocytes under the influence of activators from the vessel wall, agglutination thromb-ases develop, which occlude the lumen over considerable stretches. It is assumed that biogenic amines (histamines) are involved in the maximal dilatation of the veins.

Rewarming always occurs in two ways, that is from outside (e.g. via conduction) and from within along with the bloodstream, insofar as it becomes rectivated. Warming up from within the body is of critical importance, since warming from outside is of no use if the circulation does not simultaneously become activated; on the contrary it has a considerable damaging effect since the O_2 requirments of cell and tissue metabolism, which have been stimulated by the exogenous supply of warmth, cannot be satisfied and there is consequently a danger to the cells of asphyxia. In this respect premature rewarming may spur on the process of necrosis. *Warm blood and oxygen deficiency open the arterial vessels and relieve the cold spasm.* The gradual expansion of the arteries in the course of thawing out takes place according to the same laws as that of the blood stream; it begins therefore at the large arteries of the limbs and progresses distally into the damaged zone.

In the hypothermic region the vegetative alarm reactions to oxygen deficiency (pain) are severely upset by the cold at least for a time, so that the typical arterial spasm may continue far too long. If the circulation gets started, however, then the arterial vessels progressively expand and a state of intense *reactive hyperaemia* develops. The level of blood flow is well above normal, which one can just as clearly see in increased oscillatory deflexions as in the local warming. According to measurements by Leriche and Kunlin (1940) the temperature of the damaged zone ultimately lies a few degrees above normal. Blood pressure and blood content as well as tissue pressure increase considerably during Phase II. The veins still remain obstructed for a long time. A consequence of this is a marked congestion of the blood and the bluish-red discolouration of the limbs continues to persist for some time.

Rhythmic pulsation plays an important part in the gradual detachment of blood particle agglutinations and venous blockages, for it is much more effective than the simple increase in arterial circulatory pressure as one can see clearly microscopically (Killian 1952). The expansion of the arteries in the course of warming should not only take place through active relief of the spasm and dilatation but also to some extent passively through pressure.

At a certain borderline temperature the well-known intense thawing out pain occurs, which is sometimes extremely difficult to endure and can be very protracted. Thereafter sensations of itchiness and formication appear. A very unpleasant deep pain (periosteum pain) makes itself felt after the deep action of cold. The muscles lose their rigidity and the joints become actively and passively more flexible whilst at the same time often being painful (Fig. 22).

The more rapidly and intensively rewarming occurs the greater the pain (oxygen starvation pain); the more carefully warming-up occurs the milder are the thawing-out pains, especially when warming takes place naturally with the circulation from within. Kramer and Schulze (1944) have conducted interesting experiments in humans on the subject of *initial cold pain* and the *phase of thawing out pain,* and have recorded their occurrence along with the changes in blood contant and oxygen saturation (Fig. 23). Their experiment on the localised cooling of a finger to a temperature of -10° C shows a two-fold pain phase, namely during initial cooling and during rewarming. They found

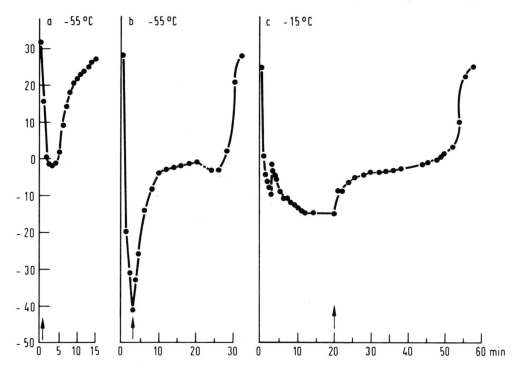

Fig. 22. Deep tissue temperature changes rabbit feet during freezing and thawing. Temperature measurements made by means of thermocouples implanted deep in the foot near the base of the toes. In each case the foot was immersed in the cooling liquid at O time and withdrawn at the time indicated by the *arrow*. *a* 1-min immersion at -55° C. *b* 3-min immersion at -55° C. Thermocouple moved slightly in foot at point indicated by dotted line. *c* 20-min immersion at -15° C. (From Pichotka and Lewis 1949)

that the pain first induced dilatation of the vessels, which leads to a cessation of the feeling of pain. The more intense the pain and the longer it lasts, the longer too is the relative vessel dilatation. If the sensitivity of the limb is abolished with novocaine a reduction in the reaction of the blood vessel system takes place both with regard to vasoconstriction and vasodilatation. The defence mechanism against the action of cold is disturbed or even abolished.

Furthermore Kramer and Schulze (1944) discovered in their experiments that a thermal equilibrium is still possible at a temperature of 0°C, perhaps even at temperatures as low as -5°C. Under -5°C intense vasoconstriction is thought to occur regularly, which leads to a considerable reduction in blood content. Such contractions in the afferent arterial vessels can no longer be abolished even by the most extreme oxygen starvation pains. Not until after the periodic vasodilatation, the purpose of which is to conserve the limb, (Aschoff-Lewis reaction, Hunting symptom) has ceased does the danger of freezing occur. Freezing does not take place immediately, however, but rather gradually, from around −3° to 4°C). Tissue damage is supposed to favour the occurrence of ice formation.

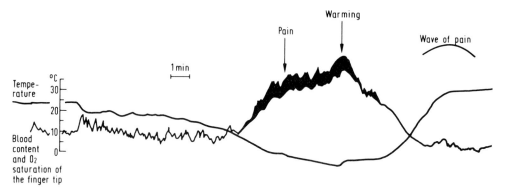

Fig. 23. Finger at -10° C (wind). *Upper curve,* temperature of the finger tip with calibration. *Lower curve,* blood content and O_2 saturation of the finger tip broadening of the curve indicates decrease in O_2 saturation, rise of the curve reduction in blood content. (From Kramer and Schulze 1944)

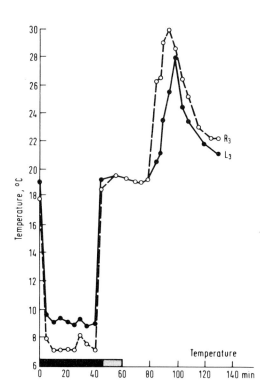

Fig. 24. Temperature curve of a finger cooled by immersion in water at 9°C (solid circles) and then at 7°C for 44 min Thereafter thawing in water at +19°C in the 44th to 59th min and then in air at 20°C. Striking increase in temperature after 80 min from an after-reaction due to vasodilation. (From Wolf and Puchin 1949)

Even when hypothermia is quickly compensated and normal temperatures attained a post-reaction of an inflammatory nature occurs, which involves further warming through reactive vasodilatation and increased blood flow, as has been shown in an experiment by Wolf and Puchin (1949), in which the thumb was cooled in ice-water and subsequently rewarmed in the air and in a water bath (Fig. 24).

Phase III

Phase III is rightly referred to as the phase of *reactive hyperaemia and hyperpulsion* (Killian 1943; Leriche 1945; Leeper 1952; Sapin-Jaloustre 1956). It is part of the overall picture of aseptic inflammation (Kreyberg 1946; Shumaker and Lempke 1951; Killian 1943, 1952) (Fig. 25).

The clinical picture is one of a deep flush, mottling of the skin and heat in the limbs. Cyanotic bluish-red zones may persist for a considerable length of time and contrast with the bluish-grey areas, which are not yet supplied with blood. The apperance of such a limb in Phase III is consequently variated and multi coloured. In 1919 Grezillier coined the expression "pied bi-ou tricolore", which was also used later by other French surgeons (Fievez 1939, Sapin-Jaloustre 1956). Since the cold leaves behind capillary paralysis with damage to the walls and a protracted disturbance in permeability, warm blood pours into a permeable vessel system so that red blood corpuscles escape from the lumen (erythrocytic diapedesis) and cause small haemorrhages and imbibition of the tissue with blood. Apart from this there are purely physical reasons for the migration of water into the damaged, acid tissue, so that even before rewarming a severe cold oedema may be present. There is a transudation of plasma through the blood vessels into the tissue (serous inflammation), which saturates it and the vessel walls themselves (especially the intima), and which may be of fateful significance (Fig. 25).

Characteristic of the rewarming phase is the *rapidly increasing secondary oedema and the abrupt swelling of the zones damaged by the cold*, which is particularly evident on the dorsal sides of the hands and feet. At the same time the skin becomes taut and shiny. When the oedema is pronounced it may of itself inhibit circulation in a mechanical

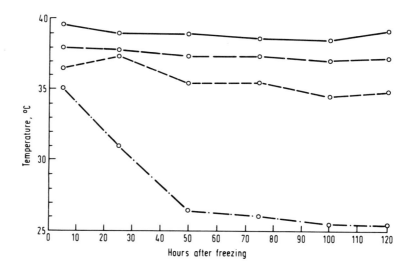

Fig. 25. Skin temperature graph of a rabbit ear, the extremities of which were supercooled for 90 s at -55°C. o--o rectal temperature; o–o proximal area of the non-exposed part of the ear; o--o distal area of the exposed part of the ear; o-.-.-o the other non-exposed ear. (From Fuhrmann and Crismon 1947)

65

fashion. The intense swelling often results in the casualty's being unable to remove his shoes, so that they have to be cut open. According to the degree of frost damage blisters may shoot up during the stage of the pronounced oedema, fill up with serum and confluate. Towards the end of Phase III the oedema becomes less pronounced, the tissue develops a spongy consistency. Not until later do the blisters begin to dry out, if they have not burst. Areas which remain waxy pale, bluish-grey or blue during the third reactive hyperaemic phase and which do not warm up with the circulation or at the most attain the warmth of the surroundings, and zones which do warm up for a brief period but then become cold again through secondary arterial vessel occlusions, are generally destined to be lost (Fig. 26). One can, however, rarely be certain about the fate of the tissue prior to 24 h after exposure to cold, and in most cases not until much later. This shows that even during Phase III one can still make no final prognosis.

Phase IV: Phase of Recovery

The clinical division into degrees of visible, manifest frost injury.

General

Many surgeons and dermatologists have attempted to develop a usable scheme for classifying frost injuries according to degrees from the clinical stand point. Perutz (1916), Wieting (1913), Dreyer (1913), Koehler (1913), Osterland (1936), Raymond and Perisot (1918), Vagliano (1948) and many others have in their time suggested a division into three degrees, Legouest (1855), and Fremmert (1880) one into five degrees and the dermatologist Ullmann (1932) has even suggested seven degrees. Most common is the one into three degrees (corresponding to burns), to which, however, was added a fourth degree of total icing-up during the Second World War. This indirectly suggests that in most peripheral frostbite cases, even when necrosis occurs, the tissue was not completely frozen ("frozen to ice") (Killian 1942 a, b; Heaton and Davis 1952; Orr and Fainer 1952;

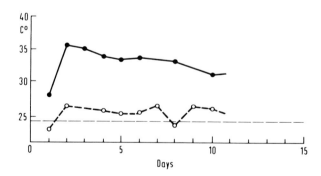

Fig. 26. Change of skin temperatures in the area of the large toe in two cases of frostbite to the large toe in men *Upper curve*, frostbite without necrosis; *Lower curve*, frostbite developing into cold necrosis; *broken line*, room temperature. (From Glenn et al. 1953)

Bell et al. 1952). Such descriptions according to degrees are basically very unsatisfactory and incorrect since higher degrees of damage are always accompanied by lower degrees.

The manifest local cold injury is categorised according to the highest prevailing developmental level without taking into account the evolutionary phases. In spite of this, the division into the degrees 1-4 with the following clinical characteristics has become widespread:
1) Congelatio erythematosa (frost erythema)
2) Congelatio bullosa with epithelial desquamation and blistering (phyktena)
3) Congelatio necroticans, gangraenosa seu excoreatica (frost gangrene)
4) Congelatio necroticans due to freezing, total gangrene of entire limbs.

Whilst 1st degree frost damage does in fact occur on its own, zones of lesser degrees of damage are always present with all the other degrees of frostbite, especially the 3rd and 4th degrees, and in general succed one another, not only in the caudal to cranial direction but also from surface to centre (Starlinger 1942, Killian 1942 a, b). Furthermore the zones of damage do not succeed one another in level planes corresponding to a segment of a limb but rather in configurations which correspond to the afferent blood vessels and inner warmer core. This is the reason why irregularly shaped areas of damage and necrosis develop (Floerken 1917, 1920 a, b; Killian 1942 a, b), (Fig. 27).

In practice one finds, therefore, that underneath zones of 3rd degree damage zones of 2nd and 1st degree damage are always present. Fortunately a necrosis may remain only superficial so that it can be peeled off or drops off on its own after mummification and drying-out and one is astonished to find tissue, which is still viable and serviceable underneath.

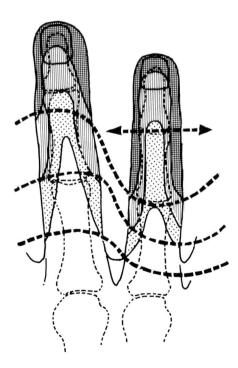

Fig. 27. Diagram of the deep action of cold; zones of degrees of frostbite

Thus bowl-like zones of damage and necrosis develop, such as one sees particularly in the case of necrosis of the heel, necrosis of the edges of the feet and necrosis of the finger tips. It is easy to be deceived, since the external condition often appears worse than it really is.

In the case of degrees of cold in immersion injuries exactly the opposite is the case. Here the external, barely recognisable damage is a very poor criterion for judging the case and it is not suited to provide information as to the nature of the internal damage (Killian 1959; Thorban 1962).

If the prolonged cooling-down of larger parts of the limb has occurred along with the local frost damage, mixed forms of visible and invisible frost injury with all the consequences may develop. Both above and below a visible frostbite necrosis one regularly finds an area which has also been damaged (Lewis and Moen 1952; Pichotka 1949; Killian 1952), a situation which must be taken into account in claims for maintenance.

First Degree Frostbite

Frost erythema is characterised by a light redness or dark redness with bluish mottling in parts, slight swelling of the skin and pressure sensitivity. It corresponds roughly to the picture of erythema solare without blister formation. This state is reached, about 12-24 h after exposure to cold, through rewarming. Due to capillary expansion and aseptic inflammatory manifestations the previously cold, pale, dry skin becomes bright red and hot (experienced as burning hot). Its temperature now lies above the norm. In this state there are generally more or less intense superficial pains and a feeling of tautness, since the deeper tissue may also become slightly swollen. In addition there is moderate dissociated disturbance of sensation. Hyperaesthesias and paraesthesias and, more rarely, anaesthesia may exist for a short time.

Zones of 1st degree frost damage generally heal up without scars even without treatment, accompanied by itchiness and desquamation of the skin. Only in a certain proportion of cases does some slight damage remain. Thus, for example, the *nails* of the fingers and toes may be lost after frost erythema or trophic disorders may develop and result in deformed hyperkeratotic nails (Moser 1942; Oehlecker 1942 a, b). As a rule the areas remain oversensitive to cold and also relatively cool. Due to permanent neuro-vascular damage, particularly of the cutaneous veins and venous plexus, there may be acrocyanosis, the flaming bluish-red colour of which is particularly ugly and disfiguring in the face and hands. In other cases abnormal pigmentation of the affected zones in the form of melanodermis occurs or the skin remains abnormally pale.

Second Degree Frostbite

It takes 24-48 h after the onset of rewarming for manifest local 2nd degree frost injury to achieve its full state of development. The more rapidly and ruthlessly this occurs the quicker the picture of manifest injury comes into being and, at the same time, the more serious is the result, at least when exposure to cold has been more prolonged and it has not been a case of rapid hypothermia of short duration. The 2nd degree is characterised by rapidly increasing oedematic swelling of the affected area. This is mostly a combination of a cold oedema, which develops on the basis of a disturbance in the electrolyte and water distribution in the increasingly acidotic tissue and an oedema, which develops in the process of rewarming. The former may be absent, the latter is due to the influy of warm blood into damaged vessel ducts and into a capillary net, which has become permeable. In the process of warming up the exposed regions reach a state of *serous inflammation with albuminexudation into the tissue* and tissue spaces. The oedema fluid may be reddish in colour due to cold haemolysis.

At the height of the *marked oedema* the characteristic blisters shoot up (hence the name congelatio bullosa). They develop on the dorsal sides of the limbs and on the face, as well as in other parts of the body, but never on the hard skin region of the inside of the hand, of the volar surfaces of the fingers or toes or on the soles of the feet. The blisters are produced by a raising of the epidermis owing to increasing hydrostatic and osmotic pressure in the oedema fluid in the relatively confined region of the skin, to be exact in the space between corium and epidermis. Their content is initially cloudy serous but then generally becomes bloody serous, so that the entire blister ultimately assumes a dark red, sometimes even blackish-red appearance. A striking discoloration also occurs in the 2nd degree frost blister as it is shrinking and drying out and may thereby occasionally deceive one into believing that necrosis has occurred. The serous content of the blisters very soon becomes opaque and purulent due to invasion of leucocytes. In contrast to burn blisters the raised skin is tougher, leathery, but nevertheless susceptible to tearing. Sometimes such blisters protrude only at the dorsal ends of the fingers and toes with simultaneous raising of the nails. Sometimes they spread over the back of an entire hand or foot especially in young people. Adjoining blisters may coalesce and form large pads (water cushions). They may also burst and the content flow out and soak the bandages. Underneath open blisters can be seen the flaming red or discoloured surface of the corium. Blisters, which are in the process of drying up, may serve as vital protection. However one never knows what may be hidden under such an epithelial swelling. See the reports of Frey (1942), Moser (1942), von Brandis (1943 a, b), Starlinger and Frisch (1944) and others. Underneath many a large blister a tissue necrosis or abscess develops, which extends as far as the underlying bone, fasciae or even a joint.

In 1944 Loos succeeded in demonstrating that frost blisters contain four times the amount of histamine-like substances as normal tissue fluid; this is to be understood as a sign of local   asphyxiation-metabolism   of the tissue. In the frost blisters the insulin values were higher than in blood serum with simultaneous hyperchloraemia and hypernatremia.

The presence of histamine points to a disturbed tissue metabolism, imperfect combustion processes due to oxygen deficiency. The whole area becomes bright red or bluish red, also mottled in parts (pied bicolore) depending on the different levels of circulation and usually becomes extremely painful (burning pain) after the cold anaesthesia has died away, as Vagliano (1948), Paunesco-Podeanu and Tzurai (1946) have mentioned in particular.

Disorders of sweating also occur and are unpleasant in the hands. The skin becomes abnormally dry and easily cracked in parts, whilst in other parts hyperhidrosis occurs, which may be tenacious (see Fig. 21).

Moser (1942) repeatedly saw hyperhidrosis in cold bluish-red hands, which was so intense that the sweat collected in visible streams in the palms of the hand and dripped off the fingers. We too have sometimes observed such cases of profuse hyperhidrosis after fresh 2nd degree cold injuries.

During exposure to cold the wide capillary network is not supplied with blood and the sweat glands are thereby disconnected. In the reactive phase and later on the sweat glands may excrete to an extensive degree as a result of increased circulation. In some cases this injury to sweat gland-innervation and -circulation may persist. In a state of hyperhidrosis the emission of warmth from the affected areas is increased and it has been established that there is a considerable delay in healing and increase in cold sensitivity.

After 2nd degree cold injuries a *disturbance of tendon and skin reflexes* may persist for some time. In other cases, however, there is a fairly persistant hyper-reflexia. Furthermore a decrease in *sensitivity to warmth and perception of warmth* has been noticed, which is possibly connected with a direct injury to the thermoreceptors and their related paths.

Occasionally one finds that the *musculature* in the area of 2nd degree frost damage has become slightly hypotonic. On occasions a fine to coarse tremor also persists for some time. These phenomena are probably based on a disturbance in the pertinent innervation of the agonists and antagonists or on a slight myositis. In the zones adjacent to the normal tissue the periosteum may show increased sensitivity to pressure and tapping. Aching pains in the limbs, slight cramps in the limbs, slight cramps in the calves or feelings of tension, which are apparently due to deficient circulation in the affected area, as a result of irritation by cold, are rarely reported. When they are present they are based on a contraction of the arteries, which lasts considerably longer than the freezing.

All blisters are subject to the threat of invasion by germs and *infection,* which must be avoided as far as possible, since it leads to a considerable deterioration of the condition. All types of suppurative processes, such as lymphangitis, thrombophlebitis, phlegmons, erysepelas, osteomyelitis, empyema of the joints may develop in the area of frost damage and necessitate early amputation due to moist gangrene. *In every case of 2nd degree frostbite there is also a danger of tetanus* and as with cases of 3rd and 4th degree frostbite prophylactic anti-tetanus treatment is a basic necessity.

The regenerative phase of 2nd degree cold injury normally lasts about 2-3 weeks. In the case of deep action of cold however complete healing may take months. Unattractive scars with scar distortions generally tend to remain only when the blisters become infected. The affected area remains sensitive to cold.

Atrophic processes in the skin cause thinning, abnormal stretching and susceptibility to damage. *A loss of the nails* of the toes and fingers almost always occurs, the substitute nails are hyperkeratotic, as are the scars on occasion and they then remain sensitive to pressure; slight trophic injuries, *acrocyanosis* or *pigmentation* occur and in many cases paraesthesias persist for a relatively long time. On the other hand deep-seated injuries to nerves, vessels, muscles or bones are generally absent in this form as long as cold effects due to immersion have not occurred at the same time. 2nd degree cold injuries very often cause trouble in subsequent winters. There are often relapses.

Third Degree Frostbite

The development of 3rd degree frostbite ensues via stages 1 and 2 and zones of the latter always surround the developing *necroses,* a characteristic of congelatio necroticans. By this stage damage is no longer confined to the superficial tissue, but rather there are layers of tissue under the frost blisters, whose viability is seriously affected, either directly due to the effects of cold or possibly due to tissue asphyxiation. Intense swelling, oedema and serous inflammation of the entire region occur. Asphyxiation-metabolism does not however occur until the thawing out period, i.e. during the rewarming phase, since tissue in a hypothermic state is resistant to oxygen deficiency. The necroses may be limited to relatively small areas, they may remain superficial without deep-seated effects, they may also, however, take hold of deeper tissue, with the result that whole portions of limbs such as the fingers, metacarpus, or even the entire hand, toes, forefoot or the entire foot are lost. Larger-scale necroses with loss of entire limbs do not occur very often, however, and are usually the result of immersion cold injuries with exceptional cooling-down of the tissue.

A *preliminary fine demarcation line* is distinguishable on the 2nd or 3rd day after rewarming, which may still shift distally in the natural warming process and through improvement of circulation with additional measures and is thus not a definitive boundary. Furthermore the externally visible, provisional demarcation line does not correspond to the demarcation of deeper tissue layers in general. One often finds that the necrosis has only a cup-shaped form so that lamellar black scabs may then be peeled off from the underlying surface. There is therefore a *sham demarcation* to which Moser (1942) has already referred. Some parts of limbs, which seem to have a doubtful prognosis, can still be saved.

Areas, whose vitality is endangered, do not warm up since circulation has completely ceased. It is possible to define the area which is not being nourished more closely by means of temperature measurements at the surface and particularly at depth and by means of arteriography, in order to gain reference points for the upper level of a necessary amputation (Leriche and Kunlin 1940). These ways of determining the matter are generally not necessary, however, since information about the dividing line between the tissue, which is still viable, and that which is becoming necrotic, is available within a few days in any case, being recognisable by the now *definitive deep demarcation furrow,* whose edges protrude like a wall and are covered with secerning granulations. At the same time the 2nd degree oedemic zones above the level of the necroses remain in a state of reactive hyperaemia and serous inflammation for a fairly long time yet, whilst the zones of 1st degree injury are already in the process of healing.

Since the necroses become dark red, brown or greyish to blue black, as long as moist gangrene does not occur, the bright picture of "pied tricolore" comes into being. Soon after *mummification of the dead tissue* and the formation of black scabs, which remain attached to the underlying surface for a good while, occur as long as no complications develop. Mummification is due to water loss and dessication and from a clinical point of view is regarded as favourable compared with moist gangrene.

The demarcation furrow extends down to the bones; distally from here the soft parts rot off if they do not dry up. X-rays show, however, that the bones keep their calcium structures for a long time so that it is impossible to decide to what extent they are

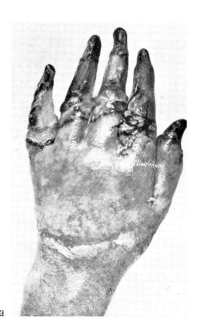
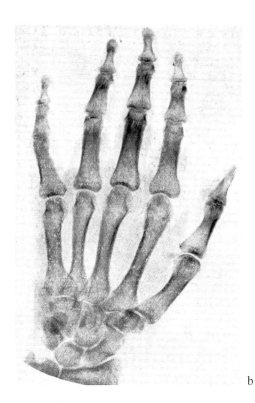

a   b

Fig. 28a and b. *a.* Severe 3rd–4th degree frostbite of the left hand with advanced necrosis of the fingers. (From Oehlecker 1942) *b.* After 14 days: the skeleton of the phalanxes demonstrate no remarkable changement

still being nourished. Therefore the X-ray does not help the clinician very much at this stage (Oehlecker 1942 a, b; Killian 1952). The bones often project freely out of the soft parts (Fig. 28a and b). The tendons, ligaments and capsules are resistant. They do in fact become necrotic and discoloured but take so long to fall off that one is generally forced to sever or remove them operatively in order to promote recovery. When the dead bones do not fall off of their own accord they can usually be removed without the use of anything more complicated than forceps a few weeks later. The entire granulating demarcation zone and the area above it (2–3 cm) are always badly nourished. If one leaves it to take its own course, *recovery will be very protracted with oversensitive, poor, thin skin.* In this area trophic ulcers develop easily. They tend to burst and recur in subsequent cold seasons. The scars are always hyperkeratotic and sometimes remain painful to pressure. Unfortunately centres of irritation often develop in this area, which grievously disturb the vegetitive functioning of the whole organism and lead to chronic pains and functional troubles. As long as they remain in existance they also as a rule lead to a spasm of the large arteries of the limbs, which has an unfavourable effect. It is therefore not expedient to leave the demarcation to its own fate.

Not only the blisters and rhagades but also the demarcation zone in particular are susceptible to the influence of pathogenic germs. The demarcation zone must always be regarded as multi-infected. Trouble is immanent when septic temperatures, acute swelling of the entire region and extreme pain develop. There is *danger of wet-type gangrene.* A multitude of septic complications including *wound diphtheria and tetanus* often have their origin here. They may still subsequently determine the fate of a limb or even endanger life.

If the course of things runs normally the oedema and serous inflammation gradually disappear; however, high albumen content in the tissue almost regularly leads to a more or less severe fibrous degeneration and scarring (particularly in the muscles) which seriously affect the usefulness of a limb and may also cause a severe disturbance in the circulation. After 3rd degree cold injury one regularly hears reports about the extreme sensitivity to cold of the region. Objectively speaking the affected limb is generally cold, the skin temperature markedly reduced. There is always trophic skin damage with loss of nails and sensitivity usually remains disturbed for years.

Fourth Degree Frostbite

Fourth degree cold injury is characterised by solidification of the tissue due to freezing. There is complete loss of circulation, cessation of metabolism and anaesthesia. The limbs feel icy cold and as hard as stone and are usually a pallid or blue-grey colour.

We are familiar with a short ultra-rapid type of freezing such as that which occurs with an ethyl chloride spray and which may be seen as a fixation of tissue in an amorphous, inert state (without the formation of coarse ice crystals) and which, if exposure is brief, may be tolerated practically without any damage. As opposed to this, however, gradual cooling leads to freezing of the free water in the cells and intersticial spares with the formation of large ice crystal needles, which apparently destroy the cells and tissue structures in a mechanical fashion in such a way that necrosis occurs. Only the latter type of freezing conforms to 4th degree cold injury and the affected tissue almost always becomes completely necrotic. As a rule therefore, total necrosis, moist gangrene or mummification occurs in the entire frozen area (Figs. 29 and 30).

Rewarming along with the blood stream does not take place in an area damaged in this way; at most a gradual rewarming up to the temperature of the surroundings occurs. In the case of a rapidly developing moist necrosis, however, one also sometimes finds abnormal heat development due to the intensity of tissue decay.

In other respects the same rules hold for the demarcation and development of gangrene as for a necrosis in 3rd degree cold injury, with the only exception that losses are much greater and affect considerable portions of limbs, e.g. the foot together with the lower leg (possibly up to the knee) or the hand with parts of the forearm.

We have often observed and described this form of cold injury (von Brandis 1943 a, b; Starlinger 1942, Killian 1942 a, b, 1943). It was confirmed in the Korean campaign (see reports of Pratt 1953; Orr and Fainer 1952; Movrey and Farago 1952; Canty and Sharf 1953).

Before we go on to internal cold injuries let us have a look at the external manifestations taking as an example a case of quadruple cold injury with deep-seated effects and partial freezing of the feet.

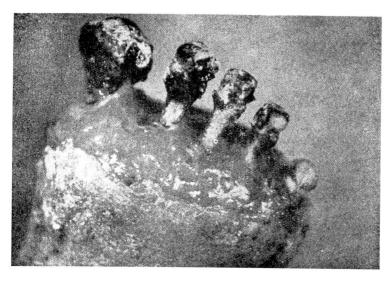

Fig. 29. Necrosis of the toes. The bone stumps can be seen to protrude from the rotting tissue and demarcation zone. (Sponholz collection, from Starlinger 1944)

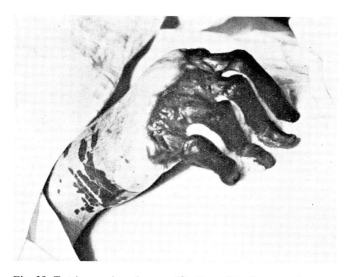

Fig. 30. Total necrosis and mummification of the fingers and metacarpal region of an old man. (From the collection of Prof. Letterer, Tübingen)

For psychological reasons a 15-year-old girl took a very large, but not necessarily fatal dose of cyclobarbital (Phanodorm) and ran into the mountains to die. She fell asleep in the open. In the night the temperature outside unexpectedly fell to minus 17°C and it snowed. The poorly clothed creature became completely numbed and suffered from hypothermia. She incurred, moreover, very severe frost damage to both hands and feet. The region of the knee joint also suffered cold damage and was also injured, for the child probably woke up again and tried to crawl to safety. The search for the girl remained fruitless for a long time. Finally she was found by the game keeper and his dog in a pitiful condition 2 days later. In hospital they immediately tried to warm up the girl in order to save her life, since her (blood) temperature had sunk under the critical limit of 30° C. Initially it was impossible to pay much attention to the peripheral frost injuries (Fig. 31a–h).

The enclosed pictures show first of all the severe 2nd and 3rd degree frost injuries to the hands with blister-formation and intense, marked cold oedema. There was complete functio laesa of the hands and sausage fingers, which led to a claw-hand and later to a monkey-hand posture. Not only the skin and the subcutaneous fatty tissue, but also the nerves and particularly the muscles of the hands and forearms were badly damaged (internal effect). The blood vessels (at least in the area of the hand) had certainly also been damaged to some extent, but after repeated bilateral blocking of the stellate ganglion the blood flow was still adequate enough to enable the hands to be preserved. The condition at various stages can be seen from the pictures. Apart from cyanotic discoloration, superficial necroses and severe functional disturbances of the forearms, hands and fingers appeared. A feeling of numbness remained. However, function later improved in the young person to such an astonishing degree that she was even able to carry out finer types of work like sewing and mending.

The severe 3rd and 4th degree frost injuries to the legs took a different course. This cold damage also led to complete functio laesa of the feet. Once there was no longer any danger to life the limbs were kept cool (but had unfortunately already been warmed previously). As much vasodilatory medication was administered as the state of the circulation could allow and blocks of the lower lumbar sympathetic trunk were carried out alternately. Fever reached over 40° C, which, with a correct regulation of warmth, in itself induces maximal vasodilation. The demarcation zone did in fact still shift slightly to the periphery, but both feet and the lower half of the lower leg became black, necrotic, mummified and had to be amputated. Luckily necrosis did not develop above the patella but on the other hand a cold vaginitis developed with such a profuse secretion as has only very rarely been seen.

In spite of the vegetative suppression induced by large doses of sleeping tablets no defence against cold injuries developed, a fact which on the one hand points to damage in the process of rewarming (premature rewarming) and on the other hand to a direct deep cold injury to the limbs.

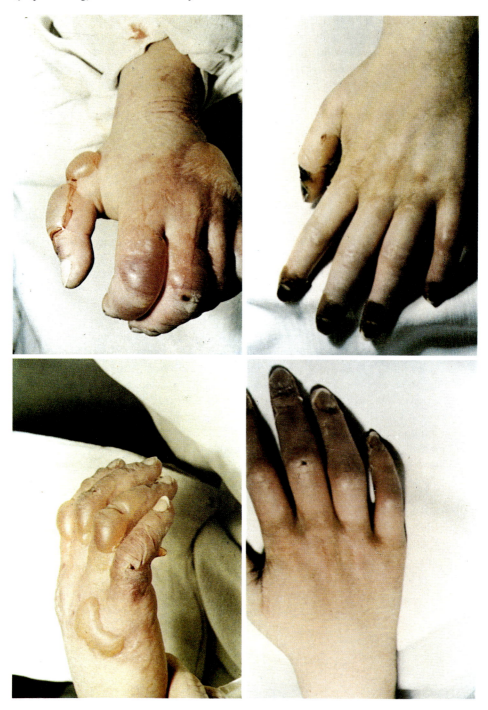

Fig. 31 a - d.

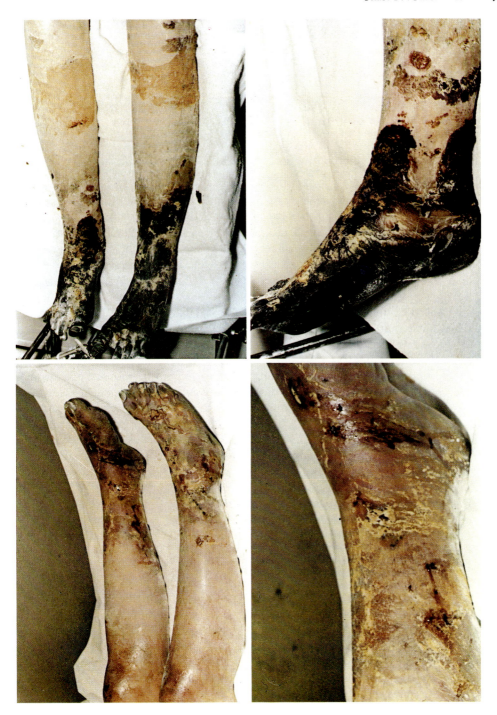

Fig. 31 a - h. Peripheral frost injuries to a 15-year-old girl, see text for discussion

77

Deepseated Cold Injuries Without Marked, Externally Visible Frostbite Sequelae (Immersion Cold Injuries)

The Problem

As early as 1947 de Bakey mentioned that in the case of the various degrees of frostbite damage is predominantly due to the action of dry cold on its own, but that in the case of *immersion-foot, trench-foot* and *trench-hand,* wet in combination with cold is the decisive detrimental factor. He even goes so far as to stress that wet plays the predominant role in this respect. This is certainly correct, since the cooling-out and cooling-down of a limb are facilitated and intensified to a considerable degree in wet surroundings.

American surgeons too have come to the conclusion that wet exacerbates the action of cold to a significant degree. This can be seen very clearly in the statistics, of the Surgeon General of the American Army, on various cold injuries (Fig. 32). As one can see trench and immersion-foot were present in 53 % of cases as opposed to 32 % banal frost injuries; damage due to wet cold being therefore clearly predominant. The proportion of severe deep cold injuries was 6 %.

The possibility of deep cold injury due to immersion or due to metal contact and repeated cooling-down and cooling-out of a limb was unfortunately neither recognised nor acknowledged by many doctors. In many cases they considered it to be impossible for deeper tissue to be damaged without the skin and its substrates showing noticeable signs of cold injury and judged these cases almost completely according to the extent of visible damage and tissue loss, although it was known that the actual damaged zone regularly extends well beyond the area of the defects and that this is the reason for the poor recovery trend after spontaneous gangrene or amputation.

The main criterion for the development of such deep cold injuries is not only prolonged exposure to cold temperatures of $0°$ C or less, but a raised conductivity of the surrounding media. This type mainly appears therefore after falling into icy water and exposure to cold in wet clothes, prolonged standing in icy cold water or cold mud and similar conditions. At the same time the temperatures do not have to be so much under $0°$ C that freezing can occur. The essential point is the gradual penetration of cold into the deeper tissue layers, which are more sensitive to cold than the superficial layers. Only in the case of thorough cooling of a limb, as the result of increased thermosteresis and collapse of the regional dimatic functioning of the circulation, can the deeper-lying larger vessels also become involved. Thus the picture of an obliterative vascular disease of an inflammatory nature develops at a later stage in the case of the latter, which is related to Buerger's disease in important aspects, but *never becomes generalised* (Killian 1959, 1962).

Bevor we go on to look at the symptomatology of these immersion cold injuries (invisible frost damage), let us have a look at the remarks of various authors on the problem, since they provide support for our view of the matter.

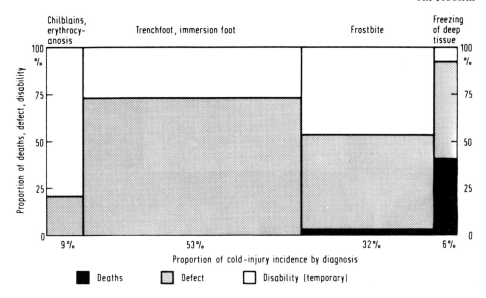

Fig. 32. Results from the American Army showing the significance of wet-cold injuries. (From Wayne and De Bakey 1958)

As early as 1902 Zoege von Manteuffel (1902 a, b) wrote in his clinical and experimental studies on late gangrene after the action of cold, that in most cases necroses and gangrene of the limbs do not occur until weeks, months or even years after exposure to cold and are due to vascular damage.

"If one is quite careful one can succeed in producing minor degrees of frostbite, which do not result in tissue necrosis, but certainly in the typical oedema and which only briefly disturb function. Repetitions and gradual gradations in the number of exposures to cold produce then a scale of injuries which have the most varied manifestations."

"Of all the types of tissues of the body which have been exposed to frost, the tissue which is the most highly organised is the first to suffer. Thus the most marked alterations to the vessels can also be seen in their muscularis. In the first days the media become cloudy. It stains poorly, some nuclei show vacuoles, at a later stage of repair hypertrophy occurs in spite of expansion of the lumen. Whilst the striated musculature of the extremities always degenerates and replaced by connective tissue, new growth did take place here in the smooth muscle of the vessels, which is quite understandable considering the lesser physiological refinement of the latter. But above all the proliferation of the intima dominates the picture of vascular changes."

These endothelial proliferations are thereafter interpreted more closely in the particular study involved as a reaction to the degeneration of the vascular wall. Alterations and new growth in the region of the elastica are also described. Zoege von Manteuffel comes to the conclusion, that there is experimental proof that cold can cause arteriosclerosis (nowadays we would say: a localised obliterating arterial vascular occluding disease of the nature of cold endangiitis).

Ratschow (1959) has since cast doubt on the correctness of these observations since he did not succeed in producing a generalised endangiitis obliterans in an animal trial without pretreatment (damaging) or sensitisation with foreign protein. Zoege von Manteuffel and Rudnitzki (1902) also failed to do this and they speak only of a circumscribed sclerosis and not of a generalised arterial occluding disease. Ratschow's strict rejection thereafter of delayed damage to the vessels and any form of late gangrene after previous exposure to cold is based on this misunderstanding. He generally conceived them to be the partial manifestation of a hereditary disease, namely a reactive inflammatory Buerger's disease. Unfortunately his erroneous beliefs very soon became prevalent inpublic assistarce medicine in spite of the fact that the very experienced surgeon Bier had in 1918 already urgently recommended that these injuries be acknowledged as war injuries even without a complete understanding of the etiology.

After the First World War Zoege von Manteuffel (1924) once more expressed an opinion on the problem of frost effects. He had encouraged his student Rudnitzki to conduct cold experiments on animals (guinea pigs).

In the report in question he says that apart from the considerable vascular obliterations (hyaline degeneration and consequent proliferation of the intima with the formation of vacuoles, new formation of elastic fibres, thickened media with connective tissue substitute, atrophy of the muscle fibres, infiltrations of the adventitia, swellings of the capillary endothelia with rupturing) *different degrees of alteration in all other tissue substrates were also able to be shown,* specifically, that the physiologically superior tissue always exibited the greatest change. Quoting verbatim: "Thus, for example, the glandular apparatus and hair follicles of the skin were destroyed.

The epitheleum showed no alterations. The muscles showed lacunae after ice-formation, then granular degeneration. In the nerves Rudnitzki (1900) found destruction of the myeline and axon cylinders with subsequent substitution by scar tissue. With respect to bone damage he mentions that the skeleton is thickened, the connective tissue is oedematically saturated with blood exudations which merge into scars. The fatty tissue wastes away.

Thus it is apparent that as early as 1924 Zoege von Manteuffel came to roughly the same conclusions as Staemmler (1943), Siegmund (1942, 1943) and many others did later on.

In order to separate the degenerative and regenerative processes from the effect of consecutive oedema, Rudnitzki elicited oedema in a number of animals by means of elastic bindings. Whilst exposure to frost only has to last for 1–15 min at a time in order to produce the changes described above after several repetitions, it was necessary to extend the application of the elastic binding each time to between 1 and 5 h in order to produce the same or similar symptoms.

The extensive review of Zoege von Manteuffel (1924) on arteriosclerosis of the lower extremities must also be mentioned in this connection since thermal influences as the cause of vascular changes together with further details about the experimental technique (Rudnitzki's results are mentioned in it). Permanent damage to the vessels after protracted exposure to mild cold is also described more closely in this report.

If cooling proceeded to a point at which muscles became hard, then gangrene of the limbs very often developed after a more prolonged period of exposure. Indeed after only a 1 to 2 h cooling period characteristic oedematous swellings of the extremities appeared. These oedemas persisted not only for days but sometimes even for weeks.

At that time Zoege von Manteuffel wrote, moreover, that after an isolated frost injury syndromes similar to arteriosclerosis developed, where as in the case of total vascular occlusion the alterations rather tended to be similar to a Winiwarter-Buerger-Edgar-Weiss' disease in humans.

Siegmund (1942, 1943) commented that *the vascular wall changes were in no way limited to the badly cold damaged, externally visible area of the 2nd to 3rd degree frost injury. They extend cranially well beyond these zones of the visible effects of frost damage into the area which has to all appearances remained healthy. In these regions the skin is therefore completely intact, but lesions have already occurred in various tissue substrates beneath.* A statement which should in itself have been sufficient proof of the existance of invisible cold injuries. But this was unfortunately not the case.

Experimental and clinical findings on the muscles and bones point even more clearly to the existance of internal cold injuries with preservation of the body surface. Thus Pichotka in 1949 found in many of his cold experiments fully developed muscle necroses which later turned into scars, whilst at the same time the skin remained intact and without visible signs of cold injury (or only minimal damage). Experimental evidence of internal injuries due to cold with preservation of the skin was particularly clear after intense cooling of the extremities. (Immersion in cold compounds.)

Apart from Zoege von Manteuffel and Rudnitzki (1924), Lewis (1941) and Pichotka (1949), as well as Thorban at a later point in 1962 have provided ample confirmation for these findings. Even Ribbert (1897, 1901/1902, 1909) and his student Kleinschmidt were aware of the fact that *the bone cells are not only highly sensitive to cold but are able to withstand the effects of cold considerably less well than the overlying soft parts or the relatively resistant skin and subcutaneous fatty tissue.* Burckhart (1915), Löhr (1921) and furthermore Boettcher (1944) made similar statements. The latter explicitly stated that, *after mild, but prolonged and thorough cooling down, bone necroses have been seen to develop before the skin shows any evidence of cold damage.*

Of considerable importance with respect to this topic is also the report of Radasewskij (1947), who traced the progress of *bone damage* at a level above tissue losses due to cold injuries and observed that it reached well up into healthy areas. It was again proved that *the bone cells suffer considerable cold injuries before there is any recognisable sign of exposure to cold in the overlying skin.*

Symptomatology of Trench Foot, Flanders' Foot and Immersion Hand

The gradual cooling-out of a limb is always noticed by the person affected but mostly ignored since the developing anaesthesia of the limb blocks out the pain. Apart from the symptoms of local cold injury which have previously been mentioned, certain characteristic signs develop in the case of thorough cooling-down and in deep action of cold, which were unfortunately only rarely paid attention to and found almost no echo in the literature.

The reports of Beckmann (1916), Sittmann (1916) and Floerken (1917, 1920 a, b) are exceptions. In his review of the cooling process of entire limbs the latter states that skin damage and local frost injuries can almost never be observed and that they develop, if at all, at a later point. Floerken's portrayal roughly corresponds to the Cold Syndrome described by Talbott in 1941. Some details are also available in the reports of White and Scoville (1945), White and Warren (1944), White et al. (1942), Ungley and Blackwood (1942), Knight (1940) and Blackwood (1944 a, b) on immersion foot, trench foot and immersion hand.

Apart from a reduction in skin sensitivity, rough dry goose-flesh over the whole limb, coldness and pallor of the arms and legs, neuralgiform dragging pains appear as the main symptom. (Floerken 1917; Killian 1942 a, b, 1943; Sittmann 1916, White et al. 1942; Blackwood 1944 a, b). A characteristic feature are peculiar, sometimes quite tortuous deep-seated pains (periosteum). In the process of loss of warmth they continue to increase up to a point at which total anaesthesia of the limb sets in. The joints and joint capsules also become painful and *tension pains* develop with movement (active or passive). As a rule the neuralgiform pains follow the course of the nerves and are similar to neuritis or neuralgia (sciatica and the like).

In 1916 Beckmann drew attention particularly to *pains of the shin-bone,* an observation which both we and Lindemann (1942, 1943) have confirmed. However, when Lindemann writes that these pains become intensified particularly at night and may also take on a pulsating character, his remarks really refer to the phase of rewarming and not the first phase of actual under-cooling. From a clinical standpoint these typical shin-bone pains lead to diagnostic problems, insofar as they are also present in other illnesses e.g. 5 day fever (Wolhynic fever), so that false diagnoses are possible.

In a state of hypothermia the tibia often becomes very sensitive to taps and furthermore there are reports of intense pains on the front edge of the shin-bone. In the initial stage burning pains are also said to be present in the soles of the feet. The pain phase is fairly prolonged since this particular form of cold damage due to immersion (cold and wet) very often occurs at temperatures of $0°$ C and above.

Progressive reduction in all sensitive qualities of the skin has often been observed, whilst deep sensitivity remains intact for a relatively long period of time. In 1942 Lindemann reported neurological findings initially of hyperaesthetic zones in the arms and legs. The ability to discriminate light touch, both sharp and blunt, was reduced and ultimately lost. The impaired areas had a glove- and stocking-form. Sometimes too, island-like zones of disturbed sensitivity, hyperaesthesia or anaesthesia developed, which were not defined according to segments or relationship to a nerve. Bevore anaesthesia develops some people experience itching, formication, or increasing numbness. Both these symptoms and the pain have been regarded as signs of oxygen-deficiency in the tissue (oxygen starvation pains according to Rein 1943), in other words-hypoxia. However, it is more likely to be a question of direct changes, irritation or damage to the cold-sensitive nerves (and nerve-ends) themselves and their vegetative components. The fact that paraesthesias, hyperaesthesias, areas of anaesthesia and also paralysis, as well as other neurovascular injuries, may persist after exposure to cold suggests the correctness of this explanation (see also our comments in the section on pathological changes in the nerves after the action of cold). Such neuralgias, neural lesions and paralyses develop most frequently in lorry drivers, pilots, seamen, fishermen, motor-cyclists and workers who are exposed to cold and wet. Their complaints are often regarded not as the result of exposure to cold but as rheumatism, periostitis or arthritis.

As a result of cooling-down the serviceability of the limbs very soon becomes reduced, a *growing stiffness* sets in. The muscles loose their elasticity and strength. They become hard and ultimately the familiar picture of the *wooden-leg with total anaesthesia* of the limb develops, of whose existance the casualty is now no longer aware (pied de bois) (Webster et al. 1942; Edwards 1951; Edwards and Leeper 1952; Sapin-Jaloustre 1956). In this state people walk in an unsure manner, tottering, legs wide apart as if on stilts, for not only is muscular rigidity present but deep sensitivity is also disturbed and, related to this, too, stereognosis, the feeling for the positioning of the joints. Movement may become ataxic. Some people tumble unsteadily when they climb down from a lorry or a horse, which is always a sure sign of the thorough cooling-down of the muscles of the shin-bone and thigh.

The symptom of muscular stiffness and rigidity is based on a change in the muscular proteins, of the myosin. It is reversible and disappears in the course of rewarming; it is therefore physically based. In addition to this there is also rigidity due to central increase in reflex sensitivity and muscle tonus, which can be got under control with narcotics.

Contrary to the reports of Beckmann (1916) the general condition of the casualty during hypothermia of the limbs is not yet noticeably disturbed in spite of considerable centralisation of the circulation. There are also no oedemas at first. These only appear after a long period in cold mud or icy water as a result of a physically based change in the electrolyte and water distribution in the tissue which has become acidy. For that reason too blisters almost regularly fail to appear.

Unfortunately this absence of externally visible symptoms very often misleads one into believing that the damage is slight whilst the opposite is actually the case. *Cold immersion injury of any form is prognostically much less favourable than the common type of cold injury, for thereafter principally delayed damage of various types may develop.*

Rewarming occurs slowly in the presence of dragging pains and anaesthesia only disappears gradually. After warming no notable changes are to be seen externally apart from an oedematic swelling of varying degrees, unless, as is often the case, localised 1st-2nd degree frost damage develops in the distal segments of the limb. It, too, may mislead one into believing that the case is harmless.

References

Allan EV, Barker NW, Hines LA (1955) Periphere Durchblutungsstörungen, 2nd edn. Saunders, Philadelphia

Ariev TV (1950a) Translation in: Frostbite. Ottawa

Ariev TV (1950b) Klin Med (Mosk) 28:3,15

Behnke CH (1950) Sammelbericht über Trauma und Stress

Behnke CH (1952) Cold injuries. In: Killian H (ed) Report

Bell LG, Stahlgreen LH, Scherer BD (1952) US Armed Forces Med J 3:35

Blackwood W (1944a) Br J Surg 31:329

Blackwood W (1944b) Br Med Bull 2:138

Blair JR (1951) Kälteschäden. Report. HOG conference, April 1951

Boehler L (1917) Med Klin 11

Boettcher H (1944) Virchows Arch Pathol Anat 312:46

Brandis HJ von (1943a) Vorträge aus der praktischen Chirurgie, vol 27. Encke, Stuttgart

Brandis HJ von (1943b) Broschüre über Kälteschäden. Encke, Stuttgart

Burton AC, Taylor RM (1946) Am J Physiol 129:565

Canty J, Sharf AG (1953) Ann Surg 138:65

Castellaneta V (1940) Zentralbl Chir 190

Davis L (1904) Indian Med Gaz 39:245

Davis L, Scarff JE, Rogers N, Dickinson M (1943) Surg Gynecol Obstet 77:561

de Bakey ME (1951) Kälteschäden. HOG converence, April 1951

Debrunner H (1941) Report of the military surgeon on 26 cases of frostbite encountered while on ski maneuvres. In: Klinik und Behandlung der örtlichen Erfrierungen. Huber, Bern, p 128

Dreyer U (1913) Zentralbl Chir 40:1628

Ducuing J, Harcourt J, Folch H, Bofold J (1940) J Chir (Paris) 55:385

Edwards JC, Leeper RW (1952) JAMA 1199

Fievez J (1939) Prog Med 67:1326

Floerken H (1915) Munch Med Wochenschr 7

Floerken H (1917) Bruns Beitr Klin Chir 106:4

Floerken H (1920a) Zentralbl Chir 47:1651

Floerken H (1920b) Die Kälteschäden im Krieg. Springer, Berlin (Ergebnisse der Chirurgie und Ortho-
pädie)
Fox (1961) Br Med Bull 17:14
Fremmert H (1880) Arch Klin Chir 25
Frey S (1942) Med Klin 44:1009
Friedrich PH (1919) Munch Med Wochenschr 129
Grattan HW (1922) HMSO 169
Greene R (1949) Lancet 689
Grezillier A (1919) Medical dissertation, Paris
Guerasimenko NJ (1950) Klinika y letchneie otmorogeniy, vol 1. Moscow
Harris, Maltby (1944) Lecture. American Academy of Neurological Surgery
Hays, Coats (1958) Cold injuries groundtype. USA General Surgeon of the Army, Washington DC
Heaton LD, Davis RM (1952) J Ky Med Assoc 50:206
Hübener A (1871) Medical dissertation, St. Petersburg
Jimeno-Vidal (1942) Wien Klin Wochenschr 55:601
Killian H (1942a) Zentralbl Chir 1763
Killian H (1942b) Arbeitstagung beratender Chirurgen, Berlin
Killian H (1943) Zentralbl Chir 70:50
Killian H (1952) Zentralbl Chir 77:105
Killian H (1959) Wehrmed Mitt 3:11
Killian H (1962) Sachverständigentagung, Bonn (Report of Ministry of Labour)
Killian H (1966) Der Kälteunfall: Allgemeine Unterkühlung. Dustri
Kirschner M (1917) In: Borchardt A, Schmieden (eds) Kriegschirurgie
Knight BW (1940) Br Med J 2:610
Koehler H (1913) Zentralbl Chir 35:1362
Kramer K, Schulze W (1944) Klin Wochenschr 192, 201
Kreyberg L (1946) Lancet 1:338
Krjukow (1914) Vierteljahresschr Gerichtl Med 47:79
Lapras A (1957) Sem Hop Paris 661
Lapras A (1959) Ann Chir 13:857
Larrey JD (1817) Mémoires du chirurgie militaire et de campagne, vol 4. Paris
Laufmann H (1951) JAMA 147:1201
Legouest (1855) Mem Med Chir Mil 10
Leriche R (1945) In: Physiologie pathologique et traitement chirurgical des maladies artérielles de la
vasomotricité. Masson, Paris, p 65
Leriche R, Kunlin J (1940) Mem Acad Chir 66:14, 196
Lesser A (1945) Ann Surg
Lewis RB, Moen PW (1952) J Med Sci 224:529
Lewis RB, Moen PW (1953) Surg Gynecol Obstet 97:59
Lindemann H (1942) Erkrankungen der Arterien durch Kälteeinwirkungen. Lecture 25 March 1942
Lindemann H (1943) Dtsch Med Wochenschr 1:154
Loos HO (1941) Zentralbl Chir 10:449
Macpherson WHHM (1908) HMSO 15
Meyer AW, Kohlschütter R (1914) Dtsch Z Chir 127/5,6
Mikat (1951) Wirtschaft Statistik 3:50
Moser H (1942) Dtsch Med Wochenschr 68:549
Movrey FH, Farago PJ (1952) Mil Surg 110:249
Mullinos, Shulman (1939) Am J Physiol 125:310
Oehlecker F (1942a) Chirurg 14:422
Oehlecker F (1942b) Chirurg 19:459
Orr KD, Fainer DC (1952) US Armed Forces Med J 3:95
Osterland (1936) Lehrbuch der militärischen Hygiene. Springer, Berlin
Partsch F (1943) Erfahrungsberichte beratender Chirurgen
Paunesco-Podeanu A, Tzurai I (1946) Kälteschäden. Masson, Paris
Perutz (1916) Arch Dermatol 123:715
Pichotka J (1949) Proc Soc Exp Biol Med 72:127,130
Pirogow N (1864) Principles of war surgery
Pranter V (1915) Wien Klin Wochenschr 28:266
Pratt GH (1953) Gen Pract 7:34
Radasewskij (1947) Beitr Pathol Anat 109:567
Ratschow M (1959) Angiologie. Thieme, Stuttgart

Raymond V, Parisot J (1918) J Chir (Paris) 14:329
Rein H (1943) Lehrbuch der Physiologie. Springer, Berlin
Ribbert H (1897) Virchows Arch Pathol Anat 147:202
Ribbert H (1901/1902) Lehrbuch der allgemeinen Pathologie. Leipzig
Ribbert H (1909) Dtsch Med Wochenschr 46
Riehl (1915) Wien Klin Wochenschr 11
Rudnitzki TJ (1900) Zentralbl Chir 237
Sapin-Jaloustre J (1956) Enquêtes sur les gélures. Herman, Paris
Sarkisov (1952) Sov Med 1:34
Shumaker HB, Lempke RE (1951) Surgery 30:873
Shumaker HB, White BM, Wrenn EL (1947) Surgery 22:900
Siegmund H (1942) Munch Med Wochenschr 827
Siegmund H (1943) Zentralbl Chir 1558
Sonnenburg E, Tschmarke P (1915) Neue deutsche Chirurgie. Encke, Stuttgart
Staemmler M (1943) Erfrierungen. Thieme, Leipzig
Starlinger F (1942) Zentralbl Chir 69:1179
Starlinger F, Fritsch OW (1944) Die Erfrierungen. Steinkopf, Berlin
Talbott JH (1941) N Engl J Med 224:281
Theiss F, O'Connor WB, Wahl FJ (1951) JAMA 146:992
Thorban W (1962) Bruns Beitr Klin Chir 207:87
Ullmann (1932) In: Handbuch der Haut- und Geschlechtskrankheiten, vol 171, p 4
Ungley CC (1949) Adv Surg 1:269
Ungley CC, Blackwood W (1942) Lancet 2:447
Vagliano M (1948) Erfrierungen. Masson, Paris
Webster DR, Woolhouse FH, Johnston JL (1942) J Bone Joint Surg 24:785
Welcker ER (1913) Zentralbl Chir 40:1625, 1768
Whayne TF, de Bakey ME (1958) Cold injuries groundtype. USA General Surgeon of the Army,
    Washington DC
White JC, Scoville WB (1945) N Engl J Med 232:415
White JC, Warren S (1944) War Med 5,6
White JC, Woolhouse FH, Johnston JL (1942) J Bone Joint Surg 24:185
Wieting J (1913) Zentralbl Chir 40:593
Wilkins RW, Hunt JS, Friedland CK (1942) J Clin Invest 21:625
Williams DJ (1923) Partitioner 171:619
Witteck A (1914) Munch Med Wochenschr 62:129, 416
Witteck A (1915) Munch Med Wochschr 12
Wolf HH, Puchin EE (1949) Clin Sci Lond 8:145
Zaretzky J (1959) Chirurgija 35:116
Zoege von Manteuffel J (1902a) Mitt Grenzgeb Med Chir 10:343
Zoege von Manteuffel J (1902b) Zentralbl Chir 63
Zoege von Manteuffel J (1924) Zentralbl Chir 51:17
Zoege von Manteuffel J. Rudnitzki TJ (1902) Grenzgeb Med Chir 10:373
Zoege von Manteuffel J, Rudnitzki TJ (1924) Zentralbl Chir 51:17
Zuckerkandl O (1916) Bruns Beitr Klin Chir 101:594

Pathological Physiology and Pathology of Local Cold Damage

The following exposition refers mainly to early injuries as opposed to delayed injuries and resultant conditions, which should be presented separately.

Changes in the Area of the Skin Due to Cold

The earliest reports on pathological changes after artificially produced cold injuries originate from Samuel (1868), Cohnheim (1873), Recklinghausen (1883 a, b), Krieger (1889), Uschinsky (1893), Volkmann (1893), Hodara (1896), Fuerst (1897), Hochhaus (1898), Rischpler (1900), Werner (1903) and Gans (1923, 1925). The experimental results proved to be fairly similar and correspond to recent results (Unterdorfer and Umbach 1977.)

Under the influence of freezing with a spray or cold-mixture extreme pallor and bloodlessness of the tissue due to spasms in all the arterial capillary vessels very soon sets in. Circulation in the affected area comes to a halt. After rewarming clearly visible reactive hyperaemia develops. As early as 20 min after freezing the first changes in the tissue and the development of *aseptic inflammatory symptoms* can be seen. The accumulation of thrombocytes in the form of colourless granular masses in the vessels was striking. Filtration processes after cold contraction of the afferent vascular ramifications took place. After three-quarters of an hour serum and erythrocytes began to extravasate from the vascular pathways into the tissue and tissue oedemas developed. After sludging congestion, stases and thrombuses, partly hyaline, partly platelet or leucocyte thrombuses, formed in the small cutaneous vessels and particularly in the veins. It would appear that the more intense and prolonged the action of cold, the more severe the thrombus development. According to Gans (1923) such thrombuses extend into the area of the papillary bodies and the subcutis.

Their significance for the pathogenesis of skin damage is evaluated in very different ways. Some authors attach crucial significance to this thrombus development in the drainage pathways, whilst others, particularly more recent workers, amongst whom are also Staemmler (1943), do not regard it as being a cause of serious cold injury in any respect, but simply a sequela of the vascular spasms with concomitant dilatation of the venoles with slowing of the blood flow and congestion in the drainage veins.[1]

Strikingly, none of these infestigators was able to establish the presence of tissue necroses in the skin, which is however related to the technique of undercooling. The fact is that all these experiments have been conducted in the form of ultra-rapid cooling with freezing, which means that a fixation of the state of tissue occurs without there being any development of coarse ice-crystals which destroy cell structures. In the case of the intense freezing of the surface of organs, e.g. liver or kidney, superficial necroses with swelling and protoplasmic disintegration, caryorrexis, and disappearance of the nuclei may, however, take place (Uschinsky 1893).

According to more recent reports of Unterdorfer and Umbach (1977) cold injuries in the area of the skin can be identified histologically even when no clinically visible signs of change are yet able to be ascertained. With moderate degrees of cold they report exfoliation fo the skin with schistasis, indistinct tissue and cell markings, disappearance of the nuclei in the layers of the epidermis, partly shrunk, partly swollen nuclei with simultaneous disintegration of the fibres of the corium. After intense cold effects they noted destruction of the elastic fibres and a striking sparcity of the nuclei of the same. The fatty tissue of the subcutis was oedematically saturated and frequently permeated with extravasations.

Rischpler (1900) and Fuerst (1897) mention in their experiments *vacuole formations in the plasma of the epidermal cells, plasmolysis, withering and disintegration of the nuclei.* The reported changes remind one of those histological pictures which one sees of the intima of the blood vessels

---

1 Nowadays the blockage of the microcirculation seems to us to be the main cause of a possible asphyxiation of peripheral tissue constituents.

or of the organelles after oxygen deficiency (Büchner 1943 a,b). At the time this aroused suspicion that cold injury in the final analysis must be a form of oxygen deficiency injury. Fuerst (1897) and Werner (1903) observed atypical mitoses, amitotic division of the nuclei and mulit-nuclear giant cells. On the other hand regenerative processes in the tissue could be seen as early as 6 h after the operation of such a cold-spray with freezing.

Staemmler (1933, 1942, 1943, 1944) and his co-worker Boettcher (1944) provided valuable additional information to these earlier investigations with the application of prolonged cold exposure periods. Up to this point only Nägelsbach (1919, 1920) had succeeded in producing *thromboses* and *gangrene* through the action of cold.

Even after fairly slight exposure to cold leucocytic infiltrations can be found in the fatty tissue. During rewarming cell particles and liberated fluid-fat may be dispersed, the latter of which carries the risk of a fat embolism in the pulmonary circulation. Such fat embolisms of the lung have often been observed in post mortems on people who had suffered from exposure. From a clinical stand-point, however, we never got to see any signs of a fat embolism of the pulmonary or systemic circulation or a micro-embolism syndrome at the Russian Front. At the same time it must be admitted that such phenomena were probably overlooked at that time, as was the case with shock-lung, since a fat embolism will only be diagnosed by someone who is aware of it. (Killian 1943; Unterdorfer and Umbach 1977).

In 1944 Boettcher found *vacuole formations with protoplasmic atrophy in the nuclei of the epidermal cells* after exposure to cold even without freezing of the skin. He observed *caryorrexis, caryolysis* and *an alveolar transformation.* He too believed that these phenomena were exclusively the result of oxygen deficiency and not the result of the separating out of the plasma colloids due to exposure as Schade (1919, 1920, 1923, 1949) suggested. Siegmund (1942, 1943, 1950) too has described such *vacuolation.* However, he also observed separation processes in the plasmatic substances in the early stages of cold injury, but considered them to be the direct result of the local action of cold.

A particularly important clinical finding is the tendency to *hyperkeratoses* and *para-keratoses* in the area damaged by cold (Fig. 33). Keratine lamellae develop on the surface of the epidermis and very often *atrophy of the skin and subcutis* is found in combination with *hyperkeratosis.*

According to the histological findings of Staemmler (1943) and Wurst (1944) the keratinisation process also extends into the *sebaceous glands* and *hair-follicles,* which actually become filled with layers of keratine-substance (Figs. 34 and 35). Both authors saw *cyst-like cavities* full of keratine substances develop and, moreover, they observed *atrophy of the rootsheaths* and therein the scanty remains of the hair. The root-sheaths themselves may also become keratinised. In contrast to this Wurst reported in his follow-up investigations in 1944 the comparatively more rare finding of the skin showing signs of deep wrinkles with copious scaling, often peeling, sometimes *as thin as parchment, very delicate and easily damaged.* We too have noticed the thick, horny-skin formations on the soles and sides of the feet which Wurst (1944) described and which tend to peel off and grow afresh.

Form the dermatological and surgical point of view there were reports of *dystrophic alterations in the area of the nails* after exposure to cold. Relevant to this topic are the earlier reports of Heller (1908), Thibierge (1911), Sachs (1927 a,b), Stüting (1930), Langenkämper (1931) and more recent reports of Oehlecker (1942 a,b), Starlinger and Frisch (1944), von Brandis (1943 a,b). Such alterations are said to occur in 75 % of cases, a figure which seems very high to us.

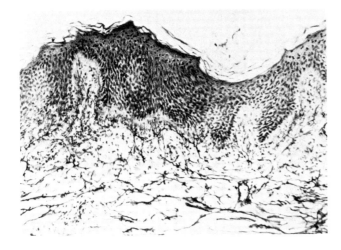

Fig. 33. Normal arrangement of elastic fibres in the skin. Weigert's elastica staining. (From Staemmler)

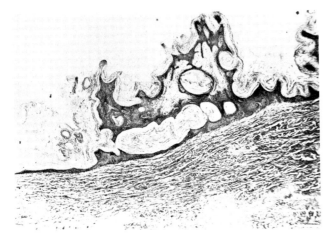

Fig. 34. Atrophy of the skin with hyperkeratosis and papillary fibroepithelial proliferation. (From Staemmler)

After cold injury the nails are thickened, very brittle, sometimes swollen and covered with deep grooves. They are irregularly formed, stunted and full of cracks. Furthermore they tend to become hyperkeratotic (Oehlecker 1942 a,b).

Hyperhidrosis has often been reported after cold injuries. A number of histological changes have been observed in the sweat glands to which Staemmler (1943) and Wurst (1944) drew attention. Apparently protoplasmic changes occur and a loosening of the tips of the sweat glands with vacuole formations, whilst the cell nuclei remain intact for a remarkable length of time. In the area of the corium an oedematous saturation of papillary bodies occurs.

Staemmler (1943) emphasises *atrophy of the elastic fibres* over large areas as a particular finding in the skin, and one which is especially evident in the area of the subepithelial, prepapillary network — for that reason the skin in the area of a former cold injury

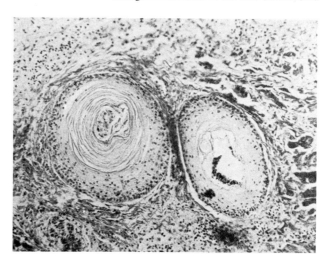

Fig. 35. Various stages of keratinisation. (From Staemmler)

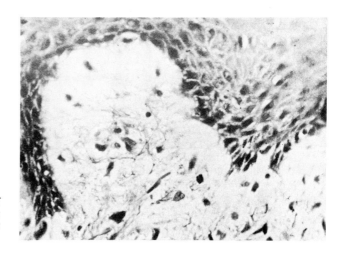

Fig. 36. Extensive fading of elastic fibres in the cutis after frost injury. (From Staemmler 1944)

can so easily be wrinkled. In other cases however it remains extremely taut, shiny and very thin for a long time (Fig. 36). Newer dates see Unterdörfer and Umbach 1977.

The alterations of the vascular system of the skin are similar to those in other regions damaged by cold. However Staemmler (1943) and Wurst (1944) noticed considerable *endophlebitis* in the venous region with granulation tissue formation. The intima of the cutaneous vessels is grossly thickened, the arterial vessels show narrow lumina, whilst the external wall-layers exhibit at most a moderate oedema. Both the muscularis and the elastica are well preserved. In the small veins of the skin region typical *alveolate endophlebitis* including lipid-containing cells was found. In contrast to the investigations of other workers, however, both authors found hardly any signs of thromboses in the lumina of the cutaneous veins.

In Pichotka and Lewis' experiments on freezing in 1949 cold necroses always coincide with deeper-lying muscle necroses. Since they could be almost completely avoided by rapid thawing both authors assumed that hypoxia, or rather ischaemia was the common cause. In their opinion the appertaining arteries and arterioles were not primarily damaged, but rather secondarily via break-down products from the regions of the muscle necrosis.

After exposure to cold the cutaneous nerves exhibit principally the same changes as are caused by cold in large nerve-trunks. In this case it is mainly a question of *disintegration of the nerve sheath with disappearance of the axis cylinders.* The disorder extends well beyond the actual area of 1st to 3rd degree cold injury. Furthermore thickening of the *endoperineurium and perineurium* was found.

It should be mentioned that carcinomas may develop in the region of old frostbite-necroses and scars with chronic inflammation. In 1977 Fee et al. reported pertinent cases. Most malignant tumours were observed in the frost damaged heel after the development of deep ulcerative processes on which Conway and Di Pirro had already reported in 1966. The earlier literature also contains reports of such carcinomas in the old scars of zones damaged by cold. Hirsch (1977), reported on a malignant tumour in a cold injury to the back of the hand.

References

Boettcher H (1944) Virchows Arch Pathol Anat 312:46
Brandis HJ von (1943a) Vorträge aus der praktischen Chirurgie, vol 27. Encke, Stuttgart
Brandis HJ von (1943b) Broschüre über Kälteschäden. Encke, Stuttgart
Büchner F (1943a) Klin Wochenschr 80
Büchner F (1943b) Mitt Geb Luftfahrtmed 7
Cohnheim O (1873) Neue Untersuchungen über die Entzündungen. Berlin
Conway H, Di Pirro E (1966) Plast Reconstr Surg 38:541
Fee HJ, Friedmann HB, Siegel ME (1977) Am J Surg 144:89
Fuerst E (1897) Medical dissertation, Königsberg
Gans (1923) Handbuch der Haut- und Geschlechtskrankheiten 3:34
Gans (1925) Geschichte der Hautkrankheiten. In: Handbuch der Haut- und Geschlechtskrankheiten, vol 1. Springer, Berlin
Heller F (1908) Z Dermatol 630
Hirsch WD (1977) Aerztl Prax 39:976
Hochhaus H (1898) Virchows Arch Pathol Anat 154:320
Hodara H (1896) Munch Med Wochenschr 14:341
Killian H (1943) Zentralbl Chir 70:50
Krieger H (1889) Virchows Arch Pathol Anat 116:64
Langenkämper F (1931) Medical dissertation, Münster
Nägelsbach E (1919) Munch Med Wochenschr 353
Nägelsbach E (1920) Dtsch Z Chir 160:2051
Oehlecker F (1942a) Chirurg 14:422
Oehlecker F (1942b) Chirurg 19:459
Pichotka J. Lewis RB (1949) Proc Soc Exp Biol Med 72:130
Recklinghausen F von (1883a) Dtsch Z Chir 213
Recklinghausen F von (1883b) In: Handbuch der allgemeinen Pathologie des Kreislaufes. Stuttgart
Rischpler A (1900) Beitr Pathol Anat 28:541
Sachs J (1927a) Dermatol Wochenschr 39:1361
Sachs J (1927b) Zentralbl Haut Geschlechtskrankh 24:748
Samuel (1868) Virchows Arch Pathol Anat 43
Schade H (1919) Munch Med Wochenschr 1:1021
Schade H (1920) Munch Med Wochenschr 449
Schade H (1923) Physiologie und Chemie der inneren Medizin. Steinkopff, Dresden
Schade H (1949) Z Exp Med 7:275
Siegmund H (1942) Arch Dermatol 184:84
Siegmund H (1943) Mitt Geb Luftfahrtmed 7:43

Siegmund H (1950) Dept Air Force 2:858
Staemmler M (1933) Beitr Pathol Anat 91:30
Staemmler M (1942) Zentralbl Chir 45:1757
Staemmler M (1943) Erfrierungen. Thieme, Leipzig
Staemmler M (1944) Virchows Arch Pathol Anat 312:437,501
Starlinger F, Frisch OW (1944) Die Erfrierungen. Steinkopff, Berlin
Stüting (1930) Zentralbl Haut Geschlechtskrankh 33:326
Thibierge (1911) Ann Dermatol 108:560
Unterdorfer H, Umbach P (1977) Aerztl Prax (Suppl) 41
Uschinsky N (1893) Beitr Pathol Anat 12:115
Volkmann R (1893) Beitr Pathol Anat 12:233
Werner (1903) Arch Mikrosk Anat Entwicklungsgesch 61
Wurst H (1944) Medical dissertation, Breslau

Damage to the Nerves Due to Exposure to Acute Cold

The appearance of anaesthetic regions during and after hypothermia of the limbs has been mentioned by a considerable number of authors. The development of such anaesthetic areas is usually combined with initial pain, so that, like Strandell (1941 a, b) and Dreyer (1913, 1914 a, b) one may speak of an anaesthesia dolorosa during the first phase. See here the reports of Floerken (1915, 1920 a, b), Scharfeter (1915), White (1943), Scherer (1934), Stopford (1918), Wurst (1944) and many others.

In 1913 Dreyer reported that anaesthetic areas were to be found in 75 % of cases of frostbite to the hands and feet. In 17 % of cases only the sole of the foot and toes were affected, in 4 % only the sides of the foot. Localised anaesthesias were also observed as was later confirmed by von Brandis (1943). In 1917 Stiefler described a burning pain, abnormal heat and cold sensations and a prolonged, singularly tortuous pain after cold injuries. He later found areas of loss of sensitivity.

Such anaesthetic regions may affect the limbs in a circular manner and sometimes assume a glove-form, cuff-form or sandal-form. Hyperaesthetic boundary zones are then to be found above those areas.

Disturbances of deep sensibility and of the thermal receptors have also been observed. In addition there is damage to the neurovasal reactions. Sorge (1929) and Floerken (1917) noticed dissociation phenomena of loss of cold and warm sensitivity. Sometimes only the cold receptors broke down. According to Stansky (1916), Schroetter (1916) and Schüller (1915) a *legging or cuff neuritis* may be found, which apparently occurs, however, in the presence of both cold and constriction. Schumaker and Lempke (1951) have also mentioned associated disturbances of sensibility in their works. The vasoconstrictor vegetative fibres are thought to be remarkably resistant and can survive when other fibre systems have long since perished. Hyperactivity of the sympathetic nervous system has also sometimes been observed, whilst at the same time the fibres related to the sensation of touch have already been eliminated.

In 1941 Stolfi and Berlozzino (1941a, b) described a peculiar straddled gait after cold injuries. These phenomena may be related to *disturbances of deep sensibility* in the lower extremities or they are the result of weakness in the adductor muscles due to partial nerve damage. Pichotka and Lewis (1949) occasionally observed similar phenomena during their experiments on muscle necroses. They also noticed a *straddled gait*, contractures and loss of the splay reflex of the toes. Bugliari and Canavero (1941) described *arthralgias* with hyperaesthetic and anaesthetic zones.

Apart from all these reports many authors, amongst them Dreyer (1913), have also described sensitivity to pressure of the nerve-filaments and of the ental origin of the nerves, manifestations of genuine *neuritis or neuralgia* (sciatica). In 1902 von Schroetter observed neuralgiform pains in the area of the tibia. As early as 1916 Stansky spoke of a trench neuritis due to wet cold that was often to be observed. Volk and Stiefler (1915) reported similar observations in the case of the nervus tibialis and the nervus peronaeus without there being any evidence of motor loss or grosser sensory functional disturbances.

Wurst (1944) found hyperaesthetic areas in the entire region of the skin after acute cold injuries, isolated areas of disturbed function and differentiated losses for touch, thermic stimuli, both isolated and also simultaneously occurring. In some cases all the sensitive qualities had been eliminated together. More detailed investigations showed that the boundaries of the disturbances very often coincided with circulatory disturbances. On several occasions a weakening of sheer strength with tremor and a tendency to muscular cramps were found simultaneously in the affected area. The regions of superficial loss however did not always coincide with injury to the musculature, Staemmler (1943) and Wurst (1944) speak of a pseudospastic paresis with slight tremor, similar to that described by Foerster and Nonne. The tendon reflexes were in the main normal, the knee jerk and Achilles tendon reflex often raised, the latter also sometimes lowered. Total anaesthesia was relatively seldom observed. Hyperaesthetic zones were more often to be found. In more than a fifth of the cases the defects persisted for months after the actual cold trauma.

A glance at the available material shows clearly that symptoms of loss of sensitivity occur much more often in cold injuries than marked motor disturbances. There is almost no one, who has suffered cold damage, that does not report a dull, numb feeling in the previously frost-damaged areas for years after and complain of sensitivity to cold in the affected limb. Only in rare cases did myogenic defects and contractures occur simultaneously.

In 1902 Zoege von Manteuffel (1902 a, b) undertook an investigation of nerve damage due to cold from a pathological - anatomical standpoint and his findings were confirmed by Remy and Therese (Sonnenburg and Tschmarke 1915), Denny quoted according to et al. (1945), Greene (1942), Siegmund (1943a-c), Staemmler (1944), Blackwood (1943, 1944 a, b), Thorban (1962) and others. Siegmund (1943 a-c) found in his experiments on the greater and smaller nerves in the more restricted and in the broader region of cold damage a *plasmatic saturation of the nerve cables, swelling of the nerve tissue, destruction of the myeline sheath and axis cylinders,* to some extent also haemorrhages in the nerves. In 1944 Staemmler delegated the systematic study of the alterations in the nerves ocasioned by exposure to cold to his students Boettcher (1944), Wurst (1944) and Hasche. Very impressive plates were published (Figs. 37–38).

They were able to carry out a detailed histological investigation of 28 clinical cases of cold injury from the 3rd to the week. In six cases no damage was found at all, in 17 cases slight damage, in two cases moderate and in three cases extreme alterations. On every occasion *destruction of the myeline sheath* was the main finding, whilst at the same time not all nerve bundles are ever completely destroyed, but rather there is always only partial destruction, and it seems to be the case that the inner regions of the nerves, as opposed to the outer lying fibres close to the perineurium, are affected to a greater extent, which does not seem to be completely understandable. Transitional states between damaged and undameged myeline sheath have often been seen. In the same bundle the fibres may be found partly preserved and partly destroyed. "Markballenbildungen" were also observed and recorded histologically. In the damaged bundles the partly granulated, partly swollen remains of myeline sheath were found permeated with fat droplets. In many cases the enlarged Schwann's cells contained fat. In contrast to these degenerative signs Staemmler and his colleagues found few manifestations of an inflammatory nature. Small lymphocytic infiltrations did in fact occur between the nerve fibres in the region of the vessels or near the perineurium, but a direct relationship to the degree of cold damage has never been found. There was an *increase in serous fluid.* The fibres were pressed asunder, a pronounced or even severe oedema was not to be found. The axis cylinders were sometimes ballooned but relatively well preserved, in other cases they were completely destroyed and had for the most part disappeared (Figs. 39–41).

The course of anatomically tangible vascular alterations does not seem to run parallel to vascular damage. Staemmler (1943, 1944), Siegmund (1943 a-c) and Schulz (1942,

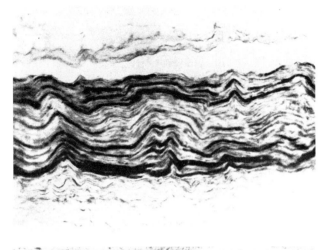

Fig. 37. Plasmatic saturation of left human peroneal nerve, after cold injury (According to Staemmler)

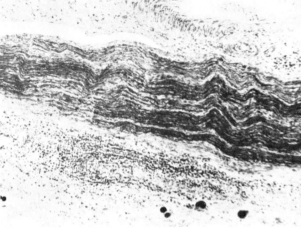

Fig. 38. Perineuritis of the perineural nerve in the same case. (From Staemmler)

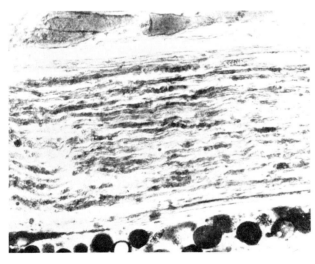

Fig. 39. Destruction of the myeline sheath in the tail nerve of a rat after experimental freezing. (From Böttcher 1944)

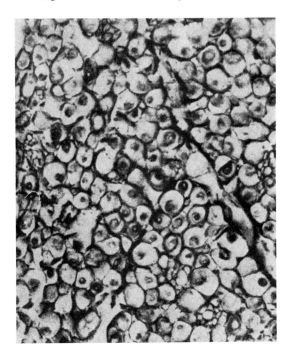

Fig. 40. Nervus tibialis r. staining of the axis cylinder according to the technic of Bielschowsky. (From Staemmler)

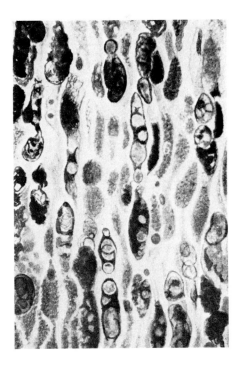

Fig. 41. Nervus tibialis l. staining according the technic of Olivencrona. Formation of medulla clumps. Markballenbildung. (From Staemmler)

1943) still believed that these lesions are caused by local nutritional disturbances, i.e. by circumscribed arteriospasms, since muscular damage was sometimes also to be seen at the same time, though muscle necroses never developed. Apparently the nerves are simply much more sensitive to cold than the muscle fibrils and may be directly damaged by cold. In 1945 Denny et al. mention on the basis of their experiments that the axis cylinders and the myeline are mainly damaged by cold. In 1942 Ungley and Blackwood speak of a *demyelinisation of the nerves.* A necrosis of the entire nerve appears to occur only after freezing (Figs. 40 and 41).

These findings were recently confirmed by Unterdorfer and Umbach (1977). In the cold-sensitive nerve cables not only does the action of cold lead to a plasmatic saturation of the cables, but frequently also to extravasations as a primary sign of damage. With more intense degrees of cold the myeline sheath and axis cylinder degenerate. A fatty degeneration of Schwann's cells takes place.

As a result of these to some extent really severe partial alterations to the nerves it seems quite understandable that paralyses have been seen to occur after cold injuries.

Alterations to the sympathetic nerves and ganglia have often been asserted and also observed; the results do not seem to be uniform or reliable (Block 1942; Sunder-Plassmann 1943). Degenerative changes to the sympathetic ganglia after exposure to cold are similar to those found in endangiitis obliterans. Plaque formation, nuclear degeneration and cell degeneration in the histological picture are mentioned. The results correspond to the findings of Paschenko (1943). These data contradict the assertions that the sympathetic nerve fibres are particularly resistant to cold.

A lively discussion about the causes of such nerve damage has understandably ensued. Nägelsbach (1919, 1920) assumed that colloidal alterations in the nerve occur, since even above 0° C without freezing symptoms of nervous loss may be observed, which

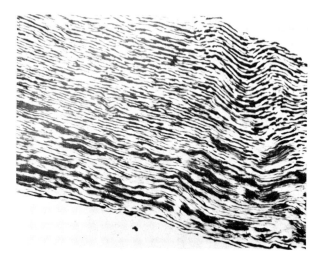

Fig. 42. Sciatic nerve in the midpart of the thigh after a 3-h immersion of the lower leg in ice-water at -2° C. Macroscopically no visible cold injuries to the skin. Clumps, vacuole formation and breaks in the continuity of single nerve fibres indicate partial damage to the nerve. Staining according to Bielschowsky-Gross. x 220. (From Thorban)

in my opinion favours the theory of a direct cold effect. He makes allusions here to the studies of Dania and recalls certain works of Trendelenburg (1917) and Schade (1919, 1920). The colloid alterations are generally reversible, only in the case of prolonged or repeated exposure to cold can permanent damage occur.

Probably the most important of the more recent experimental investigations on nerve damage due to cold were conducted by Thorban in 1962 and 1964. He wanted to explain the relationship between these injuries and delayed injuries to the vascular system which manifested themselves as cold angiitis or endangiitis obliterans of an acquired nature (see also p. 99). Let it be mentioned that after 2nd to 4th degree cold injuries vegetative centres of stimulation of a tortuous nature may develop, which may lead to late injuries similar to Raynaud's disease. Killian observed and reported on a number of such cases up until 1962.

The effect of cold on the brain for cryo-surgical purposes was studied by a whole series of investigators (Liebert and Spuler 1970; Mark-Tschiba – Erwin Hamlu 1966; Fasano et al. 1962). After induction of a cold injury in the brain with a cold probe a central necrosis was found to develop together with the formation of an intermediary zone with plaque disintegration of the tissue and around this a transitional zone to normal tissue. The authors assumed that this alteration does not only occur due to damage to the blood vessel system, but also due to disturbances of permeability and to a failure in the blood - brain barrier. Recovery took place as early as 3-4 days after. The focal and peripheral brain oedema persisted longer. The loss of the barrier-function generally extended well beyond the narrower area of damage. As is well known Brendel et al. (1965) assign considerable significance to the cold oedema of the brain. In animal experiments they were able to show that the survival time is limited in hypothermia and that a hibernation technique may not be employed for more than about a half-hour.

Changes to the Muscles Caused by Cold

The striated muscles belong without doubt to the tissues which are particularly sensitive to cold owing to their high water content - a result obtained by Rischpler as early as 1900, Marchand in 1908 and Zoege von Manteuffel in 1902 a, b. The functional changes in the striped muscles under the influence of mild cold, the increase in muscle tonus and muscular tension, the impediment of active movements, the stiffening of the limbs are in the main centrally caused, but are not as yet based on a notable alteration of the myosine. They are reversible. Muscular activity returns undamaged on rewarming. On the other hand actual damage to the musculature occurs in the case of protracted deep cooling and prolonged hypothermia of a limb. Physico-chemical alterations to the actual muscle substance now occur, which lead to stiffness. In the frozen state the affected muscles are hard and severe damage to the tissue structure with disintegration of the muscle fibrils and scar development due to the formation of larger ice-crystals may occur.

In the case of thorough cooling-down, immersion cold injuries, the superficial areas of the body, i.e. the skin and subcutis still do not as a rule show notable signs of damage or indeed any damage at all, whilst at the same time distinct muscle necroses are already developing at depth. These are in no way restricted only to an area of 3rd degree cold injury, but rather extend upwards into higher regions. Indeed muscle necroses are to be found in visible 2nd degree cold injuries.

Both Rischpler (1900) and Marchand (1908) observed a *fragmantation and disintegration of the muscle bundles with a loss of striation* after exposure to cold but believed that these injuries in the great majority of cases are not based entirely on the operation of cold, but that other causes, namely hypoxaemia or anoxia, are involved as well. Fuerst (1897, 1898), Volkmann (1893), Schmincke and Volkmann (1918) reached similar conclusions.

In a lecture in 1977 Unterdorfer and Umbach mentioned a narrowing of the muscle fibrils after the operation of cold and the development of spaces between the sarcolemma and the perimysium. These authors also noticed as did Staemmler (1943), however, that zones of well preserved fibril bundles alternate with such atrophic muscle fibres with nuclear disintegration in one and the same muscle. Furthermore a communication of Fontaine and Bollack in 1960 should be mentioned, in which they reported their observation of acute primary muscle damage in two cases of cold injuries, which spread surprisingly quickly and led by way of a venous thrombosis to gangrene of the affected limbs.

Due to the influence of cold a *waxy degeneration of the fibrils* occurs, which has been described by many authors (Kraske 1879; Horvath 1948; Brecht and Pulfrich 1948; Ullmann 1932; Rudnitzki 1900; Poensgen 1885; Pichotka et al. 1951 a, b; Fontaine and Bollack 1960. Poensgen (1885) describes a severe muscular swelling in the acute stage which is followed by atrophy of the muscle.

A detailed description of the pathological alterations to the musculature with excellent histological plates is to be found in Staemmler's monograph (1943) on local cold injuries. His investigations extended not only to the situation at the demarcation line (shin-bone preparations of persons after 3rd degree cold injury), but also to areas well above it. These observations are comparable to the results of animal experiments which Boettcher conducted in Staemmler's Institute in 1944. All these investigations show clearly that the musculature may sustain *atrophy* after exposure to cold. Staemmler (1943) has found a striking constriction of the fibrils, which lie in a network which has become too slack, so that wide gaps develop between the sarcolemma and the perimysium internum which is generally well preserved. In almost all cases the myocytic nuclei remained well preserved. An increase in number has in fact been seen on occasion, but never mitosis development. Later on the network becomes denser and increasingly encloses the narrow fibres. It is a striking fact that both well preserved and atrophied muscle bundles are to be found in one and the same preparation (Fig. 43) and that sometimes empty, swollen necrotic bundles are to be found amongst them. On occasion one also sees formation of vacuoles (Fig. 44—46).

Since irregularly distributed muscle atrophies, which develop independently of organic vascular damage and which lead to necroses, are quite often to be found between the gangrene and demarcation area, the authors thought it highly probable that these alterations are the result of functional circulatory disturbances. According to the histological findings a continuous lesion affecting the entire vascular system of a zone, which has been exposed to cold, can on no account be established. Well-preserved smaller arteries can be found amongst diseased muscle vessels. Occasionally one sees plates in proximal sections which conform with endangiitis obliterans (Staemmler 1944; Letterer 1944). These alterations must be due to something other than hypoxia.

According to Thorban's (1962, 1964) experiments it is primarily neurovasal damage, which in the final analysis, is responsible for discontinual muscle damage (necroses), insofar presumably as there are no direct effects of cold on the muscle due to deep coo-

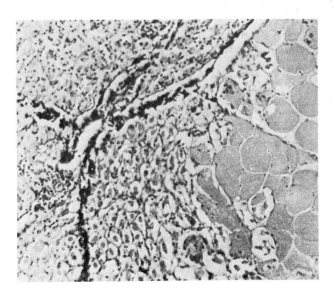

Fig. 43. Atrophy and necrosis of the fibres in the same bundle of muscle. (According to Staemmler)

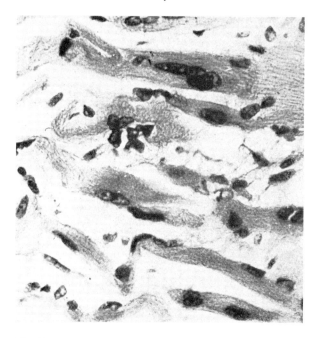

Fig. 44. So-called atrophic nucleal proliferations. (According to Staemmler 1943)

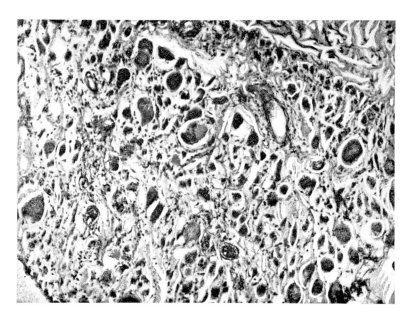

Fig. 45. Maximal irregular atrophy of muscles in the zone of amputation of the frozen leg. (According to Staemmler 1944)

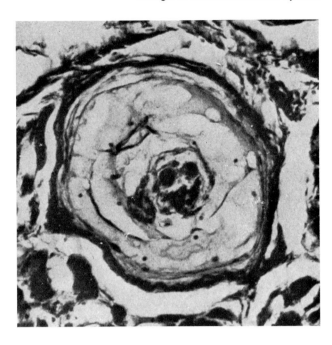

Fig. 46. Severe oedema of a muscle spindle (According to Staemmler 1943)

ling. Such ideas are not really new since scientific authorities such as Strughold (1944), Siegmund (1942 a, b, 1943 a) and others have already voiced their suspicions that cold itself can damage the autonomic nervous system of the vessels and muscles and Sunder-Plassmann (1943) referred to alterations of the regional sympathetic ganglia, which were only found in exceptional cases, however. Block (1942) too tried to find support for this theory in his experiments.

Apart from the above mentioned typical alterations in the striated muscle the pathologist Schulz (1943) found a waxy degeneration of the muscles in young men with generalised hypothermia, preparations of which he often showed me in Russia. Schulz found these strange degeneration phenomena only in winter and to be precise in 37 % of necropsies as opposed to 4 % in warmer seasons. The difference is so striking that it exceeds the limits of chance.

It is also well known that Zenker's muscle degenerations appear in various illnesses such atyphoid fever, sometimes also typhus. But the increase during the cold period justifies the assumption that cold itself may possibly be a cause here.

The findings of Schulz (1943) which at the time were regarded with intense suspicion, have been confirmed in more recent, very extensive experiments of Pichotka and Lewis (1949) on the one hand and Crismon and Fuhrmann (1946, 1947, 1948) on the other hand. Pichotka studied cold necrosis in the muscle in a sample of over 1,200 animals and reported the following findings:

At −5° C the skin temperature and that of the superficial musculature sinks to about 0° C with simultaneous loss of sensitivity and muscle strength. At −10° C skin temperatures of from −2 to −3°C were recorded and a muscle temperature of about 0°C in the deeper regions. In the superficial muscle layers the temperature approximated the skin temperature and solidification with necrotic areas developed. Exposure to a temperature of −12° C produced a skin temperature of −4° C and a temperature in the deeper muscle layers of between 0° and −3° C. A temperature of −6° C could be recorded in the superficial layers. Muscle necroses always developed under these conditions and in 20 % of cases skin necroses as well. These findings worsened at −15° C. From the onset of ischaemia a continual drop in tissue temperature similar to that of a physical body down to almost the temperature of the surroundings occured. Thereby the muscles have roughly the same temperature as the skin surface i.e. at exposure temperatures of −15° C approximately −10° to −12° C. In 100 % of cases *muscle necroses* develop at this point. In 90 % of cases skin necroses as well.

This series of experiments shows quite clearly that muscle damage together with a loss of sensitivity may develop at 0° C, that any solidification of tissue which develops at under 2° C increases the lesion proportionately. However, the results also show the clinically very important fact that *in certain areas muscle necroses develop at depth, whilst the superficial parts of the skin manifest either no signs of freezing or only minimal damage.*

Differences in the sensitivity of various types of muscle at the extremities was confirmed. The musculus tibialis anterior proved to be by far the most sensitive. This was followed by the musculus extensor longus, the musculus tibialis posterior, the triceps surae and after a much longer interval damage to the skin occurred. The extreme sensitivity of the musculus tibialis anterior, which may on its own become totally necrotic, is not in our opinion due to nutritional differences or differences in osmotic forces as Pichotka and Lewis (1949)[1] believe, but to purely physical reasons, due to the fact that this muscle lies adjacent to the shin-bone, i.e. a bone which is composed of apatitiae, which are highly conductible, and which promote a loss of warmth.

Both authors made a detailed study of the effects of undercooling at temperatures between +5° C and −40° C on groups of albino rabbits after hair removal and oiling of the rear extremities:

It was found that between 2° C and −15° C (length of exposure 30 min) 13 % of the animals died, 35 % showed total necrosis, 47 % a partial necrosis of the muscles and 5 % a superficial necrosis. On average exposure at −12° C for 30 min produced 33 % muscle necroses and at −15° C for 30 min 70 % muscle necroses. In the course of the experiments it was seen that summer and winter differences remain effective, which has so far not been able to be explained.

In an experiment on the paw of a hare Lewis (1951, 1952), made a histological study of the effects of cold lasting for between 15 min and 72 h and has published some fine plates of the results. *After 15 min he could already see the first signs of muscular lesions* − a result which conforms well with the observations of Pichotka (personal communications). Alterations in the muscle fibrils were traced up to the point of necrosis. After a 15-min exposure period definite degeneration of the muscle fibrils set in, which worsened considerably after 30 min and after typical ischaemia did not take place to this extent. Two hours later degeneration was already well advanced and oedema present. Six hours after exposure oedema and infiltration of polimorphous cells into the tissue together with extensive manifestations of degeneration are found. After 24 h necrophages develop. The maximal point of fibroplastic proliferation occurs at 72 h. After 8 days replacement of the damaged muscles with fibroplasts has taken place.

In all these experiments connective tissue proved to be much more resistant than the muscle fibrillae. Since thromboses of the vessels did not occur they cannot have been the cause of the muscle damage. For this reason Lewis and Moen (1952 a, b, 1953) assume *a primary cold injury to the musculature.* Lewis and Thompson (1951) later found on many occasions extensive muscle fibrillae necroses underneath the completely normal skin of surviving animals.

Pichotka (personal communications) moreover has voiced his suspicion that some of the necroses of the skin develop only secondarily due to blockage of the associated

---

1   Many thanks are due to Professor Pichotka for many important communications.

arterio-vascular system and occur because the necrotising musculature expels deleterious waste products. Such a possibility cannot be entirely rejected.

Supplementary comparative studies on the effects of a hypoxaemic phase turned out to be impressive. *During exposure to cold such an artificial oxygen deficiency phase had absolutely no influence on the proceedings. After exposure, however, a considerable exacerbation of lesions and increase in necroses occurred,* which was moreover completely dependent on the intensity and length of the hypoxic period.

Under such conditions the number of necroses rose from 33 % to 47 % after 4 to 6 h of mild hypoxaemia, to 53 % after 6 to 8 h and to 59 % after 10 to 12 h of oxygen deficiency.

After the destruction of muscle tissue and scar formation muscular atrophy and weakness may lead to flexion contractions in very different parts of the extremities. They were observed by Loos (1943), Scharfeter (1915), Killian (1942 a, b, 1943) and many others.

Furthermore Crismon and Fuhrmann (1947) found an increase in water content of from 5 % to 60 % in their cold experiments, an increase in salt content of from 237 to 697 % with simultaneous depletion of sodium chloride in the serum. This is a nonspecific reaction, which indicates severe alterations in osmotic relationships and in the electrolyte metabolism. Similar observations have been made in the case of burns or traumatic damage.

Since hypothermia found its use in open-heart surgery, the possibility of lesions of the heart musculature attracted attention. In 1962 Speicher et al. saw histologically a disappearance of sarcolemmic structure in the myocardium and fibroplastic proliferations in the epicardium and pericardium with adhesions, which may lead to a constrictive pericarditis with heart failure, after death in four patients with aortic valve diseases, who had been operated on in a state of hypothermia (ice slush). The authors declared that cooling of the heart should not last longer than 1 h.

References

Blackwood W (1943) Proc R Soc Med 36:521
Blackwood W (1944a) Br J Surg 31:329
Blackwood W (1944b) Br Med Bull 2:138
Block W (1942) Arch Klin Chir 1:64
Boettcher H (1944) Virchows Arch Pathol Anat 312:46
Brandis HJ von (1943) Vorträge aus der praktischen Chirurgie, vol 27. Encke, Stuttgart
Brecht K, Pulfrich (1948) Pflügers Arch 250:109
Brendel W, Reulen J, Messmer K (1965) Klin Wochenschr 43:515
Bugliari G, Canavero C (1941) G Med Mil 19
Crismon HJ, Fuhrmann FA (1946) Science 104:408
Crismon HJ, Fuhrmann FA (1947) J Clin Invest 259, 268, 286
Crismon HJ, Fuhrmnnn FA (1948) J Clin Invest 364
Denny, Brown O, et al. (1945) J Neuropathol 8:305
Dreyer U (1913) Zentralbl Chir 40:1628
Dreyer U (1914a) Beiträge zur Kriegsheilkunde. Springer, Berlin
Dreyer U (1914b) Dtsch Med Wochenschr 14:16
Fasano VA, Morgando F, Monticone GF (1962) Neurochirurgie 8:43
Floerken H (1915) Munch Med Wochenschr 7
Floerken H (1917) Bruns Beitr Klin Chir 106:4
Floerken H (1920a) Zentralbl Chir 47:1651

Floerken H (1920b) Die Kälteschäden im Krieg. Springer, Berlin (Ergebnisse der Chirurgie und Ortho-
    pädie)
Fontaine R, Bollack C (1960) Wien Med Wochenschr 110:509
Fuerst E (1897) Medical dissertation, Königsberg
Fuerst E (1898) Beitr Pathol Anat 24:414
Greene R (1942) Lancet 695
Horvath SM (1948) Am J Physiol 152:242
Killian H.(1942a) Zentralbl Chir 1763
Killian H (1942b) Arbeitstagung beratender Chirurgen, Berlin
Killian H (1943) Zentralbl Chir 70:50
Killian H (1962) Sachverständigentagung, Bonn (Report of Ministry of Labour)
Kraske H (1879) Zentralbl Chir 12
Lewis RB (1951) USA AFS AM-Report No 21-28016
Lewis RB (1952) Mil Surg 110:25
Lewis RB, Moen PW (1952a) J Med Sci 224:529
Lewis RB, Moen PW (1952b) Surg Gynecol Obstet 95:543
Lewis RB, Moen PW (1953) Surg Gynecol Obstet 97:59
Liebert KE, Spuler (1970) Neurochirurgia (Stuttg) 13:11
Loos HO (1943) Mitt Geb Luftfahrtmed 7
Marchand F (1908) Handbuch der allgemeinen Pathologie, vol 1
Nägelsbach E (1919) Munch Med Wochenschr 353
Nägelsbach E (1920) Dtsch Z Chir 160:2051
Pichotka J, Lewis RB (1949) Proc Soc Exp Biol Med 72:130
Pichotka J, Lewis RB, Freytag E (1951a).Texas Rep Biol Med 9:613
Pichotka J, Lewis RB, Ulrich HH (1951b) USA AFS AM-Report No 3
Rischpler A (1900) Beitr Pathol Anat 28:541
Rudnitzki TJ (1900) Zentralbl Chir 9:237
Schade H (1919) Munch Med Wochenschr 1:1021
Schade H (1920) Munch Med Wochenschr 449
Scharfeter H (1915) Dtsch Z Nervenheilkd 83:134
Scherer E (1934) Z Neurol 150:632
Schmincke, Volkmann R (1918) Samml Klin Vortr 785
Schroetter H von (1902) Verh Dtsch Pathol Ges
Schroetter H von (1916) Wien Klin Wochenschr 236
Schüller A (1915) Munch Med Wochenschr 62:1542
Schulz H (1943) Berichte der beratenden Pathologen
Schulze W (1942) Klin Wochenschr 646
Schulze W (1943) Arch Dermatol 184:61
Schumaker HB, Lempke RE (1951) Surgery 30:873
Siegmund H (1942a) Munch Med Wochenschr 827
Siegmund H (1942b) Arbeitstagung beratender Ärzte, Berlin
Siegmund H (1943a) Zentralbl Chir 1558
Siegmund H (1943b) Mitt Geb Luftfahrtmed 7:43
Siegmund H (1943c) Jahreskurse Aerztl Fortbild 34:9
Sonnenburg E, Tschmarke P (1915) Neue deutsche Chirurgie. Encke, Stuttgart
Sorge (1929) Aerztl Monatsschr
Speicher CE, Ferrigan SK, Wolfson SK (1962) Surg Gynecol Obstet 114:659
Staemmler M (1943) Erfrierungen. Thieme, Leipzig
Staemmler M (1944) Virchows Arch Pathol Anat 312:437, 501
Stansky (1916) Wien Klin Wochenschr 29:262
Stiefler G (1917) Jahrb Psychiatr 40
Stolfi, Berlozzino (1941a) Bull Soc Ital Biol Sper 16:153
Stolfi, Berlozzino (1941b) Zentralbl Haut Geschlechtskrankh 67:597
Stopford (1918) Lancet 465
Strandell G (1941a) Nord Med 1077
Strandell G (1941b) Zentralbl Chir 103:694
Strughold H (1944) Klin Wochenschr 221
Sunder-Plassmann P (1943) Durchblutungsschäden. Encke, Stuttgart (Neue deutsche Chirurgie, vol 65)
Thorban W (1962) Bruns Beitr Klin Chir 207:87
Thorban W (1964) Unfallheilkunde 78:203
Trendelenburg P (1917) Z Exp Med 5:371

Ullmann (1932) In: Handbuch der Haut- und Geschlechtskrankheiten, vol 171, p 4
Ungley CC, Blackwood W (1942) Lancet 2:447
Unterdorfer H, Umbach P (1977) Aerztl Prax (Suppl) 41
Volk R, Stiefler G (1915) Wien Klin Wochenschr 28:116
Volkmann R (1893) Beitr Pathol Anat 12:233
White JC (1943) N Engl J Med 228:211
Wurst H (1944) Medical dissertation, Breslau
Zoege von Manteuffel J (1902a) Mitt Grenzgeb Med Chir 10:343
Zoege von Manteuffel J (1902b) Zentralbl Chir 63

Changes in Bones and Joints

A study on the subject by Ribbert, which unfortunately disappeared into oblivion, originates from the year 1902. In it he describes his experiments on damage to the bone system due to the effects of cold.

Ribbert (1901/1902) dipped the limb of an animal in a state of bloodlessness into a cold mixture for about 10 min and soon after observed the bones become largely necrotic. A complete sequester developed, the cartilage remained partially preserved. As a rule the periosteum and the marrow survived the influence of cold without damage. The dead bone was not expelled at all, but rather clothed with a thick layer of newly formed bone substance, developing outwards from the endosteum and periosteum - a finding which has recently been confirmed by Pichotka and Lewis (1949). The sequester is therefore induced to heal.

In 1924, too, Zoege von Manteuffel and Rudnitzky observed severe swellings of the extremities after exposure to cold in the limbs of their experimental animals (ether spray used repeatedly for 3.5 - 7 min.). They were not due to oedema but rather to alterations in the bone system. Both authors obtained the following results:

The diaphyses: The tibia and fibula appeared to be covered with a thick coating of newly formed bone tissue (for weeks), so that they were almost double their normal thickness in extreme cases. In no case was hypertrophy of the bone tissue absent. The old bone cylinder showed degeneration phenomena, the osseous cells were empty and denucleated. New bone growth had also taken place in the medullary canal, if only to a slight extent. The periostal new growth developed round the old necrotic bone in regular concentric layers, showed few irregularities on the surface and histologically the picture of normal bone tissue (Fig. 47).

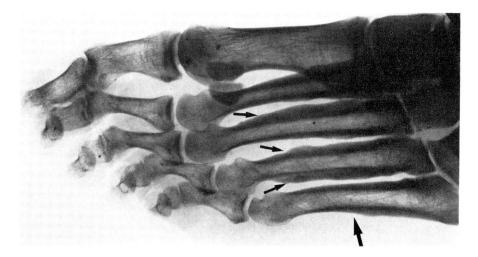

Fig. 47. Peristal reaction after repeated undercooling (winter 41/42) of the foot. Ossification around the metatasalia

The epiphyses: The alterations to the joints were different to those described. The marrow spaces extended in the direction of the glenoid surface so that the bony substance seemed to be atrophied. Resorption in the region of the articular surface reached such high degrees that the bony layer underneath the cartilage became paper-thin at some points and at other points even completely disappeared. The cartilage also showed degenerative processes, though only to a slight extent.

With regard to the causes of these alterations Zoege von Manteuffel (1924) mentions that he has found no evidence that alone the alterations to the arteriae nutritiae or the larger vessels lead to these severe, extensive alterations to the bone. Thus he assumed a *direct influence of cold on the bones* (Figs. 48 and 49).

Zuckerkandl (1916) also became involved in the problem of bone necroses after cold injuries and expressed the view that the bones mortify inside the frozen necrotic limb segments. A decalcification zone, which is recognisable on the 14th to 15th day, develops distally and corresponds to the granulation region and the hard, distally lying demarcation line. Inflammatory reactions and periostal appositions soon become recognisable above this area. At that time Zuckerkandl still believed that the bone necrosis only reached the level of the demarcation line, which proved to be erroneous.

From the series of experiments on bone injuries due to cold let us furthermore mention those of Ribbert's student Kleinschmidt in 1909.

He induced cold injuries in rabbits and rats and examined the limbs afterwards. To begin with, *the very much greater sensitivity of the bone cells as opposed to the overlying soft parts* was thereby confirmed. This means therefore relative intactness of the integuments whilst the bones have already succumbed to necrosis. New bone growth could very soon be observed, partly through an osteoid network but partly also through the deposition of thin osseous lamellae, which originate in the periosteum. Kleinschmidt found, in the presence of sufficient nourishment, a ring-shaped new growth of osseous lamellae in the Haversian canals. If this was not the case then regeneration took place entirely from the periosteum through proliferation of plethoric connective tissue.

In 1931 Löhr conducted experiments on rats. By freezing with ethyl chloride he induced artificial frostbite in the paws then found after killing a number of the animals lesions due to the direct action of cold, whilst in the case of the animals which were not destroyed, permanent bone alterations developed at a later stage.

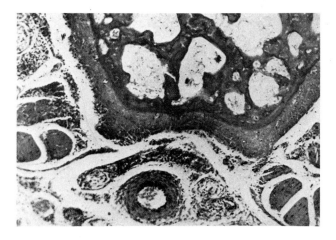

Fig. 48. Necrosis of the bone and bone-marrow in experimental freezing. (From Böttcher 1944)

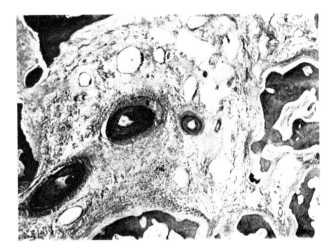

Fig. 49. Bone-marrow artery. Extreme thickening of the vascular wall, especially of the intima. Considerable narrowing of the vascular lumen (Elastica staining) x 150

In his experiments the *epiphyseal cartilage proved to be the most sensitive, the bone cells somewhat less so. The outer soft parts on the other hand proved to be by fart the most resistant,* which complied with a pattern found also by Burckhart in 1915. He noticed an extraordinary sensitivity of the bone cells, which corresponded roughly to that of the epiphyseal cartilage.

The cartilage is thought to be particularly sensitive in its superficial parts, whilst being more resistant in its deeper parts. *Shrinkage of the cartilage lining* to the size of a narrow hyaline band occurs with servere injury. Burckhart noticed, moreover, that the bony parts nearest the periosteum and endosteum are the most severely damaged. In the case of very severe frost action the bone sometimes becomes necrotic even after a long time interval.

Demarcation in the region of the bone marrow is normally well defined. The intermediary zone is narrow. The frostbite zone of the periosteum coincides with that of the bone.

In 1941/42 the pathologist Krauspe above all and his student Radasewski (1947), and also Siegmund (1942 a-c, 1943 a-c), Staemmler (1942, 1943, 1944) and Boettcher (1944) became concerned with bone alterations after cold injuries.

In 1943 Siegmund (1943 a-c) found in early cases of cold injury peristatic hyperaemia, blood stases and small foci of bleeding in the bone marrow as well as in the region of the outer periosteum. Early necrosis of the bone cells and bone substance in the region of the cortex layer as well as in the region of the spongiosa occurred.

A useful addition to his observations was made with the experiments of Boettcher (1944) from Staemmler's Institute. He obtained fairly similar results in cold experiments on animals (rat tails). *The bone proved to be extremely sensitive and is much less resistant than the covering soft parts. It could once more be confirmed that bone necroses develop even when the skin still shows no trace of cold damage* (see Figs. 50 and 51).

By examination of 23 amputation and post-mortem cases after cold injury in 1941/42 Radasewski was able to distinguish three zones of damage in the bone after cold lesions. In the gangrene area bone and marrow are completely necrotic. The vessels of the marrow in this region are obstructed. The picture is one of stasis and haemolysis. In the demarca-

108

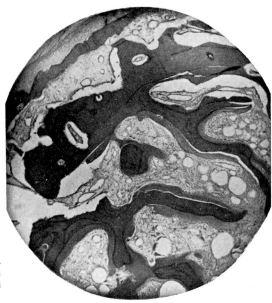

Fig. 50. Bone necrosis after cold action. Note the periostal and endostal new growth surrounding the necrotic parts. (From Oehleker 1942)

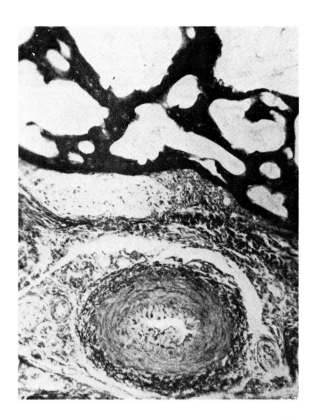

Fig. 51. Arterial contraction. Necrosis and atrophy of the muscles and bones in experimental freezing. (From Böttcher 1944)

tion area a local border between necrotic and viable tissue in the form of a leucocytic wall develops. A clear demarcation zone also develops in the bone itself. The bone cells are destroyed distally, proximally they remain at least partially preserved. The bone cells loose their stainability well into the healthy region, a documentary to their damage. The area of damage extends proximally well beyond the demarcation zone in an irregular form.

Staemmler reported that in the case of muscle necroses a direct dependence on the supply area of single bone arteries is not evident. In the main, therefore, at least with early cases, one assumes that direct cold damage has taken place and not indirect damage based on a nutritional disturbance. Obliterating endangiitis (thromboangiitis obliterans) of the actual bone vessels has only rarely been reported but it does occur. See here to the histological plates in Thorban's study (1962, 1964). In the actual reaction zone bone degeneration is thought to outweigh new development.

Some reactive processes are stressed as being particularly characteristic, for example, a tissue rich in fibre and capillaries, which originates from the bone marrow and is often permeated with haemorrhages and which expands in the direction of the leucocytic wall. Serous inflammation and alterations of the fibrous osteitis type were found. Round cells were also noticeable in the haemorrhage zone, around which lay circular deposits of fat-containing cells, which were described as fat storing mesenchymal cells, chiefly reticulum.

On the basis of their investigations Krauspe (1943) and Radasewski (1947) came to the conclusion that the reaction of bony tissue to cold is of a special nature, insofar as vessel wall alterations are much less prevalent than in other types of tissue, whereas direct cold damage is of predominant importance.

The most recent confirmation of the development of aseptic bone and cartilage necrosis and of alterations to the joints comes from Kyösola and Trasima (1974). He had the opportunity so treat and investigate 110 cases of cold injury. In 11 cases the state of pain could be relieved by sympathectomy. The demarcation and absorption of oedema were accelerated. On the other hand dextran infusions with the application of anticoagulants were unsuccessful (Figs. 52a, b).
The histological study of Rahn et al. (1977) on a rabbit's ear after local freezing and demarcation and repulsion of necrotic parts is also of interest. Not only were necrotic cartilage parts found sheathed in epithelium and a waxy deformation of cartilage parts which had been damaged by cold, but also calcification or ossification of the same. At the same time one could see signs of new cartilage development. Subsidiary findings of alterations to the vessels, hair follicles and connective tissue were also reported. After cold injuries osteoporosis and Sudeck atrophy are often observed (Fig. 53).

Radasewski (1947) attributes the high *sensitivity of the bone to cold to the good thermal conductivity of bones (apatiteae)* an opinion which we also share since Pichotka was able to establish that certain muscles which lie close to bone, e.g. the musculus tibialis anterior, may suffer particularly severe cold injuries, indeed even isolated total necrosis.

According to Radasewski three different types of reaction are recognisable in young animals:

1) On the spot regeneration.
2) Uninhibited new formation.
3) Delayed new formation.

Periosteal regeneration outweighs endosteal. Where necrotic bone is absorbed one only seldom finds signs of lacunar and vascular resorption. The bone disappears without any evidence. In the case of delayed new development, such as occurs with severe damage, it can be seen that the growth of fresh marrow only reaches a certain stage before finally the development and expansion of scanty osteoid tissue comes to a halt.

110

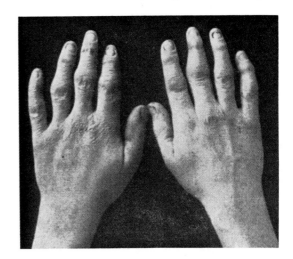

Fig. 52a. Crippled fingers after cold injury. (From Oehlecker)

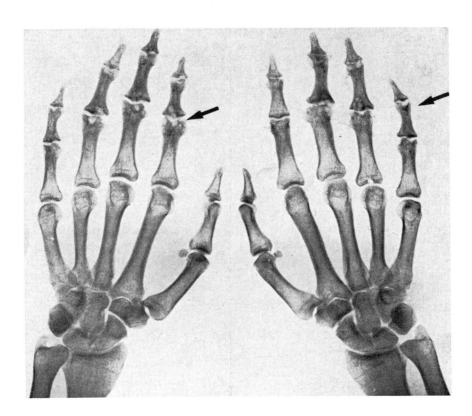

Fig. 52b. Rtg of the same case: destruction and deformation of the phlangeal joints. (From Oehlecker)

111

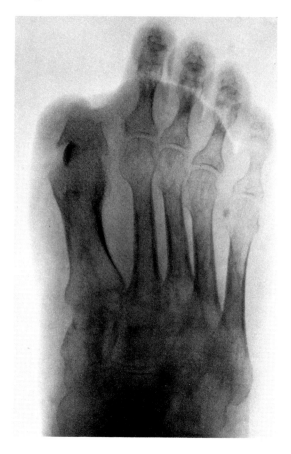

Fig. 53. Maximal osteoporosis and Sudeck atrophy after cold injury of the foot with necrosis and amputation of the 1st toe

In 1942 Moser conceded the heel bone a certain special significance, inasmuch as the bone may be preserved in frost necroses of the heel even after desquamation of the same. This observation must be limited to exceptional cases, for in general the heel bone also succumbs to osteitis and osteonecrosis, so that it is often a surgical necessity to remove large parts of the bone in order to ensure recovery.

References

Boettcher H (1944) Virchows Arch Pathol Anat 312 : 46
Krauspe C (1943) Osttagung beratender Ärzte, Berlin
Kyösola K, Trasima J (1974) J Trauma 24 : 32
Moser H (1942) Dtsch Med Wochenschr 68 : 549
Pichotka J, Lewis RB (1949) Proc Soc Exp Biol Med 72 : 130
Radasewskij (1947) Beitr Pathol Anat 109 : 567
Rahn BA, Höflin FG, Perras SM (1977) Aerztl Prax (Suppl) 41
Ribbert H (1901/1902) Lehrbuch der allgemeinen Pathologie. Leipzig

Siegmund H (1942 a) Munch Med Wochenschr 827
Siegmund H (1942 b) Arbeitstagung beratender Ärzte, Berlin
Siegmund H (1942 c) Arch Dermatol 184 : 84
Siegmund H (1943 a) Zentralbl Chir 1558
Siegmund H (1943 b) Mitt Geb Luftfahrtmed 7 : 43
Siegmund H (1943 c) Jahreskurse Aerztl Fortbild 34 : 9
Staemmler M (1942) Zentralbl Chir 45 : 1757
Staemmler M (1943) Erfrierungen. Thieme, Leipzig
Staemmler M (1944) Virchows Arch Pathol Anat 312 : 437, 501
Thorban W (1962) Bruns Beitr Klin Chir 207 : 87
Thorban W (1964) Unfallheilkunde 78 : 223
Zoege von Manteuffel J (1924) Zentralbl Chir 51 : 17
Zoege von Manteuffel J, Rudnitzki TJ (1924) Zentralbl Chir 51 : 17
Zuckerkandl O (1916) Brund Beitr Klin Chir 101 : 594

Vascular Changes

Relationship Between Peripheral Reactions to Cold and Overall State of the Circulation

The impression that cold reactions, especially the initial ones, have been presented and evaluated in very varied ways is in our opinion due mainly to the fact that their dependence on the overall state of the circulation has not been sufficiently taken into consideration. Either from the experimental or from the clinical standpoint; although Krogh (1924), Rein (1931) and others have already referred to this important factor.

Reactions in the service of the physical regulation of warmth with the purpose of increased output or retention of warmth largely prevail over exogenous factors (Rein 1931, 1943; Killian 1942 a, b, 1945; Grosse and Brockhoff 1950; Vogt 1953; Schneider 1955). They may alter the picture of a vascular reaction considerably in the peripheral zones in spite of the fact that this very area has independent reaction mechanisms at its disposal. For this reason, reactive cold reactions during a phase of freezing or shivering, or during and after a depressive circulatory condition, turn out differently than those during heavy muscular activity, warming-up and a stimulated state of circulation which are suited to postpone a centralisation of the circulation during exposure to cold.

As is well known the rabbit ear offers good subject matter for the study of alterations in the circulation. A contraction of the arterioles and the arterial capillaries induced by local undercooling can be directly observed. In the case of a generalised cooling of the animal a reflex contraction of the vessels follows relatively independently of external local influences. The number of perfused capillaries is not thought to be noticeably altered thereby and the colour also only slightly, but alone the state of the arteries and arterioles in the sense of a contraction. The veins and venules show only a brief contraction then a slight dilatation (see in comparison the results of Tittel 1944; Meiners 1952; Schneider 1943, 1952, 1953, 1954).

In 1931 Rein was able to demonstrate with the use of his thermostromuhr that powerful alterations in circulation are, caused by limited local cooling, e.g. through laying a piece of ice on the forehead (trigeminal region). Particular importance is attached to his experiments on reactive vascular expansion as a function of the general state of the circulation.

After artificial cooling the course of rewarming was traced thermo-electrically. On average it increase from 7° to $13^{\circ}C$ after 1 h. A warming reaction in the fingers only appeared when the rest of the body was well protected from cold and there was no shivering. Otherwise the vascular spasm increased namely, the fingers became colder, all rewarming stopped. These results have been confirmed by Lewis (1932, 1938), Weisswange (1944), Jarisch (1939, 1943), Ranke (1943), Fuhrmann and Crismon (1947).

The periodic heating phases of hypothermic peripheral limbs (particularly clearly seen in the thumb and large toe), i.e. the Aschoff-Lewis reaction, showed diurnal and seasonal fluctuations corresponding to changes in vasomotor tonus. In 1944 and 1948 Kramer and Schulze succeeded in showing that this reaction also develops differently with disturbances in heat regulation, for example, with hypothermia. Thereby magnification and broadening of the thermic amplitudes occur and periods become less frequent. Freezing or shivering, a deficit in heat regulation with reactive increase in vasomotor tonus on the other hand leads to acceleration and increase in the periodic heating phases, whose amplitudes are then smaller, however. In a state of oligaemia periodic vascular dilatation with the purpose of conserving the endangered tissue still takes place: with total ischaemia this phenomenon disappears, however. The tissue or limb cools down thoroughly like a physical body.

Alcohol in small doses produces an increase in this phenomenon through its central action and a reactivation in the case of extinction, insofar as this is still possible at all, (compare Killian 1966)

In 1931 Lewis gathered thermoelectric observations concerning the distribution of temperature. The fingers showed the lowest temperatures and must be regarded as particularly sensitive to temperature change. In the face the red parts, i.e. the tips, the ears, nose and cheeks were strangely enough the coolest. They showed low temperatures and are therefore relatively at risk in cold. According to Stray (1943) the ear is the coldest, followed by the cheeks and nose. In spite of relatively good circulation the region of the check-bone is also a relatively cool region. We refer to Ipsen's monograph (1936) in which more detailed information about the distribution of temperature is to be found.

The temperature of the tissue runs parallel to the flow volume at any given time. According to Kramer and Schulze (1944, 1948) registration of flow volume, blood content and finger temperature by means of the light absorption technique with exposure to cold shows that both run parallel whilst blood content on the other hand does not (Figs. 54 and 55).

The hypothermic region becomes a centre of stimulation which causes the afferent pathways (arteries, arterioles, arterial capillaries and precapillaries) to contract. The contraction persists as long as stimulation continues. Now, it is characteristic of cold damage that stimulus formation persists for a long time and may lead to a lasting spasm of the afferent pathway up to the large arterial trunks of the extremities. The constriction of the arterial afferent pathways in the second phase of cold exposure may be interpreted as a useful reaction, since it serves to protect the entire body against cold.

Phases of Cold Reactions in the Vascular System

According to Moser (1942), Ratschow (1933, 1936) and others the vascular cold reaction in humans proceeds in three phases according to the following scheme:

1) Stage of pallid skin with onset of anaesthesia.
2) Stage of blue-red skin with swelling and patchy cyanosis due to isolated secondary dilatation of the terminal pathways of the venous capillaries and plexus.
3) Stage of bright-red skin.

This division is not at all satisfactory and to some extent contradicts my own clinical experience as well as that of many other authors who have witnessed the development of fresh cold injuries or have conducted cold experiments. A primary dilatation is fleeting and is followed initially by a phase of bright redness, then by a fourth stage of waxy pallor with total ischaemia and finally the fifth stage of the secondary reaction with blue-red or blue-grey discoloration.

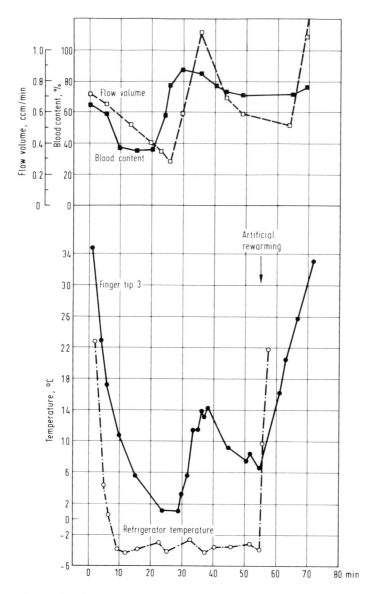

Fig. 54. Simultaneous registration of finger temperature, flow volume and blood content (light absorption) at an external temperature of -4°. Flow volume and temperature progress in a synchronous and parallel manner, not, however, blood content. During rewarming flow volume does not increase until finger temperature reaches 22° C. (From Kramer and Schulze 1944)

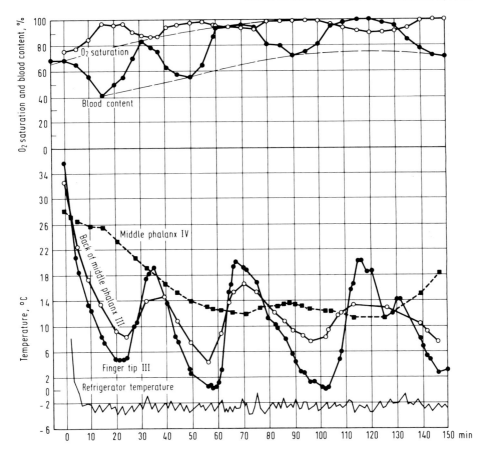

Fig. 55. Ogygen saturation, blood content (light absorption measurements) and finger temperature at -3° C. Blood content increases in each case 10 min before the rise in finger temperature. Mean blood content rises during exposure to cold. Note the Aschoff-Lewis reaction (Hunting phenomenon). (From Kramer and Schulze 1944)

Within the framework of cold reactions Stray (1943) concerned himself especially with changes in skin colour and found that between 0° and 5°C a reddish flush develops within a few minutes. Goose-flesh on a pale bluish background already develops at +22°C, reaches its maximum at between +14,5° and +13,5°C and disappears at +7°C. It reappears during rewarming at about +7°C. A reddening of the skin between single follicles begins between +19° and +20°C in humans. The skin colour is then an inhomogeneous reddish blue. At about +16°C it becomes blue red, at +14,5°C bright red, later increasingly lobster red up to +7°C. Stray like ourselves interprets this sudden alteration of colour not in terms of high flow velocity in the arterial side but as an *arterialisation of venous blood*, which already takes place at a temperature of +10°C. At +9°C an approximation of the O_2 content of the venous blood with the arterial has already taken place (Brown and Hill 1923; Goldschmid 1950). Craigh (1945) describes this state as *"pale reaction"* in mild cold and distinguishes it from *"white reaction"*, e.g. in the forearm of the human without the presence of gooseflesh and with total anaesthesia in severe cold of about minus 4°-5°C.

117

Neither the stage of bright redness nor that of the initial blue-red skin as yet gives cause for alarm. The sudden appearance of a waxy pallor due to ischaemia with total anaesthesia on the other hand always signifies acute danger of freezing. This was also confirmed in the most recent American reports from the Korean War and emphasized by Sapin-Jaloustre (1956).

Transient Dilatation as an Initial Reaction

Lewis noticed a *fleeting dilatatory reaction* in the capillary region of the surface areas to cold exposure. Later on a swelling or weal-formation possibly follows in a zone which becomes recognisable in a dilatation of the small cutaneous vessels, the terminal arterioles, capillaries and vessels of the subpapillary plexus. This transient dilatatory reaction is generally limited to the zone which has been exposed to cold and is independent of the associated sensory innervations, since severing or degeneration of the regional nerve cables did not alter the reaction. An artificial blood blockage also made no noticeable impression. Lewis believed that this initial transient vasodilatation is the result of the direct influence of cold on the vessels and that it belongs to the first phase of the "triple response" phenomenon.

In our capillary microscopic investigations on frog tongues in 1925 we occasionally saw fleeting dilatation in the presence of every banal stimulus, which is completely unspecific. It seemed to be fairly meaningless from an experimental and clinical point of view.

Krogh too saw *initially a fleeting dilatation of the capillaries* in the frog tongue with exposure to cold at $+2^{\circ}$C. Most authors have always only been able to recognise an initial vasoconstriction of the small arterial vessels with exposure to cold.

In fact reports on initial cold reactions vary so much that it is really difficult to make sense of them. This is probably due to variations in technique, differences in the type of animal and differences between cold-blooded and warm-blooded subjects.

Vasoconstriction

Vasoconstriction is the essential main reaction to cold. It has been experimentally and clinically confirmed thousands of times.

Whilst Siegmund (1942 b, 1943 b, 1950) was only able to observe a contraction of all vessel segments with the capillary microscope, Kreyberg (1949) saw a *single spasm of the terminal arteries and venules of the skin* with exposure to cold (ice water) on the skin of a rabbit, and simultaneously dilatation of the superficial venous vessels, in which the blood was literally confined. Not until hours later did the spasm weaken and fresh blood flow into the area again. The blood supply was once more severely reduced 18-24 h later.

The experiments of the students of Schneider (1941), Tittel (1944) and Meiners (1943) on the rabbit ear are muche more informative. Their results are summarised in Table 6, p. 120.

This shows how important it is to differentiate between the reaction of the frostbitten regions themselves and those outside the frozen are (Fig. 56). It seems to be significant that the initial reaction of all the blood vessels in the frozen area, arteries, veins and capillaries, is to contract.

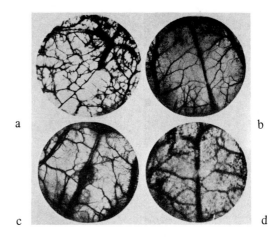

Fig. 56a–d. Middle artery of a rabbit ear. A circular portion of the ear was frozen at the level of the dividing point of the artery. a At the point of freezing the vessels are paralysed, the afferent vessel closed by spasm. b The same after sympathicus transection 3 days before the trial. The marginal spasm at the periphery of the site of freezing is still present, the general spasm is absent. Local mechanical stimulation does, however, still lead to the development of a constriction ring. c Three days before the trial the artery was pinched. The spasm extends as far as the point of pinching, but no further. d Sympathectomised ear. In the paralysed region is an agglutination thrombus. The marginal spasm is not sufficient to exclude the damaged area from the circulation. Embolisation of the distal ramifications occurs later on. (From Meiners 1952)

After the exogenous cold action has been withdrawn all the blood vessels in the actual frostbitten area dilate to a marked degree, cease to react to any stimuli, and can only change their lumina passively as a reaction to pressure. The active vasoreactions and regulation are therefore no longer present.

After initial capillary contraction maximum capillary dilation and complete paralysis are soon observed. The blood ceases to flow in the capillaries.

In the *neighbouring area* the arteries first dilate during the time of exposure to cold as if in an attempt to warm up the area, then arterial spasms occur around the edges and spread well into the healthy area (secondary arterial spasms). This spasm of the arteries more or less cuts the frostbitten area off completely from the main circulation. The relaxation of the spasm is accompanied by an increase in the motility and sensitivity to stimuli of the afferent arteries. *An increased tendency of these arteries to contract remains for a long time after the cold action has ceased,* so that fresh spasms with signs of defective circulation may occur at a late stage.

It was particularly difficult to explain the bluish-grey cutis marmorata due to secondary filling of the capillary area, for after the formation of an arterial spasm the area first becomes anaemic. The only possible explanation for this is that there is a secondary filling from the neighbouring areas, corresponding to the pressure gradient and possibly also a reflux phenomenon of the blood, which the author was often able to observe in the capillary area when the circulation had stopped. This can only be simply a pressure passive seeping back of the blood into the dilated, totally paralysed venous capillaries. The blood corpuscles do not move, they completely fill the capillary lumina and are deprived of oxygen. This accounts for the dark blue colour, which is the result of greatly reduced

119

Vascular Changes

Table 6. The effects of cold on blood vessels according to Tittel (1944) (rabbit ear, effects of cold with CO_2 snow) after special microphotogram

Arteries, arterioles		
Preliminary control short-term cold action	After 30 s	Beginning of arteriospasm in the affected area
	After 45 s	Secondary spreading of the same
	After 1 min	The same
	After 4 min	Maximum spreading of the arterial spasm
	After 5 min	Beginning of the relaxation of the spasm, narrow bridgings, formation of the frostbite halo, which becomes more pronounced.
Preliminary control more prolonged cold action	5 min	After arterial blood vessels within frostbite halo greatly contracted, but outside area dilated! Increased filling of the cold damaged arteries and simultaneously increased tightening of the non-affected area. 2 min after cold action formation of a secondary spasm of the afferent arteries with pronounced dilatation of the frostbitten arterial blood vessels, finally maximum contraction of the afferent arteries. Spasms, total vascular occlusion, increased motility of the non-frostbitten arteries; alternation between expansion and contraction, increased tendency of these arteries to contract. 17 min after cold action: gradual relaxation of the spasm; links between non-damaged arteries and frostbitten arteries become visible. 20-25 min: on the edge of the frostbite halo a tightening of the blood vessels in varying degrees, clear delineation of the frostbitten area with maximum dilatation of all frozen arteries.

Veins (peripheral veins and rabbit ear)		
Preliminary control short-term cold action 1 min		After 1 min. localised in the frostbite halo contraction of all blood vessels (including veins). After thawing: a visible total contraction of the veins: development of secondary spasms of the arteries, then the beginning of the relaxation of the venous spasm. After 1.5 min: relaxation of the venous spasm; the veins become completely free, then pronounced dilatation of veins and also of arteries in frozen area. Maximum dilatation of the veins, formation of frostbite halo.

Capillaries		
Preliminary control relatively slight capillarisation, then cold action 10 min		After: pronounced capillarisation and capillary dilatation. Heavy exudation and erythrocytic diapedesis in the tissue. The capillaries are filled with a granular brownish mass. The blood vessels are not clearly defined. At the end of a capillary sometimes loss of a drop of blood. The blood vessels are covered in a reddish substance and raggedly defined. Blood comes to a complete standstill! Total capillary stasis.

120

Table 6. continued

Capillaries	
Total freezing of an ear	2 min after: blurred appearance of blood vessels, the beginning of a secondary filling of the blood vessels; secondary spasms of the afferent arteries. After 45 min: the arteries are free again but narrowed. After 55 min fully developed oedema

haemoglobin. Due to the stasis the erythrocytes which have gathered, become congested and clogged, there is a clumping and sludge formation until the capillary lumina are completely blocked. This also leads to exudation and diapedesis of the red blood corpuscles.

As part of a reflection on the physiological bases of blood supply to the organs, these results of Tittel's (1944) and Meiner's investigations of 1952 prompted Schneider to make the following comment: *As a reaction to localised cold stimuli there is an immediate, maximum contraction of the small arteries and arterial capillaries affected by the cold. The area becomes anaemic. The afferent arteries in the surrounding area, however, dilate.* This dilation can be explained on the one hand by a sudden increase in resistance at the periphery while the afflux and pressure remain constant, but it can also be considered as a practical reaction of the body to warm up the cooled area again. This appears to cause short-circuiting. If exposure is prolonged and the cold stimuli become stronger a *reversal of this reaction* can be observed, namely in the more restricted frostbitten area the *capillaries dilate and become paralysed,* whereas the afferent arteries and arterioles as a reflex reaction contract maximally. According to the view of Shumaker and Lempke (1951) the critical vasoconstriction consists of three different components:
1) Long-term local vasoconstriction as a result of direct exposure to cold (cold stimulus).
2) Local reflex vasoconstriction, which is conveyed by the sympathetic nervous system.
3) General vasoconstriction which, operates via the hypothalamus, and is triggered off by the loss of blood temperature.

It is probably the similarity of these three processes which makes the arterial spasm due to cold so intractable. The reduction of the blood supply leads to a drop in capillary pressure, so that the fluid content of the tissue decreases, and it shrivels. In the initial stage this can be seen in a plethysmogram. In the course of vasoconstriction a filter mechanism in the terminal vessels can be observed. The smallest arterial vessels do not close completely at first. After the erythrocytes have been filtered off they they are partly filled only with plasma, until the blood flow is completely interrupted. Under the microscope the erythrocytes disappear and at the same time the tissue becomes cloudy.

As small amounts of oxygen are still dissolved in the circulating plasma at this stage a certain minimum of oxygen is still being supplied, which is, however, by no means sufficient after a time. According to Rein (1931, 1943) 0.23 % to 0.3 % volume of oxygen are contained dissolved in the plasma water. *Oxygen absorption and the release of haemoglobin from the blood corpuscles is only ever possible in either direction by way of hydrosolubility in the plasma,* a fact which we have referred to many times. (See, for example, Killian and Doenhardt 1955 in the corresponding section on oxygen supply.)

Irradiation and Consensual Reactions

It is not difficult to show that the cooling of a small area, e.g. the lower part of the arm, after a short time causes distal vasoconstriction of the capillaries at the perionychium and proximal cubitalis-brachialis.

This manifestation has been observed by many authors and clinicians, among others by Müller (1918), Weiss (1921), Krogh (1924), Lewis (1927), Burton and Taylor (1946), Burch et al. (1947), Bader and Mead (1949), Kramer and Schulze (1948).

The reaction ceases after novocaine blockage, which led one to assume a nervous influence. Consensual reactions on the other side have been regularly observed and it is without doubt not only the larger but also the smallest blood vessels which are affected. These co-reactions must occur via the autonomous nervous system since a removal of the sympathetic ganglia and tracts in question inhibits this phenomenon. The consensual reactions change immediately according to Kramer and Schulze (1948) if the co-reacting side is itself exposed to thermal stimuli, which is shown by the changes of the Aschoff-Lewis reaction.

Burton and Taylor (1946), Burch et. al. (1947) and others have used consensual cold reactions on the contralateral hand or foot (in a plethysmogram) as a test for the cold reaction range of an individual (Alaska cold test). Men, in whom the blood had temporarily ceased to flow in the fingers apparently proved to be resistant and were able to work outside with bare hands at very low temperatures, which other people could not manage under the same conditions. Such tests do not, however, suffice to enable conclusions to be drawn about the cold tolerance or resistance of an individual, and subsequently to select persons who would be suited, for example, to going on arctic expeditions.

State of Primary Bluish Redness and the Stilting Phenomenon

While the arterial blood flow is throttled, the venous capillaries and plexus, however, are in a state of relaxation (paralysis) and maximum dilatation due to the cold; a slowing down of the circulation in this area must result, which finally leads to a congestion of the red blood corpuscles. The blood only moves very slowly through the venous capillaries in accordance with the new situation and also short circuits. The blood which moves very slowly or has even come to a standstill in the veins is deprived of its oxygen, which is only poosible, however, if the tissue metabolism has not completely stopped. The degree of cold limits the reduction of oxygen. The blue marmoration and bluish discoloration of the skin is therefore caused by the dilatation of the veins with the appearance of congestion and too high a concentration of reduced blood.

In our opinion this process is only a primary venous relaxation, caused purely by the cold, which vasodilating substances have still no part in worthy of mention, as the condition required for their formation do not yet exist at this point.

122

Bright Red Stage

The state of bright redness after exposure to cold forms when the arterial blood supply is throttled, i.e. oligohaemia.

Larrey (1817) reports is his war memoires as a surgeon that *all those suffering from cold injury have bright red venous blood.* Cadaveric ecchymosis could be distinguished on the corpses but they were bright red in colour. Bright redness is a sign of highly saturated oxyhaemoglobin. The bright redness of the 3rd stage is, therefore, primarily the result of a lack of oxyhaemoglobin reduction, poor use of the oxygen supplied, due to a decrease in local cell metabolism. According to Barcroft's graphs there is also a decrease in the dissociation of the oxyhaemoglobin as the temperature drops. This finally leads to a *compensation of the arteriovenous difference.* In addition the rate of flow in the contracted arteries, arterioles and arterial capillaries, and also to some extent in the short-circuited draining veins, is accelerated during this phase, so that the time in which the oxygen is released from the blood is decidedly shortened and the oxyhaemoglobin reduction decreased. According to my own observations only the blood in the actual main areries then still flows for a time.

These ideas also support the observation that during the stage of bright redness due to exposure to cold wounds only bleed slightly and the oxygen saturation of the venous blood shows a value of almost 100%. If a limb in such a cold state is then exposed to a temperature over +6°C the tissue metabolism begins to function again and oxygen still present in the blood is rapidly devoured.

Experiments carried out in connection with these problems by Staemmler in 1942 and 1944 and by Boettcher in 1944 after the models of Natus (1910) and Ricker (1924, 1927) on the mesentery and on the pancreas of rats and rabbits have produced results which we have reproduced briefly in Table 7. They are in good agreement with the experiments of Schneider and his pupils, Tittel (1944) and Meiners (1952) (see Table 7).

Table 7. The effects of cold on the blood vessels of the pancreas and the mesentery according to animal experiments by Staemmler (1943)

Cold stimulus	Terminal vessels as a whole	Capillaries	Precapillaries	Aterioles	Arteries
Slight cold stimulus	Slowing of circulation	First dilatation	Partly dilatation	Slight dilatation	Increase of blood supply
Medium and strong cold action	Upto stasis	Contraction, possibly 2nd dilatation	Contraction, partly dilatation	Contraction with spasm	Max contraction with spasm
Blood	Plasma extravasation oedema	Filter process, separation of cells and plasma, metataxia	Blocking mechanisms		

In 1943 Staemmler observed in the area of the capillaries and precapillaries with their sphincters the existence of *blocking mechanisms and filter processes.*

The cells are separated from the plasma and metataxia can be observed (sludge phenomenon). Staemmler also noticed blockages in the region of the arterioles. He did not, however, observe a total circulatory blockage of the blood vessels. This state in the terminal vessel area was gradually followed by the development of damage to the walls. Peristasis and stasis are formed. Following Staemmler's investigations, in 1944 Boettcher closely followed microscopically and macroscopically tissue changes in rat tails.

At first the tail turned pale all over due to the cold, then came the state of bright redness with a transition to a *bluish-red discoloration.* He therefore found macroscopically a *three phase* sequence of reactions. During the blue phase the tissue as swollen. When the cold action was withdrawn reactive hyperaemia could be observed. Repeated exposure to cold at certain intervals of time finally resulted in the tip of the tail remaining deep red, but turning pale as a reaction to cold stimulus. In each of the following experiments the blue discoloration appeared more quickly. Whereas the peripheral parts showed a dark discoloration, the proximal parts remained pale.

In the state of paleness small wounds almost stopped bleeding and also in the state of bright redness or dark discoloration the bleeding hardly increased at all. This clearly proves the maintenance of a maximum narrowing of the arterial pathway throughout the secondary period. In the more restricted area of the capillaries amongst the terminal vessels, the contraction phase remains fairly short and is followed by the relaxation of the small blood vessels. A histological investigation of the tissue at the tip of the tail showed bloodlessness. The capillaries appeared to have collapsed and were flat, they were hard to recognise because the cell content was missing (filter phenomenon). In the middle part of the tail Boettcher found the *arteries to be maximally contracted* but with changing lumen and still containing blood. The veins were dilated, and full of blood, around the tail root only the main arteries contracted, *the veins were maximally dilated and full of blood.*

Quite a number of authors have tried to follow the process capillaroscopically in man: Bruns and König (1920), Krogh (1929), Ariev (1939 a, b), Lewis (1928/1938), Siegmund (1943 b), Häussler (1943), Quintanilla et al. (1947), Kreyberg (1949). After loss of temperature a paleness of the skin due to a contraction of the small arteries, arterioles and arterial capillaries to within the venous area was observed. In 1943 Siegmund observed in the capillaroscope primary contraction of the pathway of the papillary body, of the subcapillary plexuses and of the corium plexus. Only after longer exposure at lower temperatures did he find secondary dilatation of the terminal vessels with acute slowing down of the circulation.

According to the information provided by Boettcher (1944), recovery is still possible after peristatic hyperaemia. This, however, depends on the duration of exposure. It has, at least, been shown that, with cases of chronic bluish-red discoloration of the skin, after a warm bath a change in colour to bright red can be observed, which proves that the venous blood vessels are still not completely paralysed as they react to loss of temperature. The fact that areas that were previously blue become bright red is certainly connected to some extent to the increase in the rate of capillary circulation and the decrease in the release of oxygen. If a cold stimulus is applied locally to a bluish-red spot which has been chronically damaged by the cold (acrocyanosis), e.g. if a piece of ice is placed on it, one will likewise observe a bright red discoloration which the capillary microscope reveals to be caused by active constriction of the vascular lumina and an increase in the flow velocity.

Waxy Paleness

The waxy paleness of the skin (nose, cheeks, ears, fingers, toes, hands, feet) which normally appears suddenly in heavy frost after the state of bright redness or bluish red marmoration is clearly the result of a *complete spastic occlusion of the arterioles and arteries with maximal narrowing of the large arteries of the limbs,* the latter remaining,however, still open. Experimental as well as clinical experience has shown that not only ischaemia occurs but that the circulation in the frozen area comes to a complete standstill. In this state the veins are drained until they are almost empty, they contain no or only a very few red corpuscles, and only plasma. The tissue, which is no longer supplied with blood, receives, therefore, no oxygen, and cannot release any more metabolic waste products or CO_2. This tissue metabolism ceases to function as long as the acute cooling lasts. The tissue no longer consumes oxygen either, or at the most only slight traces. It is preserved in this state. There are, however, limits to this freezing, as it is not tolerated by the cells for a longer period.

Every transition to the state of waxy paleness means clinically that there is danger of freezing, necrosis or death from exposure, which makes it essential for protective and counter measures to be taken.

Evidence of an Arteriospasm from an Arteriograph and Other Test Methods

As far as we know arteriographs were first used to study vascular change after exposure to cold by Leriche and Kunlin in 1940. They only ever found one *lasting arteriospasm* of the large and small arteries of the affected limb. Leriche (1945) was the first to succeed in showing *vascular occlusion after cold damage.*

In 1941/42 Laewen (1942 a, b) also found a spasm of the arteries arteriographically. On the arteriogram it almost reached the demarcation line. In 1941/42 Jung and Fell (1942 a, b) analysed ten cases of severe frostbite using oscillogram and arteriogram simultaneously to show the therapeutic possibilities of performing a sympathectomy in such cases.

There were cases which came to be arteriographed between the 4th and the 25th day and 2 months after the primary frostbite. An acute spasm of the afferent arteries was always diagnosed. That it was a genuine spasm and not a case of organic vascular change could be proved by the fact that after the influence of the sympathetic trunk had been eliminated by periarterial or periganglionic novocaine blocking or by gangliectomy a marked widening of the arteries could be observed almost to their normal calibre. In accordance with this in all ten cases poor circulation and a very fine pattern of the constricted large arteries with their branches was found.

In a comprehensive study Breitner and Wagner and later also Judmaier (1949) investigated cold injuries arteriographically. The carefully compiled clinical and radio-

125

graphic analyses revealed the same conclusions as those already reached by Leriche et al. Most of the cases investigated were cases of 3rd degree frostbite in *its advanced stages*. It could be seen that the superficial arterial vessels did not always react in the same direction as those deeper down. The dominant reaction to cold was once again the maximal contraction of the afferent arteries. It remained for *months, sometimes even for years* and only began to disappear very slowly. *Changes to the vascular walls and occlusion of the lumina were occasionally recorded arteriographically too.* Breitner and Wagner also observed in the *afflux area above the actual frostbite spastic constriction of the blood vessels and the same time in the region deeper down damage to the vascular walls* – a finding which is of great significance for immersion foot. In 1947 Shumaker et al. used the arteriograph to investigate cold injury patients in order to establish the extent of the circulatory disorders. In 1953 Piroszinski and Webster did the same. Recently a considerable number of American surgeons have used arteriographs systematically to discover to what degree blood is being supplied to the tissues as this determines the point at which an amputation must be made. (See here the report made by Webster et al. from the Korean campaign of 1955.)

A further important way of investigating cold injuries in their various stages and particulary in the advanced stages is to use the oscillographic method according to Recklinghausen (1883 a, b), which is generally carried out today in Germany with the apparatus designed by Gesenius and Keller. It is true that it is not exact, but it does provide relatively reliable information on the circulatory condition of a limb.

Subsequent to their arteriographic studies Wagner and Judmaier found on the oscillogram in all their cold injury cases already outside the actual frozen area a considerable decline in the oscillographic curve with very small deflections, which clearly revealed a deterioration in the circulatory condition. These circulatory changes should not immediately be related to direct damage to the vascular wall, they are an expression of the permanent cold spasm unless an arteriographic restriction of the lumina, roughness of the vascular walls or even blockages of the blood vessels have been observed.

As a complement to oscillography Breitner (1932, 1943, 1944 a, b) exposed the damaged extremities to a warm-cold stimulus and then carried out once again ascillographic checks to obtain an impression of the spastic state. It could be seen, however, that with a prolonged spasm the circulatory change remained minimal after this warm-cold stimulus and that the range of reaction was remarkably poor. If one succeeds in successfully restricting or eliminating the influence of the sympathetic nervous system, the responsiveness returns to a large extent, which must be seen as further evidence of the fact that it is first of all only a functional change and as yet not organic damage.

Recklinghausen's (1883 a, b) *oscillography* is of little practical use for new cold injuries. In the stage of reactive hyperaemia the afferent pathways are dilated and increased oscillation is then to be found. In the actual frostbitten area one cannot usually apply it in early cases either because of the development of reactive oedemas in the region or because blisters or granulation make it impossible to place the cuff on the affected area. The oscillation waves are generally increased in all inflamed parts. If an oedema is present, the values are mostly lower and cannot be used. As most cold injuries occur on both sides one has no means of comparing with normal conditions.

Häussler and Lotsch used the *Moskowitsch test* to check the circulatory condition after cold damage. A state of reactive hyperaemia is created by stopping the blood flow

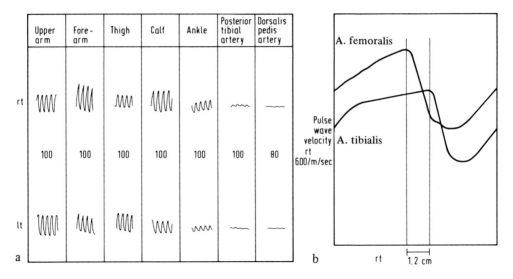

	Upper arm	Fore-arm	Thigh	Calf	Ankle	Posterior tibial artery	Dorsalis pedis artery
rt							
	100	100	100	100	100	100	80
lt							

Fig. 57a. Acquired, circumscribed cold endangiitis due to immersion. No generalisation of the arterial obliterating disease. Poor oscillographic values in both lower legs and feet, with normal pulse wave velocity (6ms) in thigh to ankle region. (Killian 1963)

Fig. 57b. Pulse wave velocity, from the same case. (Killian 1963) Distance A. femoralis: A. tibialis 50 cm

for 10 min. The hyperaemia test had already been used by Lewis, Ratschow and others to test different kinds of circulatory disturbances and it was on Jarisch's advice that it was applied to the study of cold damage. As far as the technique is concerned we refer to the descriptions in Ratschow (1953, 1959) and Ipsen's (1936) monographs. Judmaier (1950, 1952 a, b), too, used this hyperaemia test to diagnose frost damage and circulatory disturbances. In 29 cases of frostbite Häussler (1943) was able to show by means of the Moskowitsch test, after varying lengths of time, how far up into the apparently healthy area above the frostbite circulatory disturbances could still be observed. The blood supply was blocked in the upper arm and the thigh area in the normal way with a sphygomanometer cuff for a period of 7 to 10 min.

It turned out that in the case of 1st degree frostbite, which had occurred up to 6 months earlier the reactive reddening was always normal in degree and extent. There was no circulatory damage. In the case of 22 patients, however, with 2nd and 3rd degree damage dating back to 1940/41 or 1942/43, in other words up to 2 years earlier, severe circulatory damage sometimes up as far as the knee was discovered. The redness reached far into the apparently healthy tissue and showed a segmental edge. According to Jarisch and Häussler the results of the Moskowitsch test are apparently sometimes paradoxical. Judmaier (1949) explained this phenomenon by the fact that some small arteries and capillaries are not affected by the damage and changes to the vascular walls, which was later confirmed by the histological investigations of Staemmler and his pupils.

Within the framework of studies on the effects of fever during cold injuries Schwerner (1944) carried out comparative investigations on my behalf using different functional methods to test circulatory damage above the actual frostbitten areas.

127

In 66 patients with older bilateral cold injuries to the lower extremities the oscillation curves were first of all recorded applying varying degrees of pressure at each point of measuring. In the lowest third of the thigh a marked deterioration in the circulation could usually be observed. In isolated cases the oscillation waves were greatly limited. The differences were, however, on the whole slight compared with the findings of Breitner and Wagner and also the oscillograms of Philipides on cold damage, and showed that oscillography alone cannot provide sufficient information on the true circulatory condition. Other functional tests must also be adopted.

Subsequently skin temperature measurements were carried out according to Ipsen (1936) and using the Moskowitsch test on the same patients of Schwerner (1944). A tourniquet was placed on the affected extremity at a high (proximal) position for 10 min and then 15 min after it had been loosened the increase in temperature and the extent of this increase were measured. Once again it was revealed that the rewarming process occurred only slowly far into the apparently healthy area and the initial temperatures were normally not reached again. They remained on an average 0.2° C below the norm. Sometimes the deflections were considerably more marked. By way of comparison Schwerner (1944) carried out cooling tests on the same patients. The damaged area was cooled for 10 min to 16°C, skin temperature and the process of rewarming after drying was observed as Ipsen (1936) had recommended. Normally in the area of the hand and the forehead the original temperature is already reached again after 5–6 min. With cold injury patients, however, it remains on an average 5°–6°C lower. Such extreme deviations prove that this test is considerably more sensitive than some of the other test methods used with cold injuries.

As a pendant to this the test in which artificial ischaemia is produced for 10 min, previously used by Ratschow, was carried out on the same patients of Schwerner (1944), and the natural process of rewarming under the bed covers was observed. The initial drop in temperature and the rewarming were checked after 10 and 15 min. Of 52 cases 30 did not reach original temperature again, which likewise indicates the presence of circulatory damage.

Today a considerable number of other functional investigation methods are available for the determination of the extent of cold damage to the vascular system at early and advanced stages. The number of monographs on this subject is vast. We refer to the work of Kappert et al. (1948), to Abrammson's monographic account (1944), to the monographs of Ipsen (1936), those of Allan et al. (1947), and of Strout (1945), as well as the angiological work of Ratschow (1959), Marx et al. (1956), in which more recent methods of investigation are described in detail (the most important references can also be found there).

We must restrict ourselves to mentioning just a few of the more recent methods of investigation, which, for the most part, have not yet been used to determine the circulatory condition after exposure to cold or cold damage:

1) Photoelectric oscillography.
2) The application of thermal conduction probes.
3) The determination of pulse rate optically or with Bueke and Brecht's Infratinabnehmer.
4) Rheography according to Polzer and Schuhfried.

5) Plethysmography.
6) Photoelectric plethysmography according to Matthes with simultaneous determination of blood saturation (according to Kramer and Schulze 1944, 1948).
7) Serial aortography and aortokymography.
8) The fluorescin methods.
9) Tomo-oscillography according to Eyrup.
10) Ultrasonic flow measurement with Doppler's flowmeter.
11) Quantative measurement of blood supply with Barbey's vasoscript.
12) Phlebemphraxis plethysmogram.

In a very simple manner Aldrell and McClure injected 0.2 ml isotonic saline solution intradermally and evaluated the resorption delay in the damaged area.

Stage of Secondary Bluish-grey Discoloration

The conditions responsible for the dysfunction of local tissue metabolism due to oxygen deficiency and the formation of vasoactive substances are not present until a limb in a state of olgaemia or ischaemia begins to warm up.

If vasodilating substances such as amines form, then secondary dilatation of chemical origin of all the terminal venous capillaries and the plexuses can be observed. Lewis apparently believed that this was first caused purely by cold paralysis. As far as we know, however, he was later persuaded by the convincing arguments of Krogh (1919), Castellotti (1929), Beecher (1936) and many others of the fact that secondary dilatation with bluish grey discoloration after an anaemic pallor of the skin was due in the main to vasoactive substances (H substances).

These amines, for example histamine, are probably formed by the decarboxylation of the histidine accompanied by oxygen deficiency. It is not until now, in the course of the formation of acute reactive hyperaemia that marked oedemas and blisters develop due to disturbances in the permeability and the tissue becomes over heated because of inflammatory symptoms.

The secondary warming during the phase of reactive hyperaemia after cold action can be easily recognised in a comparative experiment on the rabbit's ear. Whereas on the non-damaged side the temperature returns to normal values of about 26° C the tissue temperature of the cold damaged ear (90 seconds — 55° C) after 120 h still remains around 36°C. (See Fig. 25).

Effects of Cold on Lymph Flow

Langohr et al. (1949) studied the effects of cold on the blood and lymph flow with special methods. They always found that the arterial blood flow and the lymph flow to be reduced, according to the degree of the physical action (flow measurements of the arteria cubitalis). During the thawing out it increases again. In the case of advanced frost damage heat encouraged and cold inhibited the lymph flow. In each case the reactions of the lymph flow were delayed compared with those of the blood-stream. The maximum reactive blood flow coincides with the formation of the lymphatic oedema. The protein concentration of the lymph increases considerably when heat is applied and the circulation returns. This can lead to coagulation of the lymph and blockage of the lymphatic channels.

Electrolytic Changes

As early as 1892 Koch found that the electrolytes present in solution in the tissues and fluids undergo changes in concentration and distribution due to the effects of cold, and this can cause considerable internal disorders. Although information has been obtained to some degree on electrolytic changes in tissue and in blood within the framework of experimental studies on hibernation and observations during hibernation or after cold injuries (see data in my monograph "Kälteunfall" 1966 and in Veghelyi's monograph on hibernation 1960) far less is known about such changes in local cold damage to tissue. It seems to be fairly certain that the electrolyte concentration changes in the cells and the extracellular area are the result of the tissue acidosis as they can be reduced or prevented to a large extent by compensation.

Today much greater importance is attached to electrolyte concentration changes in the cells which Killian drew particular attention to at the Swiss surgeons's conference in 1958. The decrease in the potassium concentration in the cells is especially noteworthy (apparently about 30 %, possibly more) accompanied, as it is, by an increase in the extracellular area of the tissue fluid, the lymph and in the blood. After this, however, there is a considerable, continuous loss of potassium, as it cannot be retained in the kidneys. Hypokalaemia cannot, therefore, be prevented by a renal blockage.

Sodium and calcium act in the opposite direction, in time they become considerably enriched in the cells after cold action, which for 2nd to 4th degree cold injuries and internal cold injuries is certainly of significance. On the other hand there is a drop in the sodium concentration, and also in the calcium concentration in the extracellular areas. In contrast to this in 1947 Crismon and Fuhrmann found a considerable increase in the salt content in the oedema fluid. The rise in the salt content apparently exceeds by far during the hyperaemic phase of a cold injury the increase in the water balance of the tissue. Crismon and Fuhrmann considered this phenomenon not only to be the result of cold ischaemia but also of pathological permeability for sodium chloride.

The increase in the calcium and sodium concentration is continuos according to the length of the exposure so that values can be reached which apparently cause irreparable damage to the cells. For calcium a concentration increase of up to 70 % was registered.

The behaviour of magnesium is apparently of little significance for local cold injuries.

An increase in the disturbance of the permeability in one direction and of the osmotic force is associated with these precesses and is noticeable in the frostbitten area.

In the case of ultra rapid cooling and freezing of the tissue the phase of electrolytic changes and osmotic increase is literally by-passed. Here acute disturbance of the water distribution is not found either, which must have a favourable influence on the preservation effect.

130

Primary Acidotic Cold Oedema

An oedema is generally not yet to be found on limbs which have only recently suffered a cold injury, one is more likely to encounter the opposite, namely dehydration with hard, dry, non-elastic skin. This, however, is a question of the rate of progress and particularly of duration of the cold action. The longer limb takes to cool down, and the longer it lasts, the more quickly the tissue is likely to be increasingly impregnated with oedemas.

In 1915 Smith et al. found a slight, progressive, oedematous swelling of the subcutis in animals during 2 to 3 days of permanent exposure of the limbs to mildly cold mud. According to the ideas of Kreyberg (1946, 1949) this is apparently due to the fact that the resorption is delayed and hindered, a view which, however, could not be upheld. Dry cold caused considerably less damage than damp cold, since the element of cooling was far less pronounced due to the far greater conductivity of water. After thawing out at 37° C the oedema spread rapidly.

These observations show that one must differentiate between a *primary cold oedema* and a *secondary, marked oedema,* which forms relatively quickly, sometimes even vehemently in the course of the rewarming process. Blisters nearly always occur with the latter.

Lewis's plethysmographic measurements of cold oedemas of 1924 showed these differences impressively.

Only a rather gradual swelling of the skin and subcutis to 15 % of the normal volume within 3 h was the result of cooling the extremities to plus 5° C. It is due to a change in the water distribution. The position is of importance, as more acute swelling occurred on an arm which was hanging than on one held in a horizontal position. A kind of reflux congestion must be involved.

The cause of these primary oedemas seems to us to be hyperacidity of the tissue, local acidosis in the exposed area, since acid tissue attracts water.

As early as 1933 Staemmler found *lasting acidosis* in his experiments and drew attention to the noticeable drop in the alkali reserves. In 1933 Geiger came to the same conclusion. The findings have since been confirmed on many occasions. Acute acidosis is today even included among the causes of death due to general loss of temperature and it is regularly controlled during hibernation with or without a pump oxygenator for heart operations. (For further information see in "Kälteunfall" the section: "Causes of death due to loss of temperature" Killian 1966)

One became aware of the hyperacidity of the organism mainly as a result of cooling experiments (Ducuing et al. 1940). Here acidosis is caused by fixed acids flowing into the bloodstream. It must be remembered that during artificial hibernation the tissue temperature on an average is not lower than $29°-30°C$, in other words, a long way from the zero mark. To what an extent, therefore, must acidotic changes to the peripheral tissues be felt, since these almost reach freezing point or even lower values after exposure.

According to Veghelyi (1960) in almost every case of cold injury acidosis is present. It is by no means of respiratory origin, but purely metabolic, since CO_2 retention does not occur (Rosenhain and Penrod 1951). A disturbance of the intermediary metabolism and inadequate burning of carbohydrates in the muscles is assumed and yet these processes have still not been sufficiently clarified. Some authors believed that the defective oxidation process was caused by too low oxygen pressure in the tissue due to cold.

131

Since, however, the muscles are rich in glycogen, Schneider attributes far less significance to this factor in the muscles than, for example, in the brain, which is very sensitive to too low a O_2 partial pressure.

The view which generally prevails today is that *adenosine diphosphoric acid and adenosine triphosphoric acid,* which release phosphoric acid when they are broken down, are responsible for this acidosis of metabolic origin. *Creatine phosphoric acid* can also be broken down into creatine and phosphoric acid. *Pyuric acid and lactic acid* must also be considered here, since only a small amount of these acids is burnt up in the muscles, the main part being completely burnt or resynthesised by the liver. Under the conditions of cooling down the organism has to sacrifice its oxygen but this is later made up again (Rein, Schneider 1943).

Compared with these organic, fixed acids the acid intermediary products from the lipometabolism (acetoacetic acid and betaoxybutyric acid) probably do not play an important part at all in the acidosis of localised cold injuries accompanied by an O_2 deficiency. The same applies to the amino acids although they are of significance in the reactive changes to the vascular system after cold action.

Formation of Secondary, Reactive Oedemas

Every natural thawing out of cooled tissue takes place partly from the outside, partly from inside via the arteries, along the main blood vessels and their ramifications. The rewarming process via the bloodstream is dominant unless the exogenous heat input is artificially increased. During spontaneous thawing the distal regions, such as the body surface still remain relatively pale or with bluish-red blotches until the arterial blood vessels reopen in the direction of the periphery. Finally the whole area way outside the frostbitten area is supplied with a maximum of blood, it becomes bright red, hot and swollen. Hyperpulsation can be observed as part of a developing aseptic inflammation, which Kreyberg drew particular attention to in 1946 and 1949, although the main arteries and the main ramifications mostly persist in a state of moderate contraction. One does sometimes find, however, even during the phase of reactive hyperaemia dilation of the arteries and an increase in the blood supply at least as far as the actual damaged area, which later disappear to be replaced for a longer period by secondary narrowing.

In the region of the *terminal vessels,* especially in the *venous thigh* the blood vessels reveal *maximum paralytic dilatation.* Their ability to contract has been lost. If the blood begins to flow again the vessels submit passively to the increasing circulatory pressure, and become extremely full as long as they are not blocked by sludge, congestion or agglutination thrombuses.

The actual *secondary oedema,* the acute swelling of the limbs with the appearance of blisters, in 2nd to 4th degree frostbite, does not generally form immediately after thawing but not until 12–24 h later, in any case not until *larger quantities of fresh blood have pured into the vasoparalytically damaged capillary area, which is a sign of abnormal permeability.* In his description of serous inflammations Eppinger claimed that intermediate stages of protein catabolism, the amines, are strong capillary poisons and make the vascular wall abnormally pervious to protein. Signs of albuminuria become visible in the tis-

sue, which according to many authors is the basis of many different kinds of late sequelae due to the effects of cold, (especially of the blood vessels).

After blockage of the blood vessels reactive hyperaemia with a decrease in vascular
tone occurs, which corresponds to dilatation. It is attributed to nutritional reflexes (Hesse and Fleisch), which are only partly nervous. They are largely direct, localised and of
chemical origin, the result of a sudden accumulation of acetylcholine, adenosine, histamine etc., which apparently have the effect of mutual potentiation. They are responsible in the initial reaction phase for capillary dilatation. The arterioles, which are of
decisive importance for nutrition and intake, are not reached, however, by these vasodilators, at least not before passage of the liver and therefore the above explanation is unsatisfactory. According to the investigations of Hesse and Fleisch a nutritive widening
of the local arterioles is the nervous effect of a local irritation of autonomous elements
and is transmitted intramurally independent of the central areas.

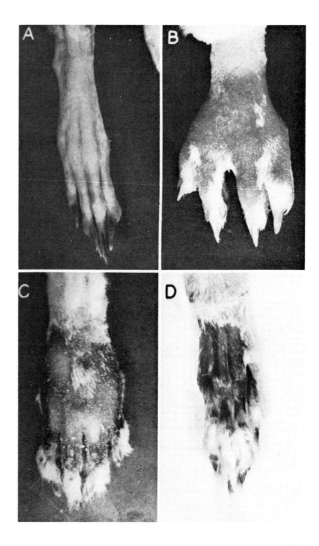

Fig. 58 A-D. Experimentally induced cold oedema with transition
to gangrene in the foot of a rat.
The enormous secondary cold oedema after brief cold damage at
-55⁰ C can be seen. (From Fuhrmann and Crismon 1947)

Such vasoactive amines can only form during a phase of relative oxygen deficiency, which leads us to assume that they come into existence not during the cooling phase but mainly during the rewarming phase. Actually reactive hyperaemia due to cold fits well into the whole framework of biological processes, as it leads primarily to oligaemia or ischaemia, i.e. to a blockage of the bloodstream.

In the secondary hyperaemic phase the blood vessels are filled to a maximum and dilated. On the venous side the dilatation is partly passive according to the experiments of Shumaker and Lempke (1951). However, genuine cold paralysis of the venous region can be observed in some places, encouraged by the effect of the amines. It must be mentioned that in the 4th and final phase a disturbance of the thermal regulation remains, as was established by Mallet et al. in 1946, which indicates increased hypotonia of the sympathetic nervous system, since, according to Ducuing and Harcourt (1915), and others, the reactions of the vascular system return to normal after a blocking the sympathetic trunk.

Crismon and Fuhrmann (1947) experimentally on rabbit ears the pathogenesis of the cold oedema, the acute increase in volume and weight, the increased tension of the skin, and the development of blisters (2nd phase of the plethysmogram; Fig. 58). In the subcutaneous tissue oedema pressure values of plus 25 cm water were found. Unfortunately

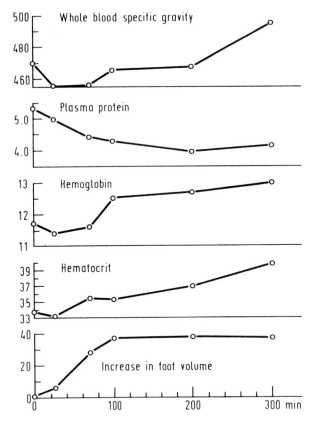

Fig. 59. Time course of changes in the entire blood in an animal (rabbit) after 3-min exposure of the hind foot at −55°C. Measures include: specific gravity, plasma proteins, haemoglobin, packed cell volume and foot volume and foot volume. (From Fuhrmann and Crismon 1947)

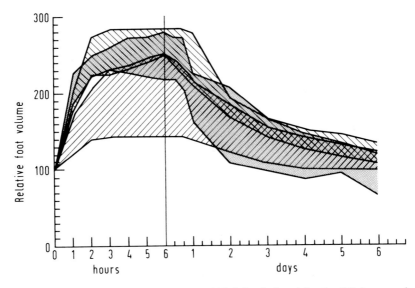

Fig. 60. Volume changes in rabbit feet after exposure at -55° C for 1, 2 and 3 min. (Minimum and maximum. *Area shaded right,* 1-min immersion; *area shaded left,* 2-min immersion; *area spotted,* 3-min immersion (From Fuhrmann and Crismon 1947)

the hydromechanical pressure values of the oedema were not measured separately within the fascial sheaths of the extremities, even though it is well known that an increase in pressure here, e.g. due to arterial haemorrhage, can cause great damage (complete ischaemia and gangrene). The processes are particularly dangerous in the area of the calf (Figs. 58–60). The reactive oedema is never restricted to the frostbitten area alone, but moves systematically to the low pressure areas, i.e. in a proximal direction.

In 1947 Fuhrmann and Crismon discovered that besides a high Na C concentration in the *protein content* of the oedema fluid and of the bladder contents can be as much as 4.3 %. At the same time the *protein content* of the circulating blood volume decreases. The *haematocrit* value increases.

The migration of fluid containing protein from the damaged capillaries to the tissue space could easily be followed under the *fluorescence microscope*:

Crismon and Fuhrmann reported in 1947 having observed that as long as tissue remained in a cooled or frozen state no increase in fluorescence occurred. It began during thawing, reached its climax during the reactive hyperaemic phase around the second day and corresponded to the formation of a marked oedema. The authors captured the migration of the fluorescent fluid from the tiny blood vessels into the tissue space on a photograph. Regularly after 2 x 24 h the interstitial fluorescence ceases because at that point the secondary blocking of the vessels due to agglutination thrombosis is completed and the circulation interrupted once again. This occurs 50 to 55 h after exposure.

In 1944 Lange and Boyd also carried out experiments with fluorescence for purposes of diagnosis and prognosis.

After intravenous injection of the substance only a pale green lightening of the tissue in the normal tissue areas was found. In the presence of an inflammation, however, in

135

other words during the reactive hyperaemic phase a bright yellowy green discoloration was visible, which was caused in the main by the appearance of extravascular fluorescence. When the rabbit had been cooled (at minus 30°C for 30 min in an alcohol bath) the fluorescence disappeared completely within an hour, which proves that for that time the circulation came to a complete standstill. Afterwards it increased rapidly and after 4 h, in accordance with the acute permeability, hyperfluorescence could be observed. Pressure applied to the afferent blood vessels was to no avail, which proved that the fluorescent fluids were outside the bloodstream. Maximum fluorescence coincided with a maximum of oedema formation, heat, redness, capillary dilatation, an excessive pulse rate and heavy blood flow. If there is capillary damage, fluorescence only disappears very slowly. This hyperfluorescence disappears in some cases after between 48 and 144 h as shown in Crismon and Fuhrmann's (1947) experiments. Here gangrene mostly developed. The behaviour of the temperature of the skin and tissue corresponded to the outward appearance.

During the hyperaemic stage and the formation of localised marked oedemas there is a sharp rise in the local temperature, which after the 50th h may begin to drop again (secondary thrombosis).

The skin then cools down because of a lack of blood supply until it has reached the outside temperature.

Between 1946 and 1949 Kreyberg also used an intravital stain with lithium carmine to study the cold injury oedema. He discovered that it showed a change in character after the 12th h, since it was not until this time that lithium carmine left the bloodstream, entered the frostbitten area and appeared in the intersistial tissue.

According to Kreyberg only the secondary oedema is caused by damage to the capillary wall, the primary cold oedema during the actual exposure he believed to be the re-

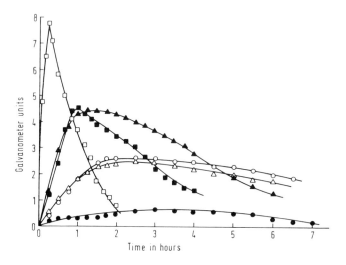

Fig. 61. Graphic representation of the intensity of fluorescence of rabbit ears after exposure at -55° C for 90 s. Fluorescine injection occurred at zero time; □, normal ears – precontrol (6 animals); ■ immediately after exposure to cold (5 animals); ▲, 1 later (4 animals); ○, 1 day later (3 animals). △, 2 days later (3 animals); ●, 3 days later (2 animals)

sult of disturbed absorption, (in our opinion acidification of the tissue with disturbance of the electrolyte and water distribution. Primary cold damage, see above).

Oedemas rich in protein are said to appear earlier in man than in animals (Kreyberg 1946, 1949), and there are not only apparently differences between man and animals (warm-blooded animals) but also between warm and cold-blooded animals. It is a well known fact that in the frog a disturbance of the permeability is not the reaction of the blood vessels to cold, so that neither secondary hyperaemia nor oedemas follow.

Manifest Findings Concerning the Vascular System After Cold Damage

In the earliest pathological reports on cold injuries information on changes and damage to the blood vessels can already be found. From Boettcher's short historical summary of 1944 it can be seen that Krieger as early as 1889, Hodara in 1896 (a,b), as well as Volkmann in 1893 and Fuerst, the latter in a dissertation in 1897, have all published their observations on vascular damage during cold injuries. These were followed by a series of studies by Rischpler in 1900, Rudnitzki in 1900, Zoege von Manteuffel in 1902 (a,b), Marchand in 1908 and Ricker in 1924. Reports were made by Schade in 1920 (see the handbook for pathology, 1926), by Nägelsbach in 1919, 1920, by Hellmuth in 1930 (a,b), Ceelen in 1932, Lindemann in 1942, Block in 1942 and 1943.

At the turn of the century in the Estonian area, Zoege von Manteuffel and Rudnitzki (1902) studied juvenile or advanced stage gangrene after cold injuries; they were often able to see whole limbs suddenly become necrotic months or years after cold damage. Their observations lead to a series of experimental investigations which revealed that many physiologically highly developed and differentiated tissues may suffer from exposure to cold. Acute changes and destruction do not only occur on the body surface but also to the blood vessels. Zoege von Manteuffel described as early as 1902 (a,b) proliferation of the intima with hydropic and hyaline degeneration, new growth of elastic fibres, a thickening of the media due to fibrous proliferation, atrophy of the muscles and infiltration of the adventitia. The capillaries showed a swelling of the endothelium and lacerations.

Subsequently studies were carried out on cold injuries by Staemmler in 1942 and 1943, Siegmund in 1943 (a), Krauspe in 1943, Schulze in 1942, Büchner in 1943 (a,b) and Letterer also in 1943 and organic vascular changes not only in the actual frostbitten area but also in the surrounding area were observed and described.

As is well known, the occurrence of the latter was strictly denied by Ratschow and his pupils, von Fuschsig, Fontaine and Bollack (1960). If in the case of gangrene occlusive vascular changes to the afferent arteries were observed in the area above the cold injury, Ratschow took this to be a sign of the beginning of constitutional endangiitis obliterans or early sclerosis, a theory which led to many cases of false diagnosis in the field of social medicine. The more recent investigations of Hager and Hofstedter (1977) see below, support our views.

In 1941/42 histological sections were prepared from fresh cases of 2nd and 3rd degree frostbite. The arteries were always in a state of maximum contraction, the veins always in a state of maximum dilatation and total thrombosis (Fig. 62). See here the Figs. in my work of 1942. This finding compares favourably with that published by Block in 1942 (Fig. 63).

Staemmler's call for a distinction to be made between early changes which are predominantly of functional or purely physical origin and secondary damage to the vascular system and the tissues is completely justified.

In his lectures at the conferences of consultants (in the Military Medical Academy 1942/43) Siegmund (1942 b, 1943 b) expressed the belief that oxygen deficiency and

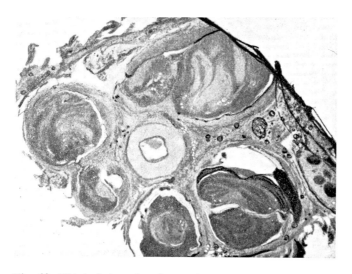

Fig. 62. Histological section from a frostbite focus. In the centre a maximally contracted artery, adjoining several maximally dilated and totally thrombosed veins

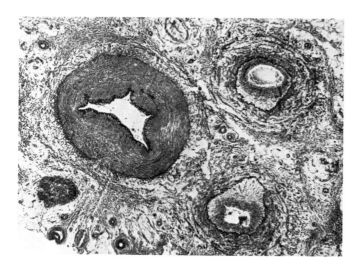

Fig. 63. 30-years-old man. Angiitis obliterans 1 year after frostbite. Beside the severely altered artery two extensively thromboangiitically constricted veins. (From Block 1942)

asphyxiation metabolism of the tissue *during exposure* must result, since the arteries react with spastic contraction, in other words oligaemia or ischaemia must occur. This spasm is indeed very intractable and often difficult to cure (we nevertheless doubted the accuracy of this interpretation).

In 1944 Staemmler observed that the larger arteries here and there degenerate into a spastic state, which coincided with some practical surgical experience. Such angiospasm can occasionally be seen spread over large areas during vascular operations or after injury to the arteries. The vasoconstriction literally creeps upwards from the affected area and is thoroughly intractable. A state of maximum contraction is gradually reached. We have often tried to relax the vasospasm. Besides brushing on strong anaesthetic solutions, we have also attempted to overcome the angiospasm by injecting different substances into the lumen but the results were not satisfactory. After suture of a vessel it can take up to 24 h before the vasospasm above the injured area gradually relaxes.

In 1943 Jarisch pointed out that such vasoconstriction can also be observed on isolated vascular specimens and that it can, according to the investigations of Monier, develop as the result of impulses within the vascular arterial wall. Compare here my remarks on the so-called arterial distension disease at the surgeons' conference in Munich in 1951 (acta chirurgica helvetica). Here nutritive stimuli were mentioned, which play a critical part in the whole pathophysiological field. Jarisch (1943) also drew attention to the fact that such arterial spasms which have a tendency to spread are not only observed after physical damage such as frostbite but also after poisoning, e.g. with lead, nicotine or ergotamine.

In his histological specimens and sometimes also capillaroscopically, Siegmund found maximum bloodlessness and contraction of all the arteries, arterioles and arterial capillaries. He even speaks of contractions on the venous side. Not until warm blood had flown into the previously damaged area did the blood vessels become extremely full and the terminal vessels dilated. The veins, in which stasis had formed, became particularly full. At this point the endothelium still showed no sign of damage. Here exudation first began and plasma passed through the vascular walls. Finally a relaxation could be observed, also a swelling and lifting of the endothelium due to the influx of a liquid containing protein into the subendothelial spaces (endothelial vesication). Impaired development of the basal substance could also be observed. The fibres of the vascular walls are driven apart by the oedemas rich in protein.

This corresponds to a state of albuminuria of the vascular wall, in other words to the clinical picture of Eppinger's serous inflammation, which can be compared with Schürmann's dyshoria. A clotting of the emigrated plasma, and the formation of collagenous and elastic fibres (at the same time preserving the endothelial layer) do not occur until this stage.

Ducuing et al. reached similar results in 1940 from their experience of the Spanish Civil war. They, too, found changes to the intima of the arteries after cold injuries, which have since been confirmed time and again (Figs. 62–64).

Siegmund stressed the fact that changes were by no means restricted to the severely damaged area of a 3rd degree cold injury, but also reached far beyond the region of visible frostbite up into the apparently healthy area.

He attached utmost importance to the fact that the vascular wall and its contents presented a physiological whole (as recently Hess 1977, too), and that the changes apply

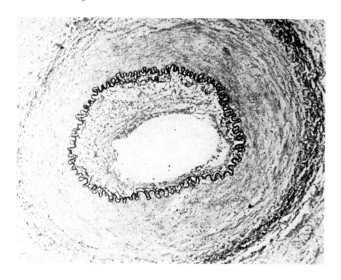

Fig. 64. Arteritis in the demarcation area. Almost purely exudative inflammation of the intima

to both parts, the reactions being felt reciprocally. Clotting processes within the vessels affected the walls and catabolic products of the latter in turn have an effect on the contents of the blood vessels.

Only two works of more recent date on morphological changes after local cold action have become well known:

Gottschalk et al. carried out cold experiments on dogs and found that the damage was not only dependent on the degree of coldness but also on the duration of the action and the localisation. A similar histological picture can be obtained in the tissue, according to the substrata, to that of the haemorrhagic infarction with necrosis after 4 days. After 10 to 14 days the necroses proved to have cleared up and within 4 to 5 weeks scars formed showing no signs of irritation. They found the capillaries, arterioles and venules damaged, in some cases destroyed, as a direct result of exposure. The medium-sized arteries proved to be considerably more resistent and the main arteries remained intact. Vascular ruptures due to cold action were not observed.

In 1968 Gracey and Ingram confirmed that the small blood vessels are particularly affected and the occurrence of perivascular plasma exudation combined with sludging and reduced microcirculation, which can stop completely.

The organisation of subendothelial clotted plasma, which contains red corpuscles, leucocytes and fat droplets takes place relatively quickly inspite of fibrinolysis. According to histological findings there is a transformation into slack, fibrous connective tissue, which can make the damage or the occlusion irreparable.

Mantscheff (1943) assumed destruction or lacerations of the capillaries as the result of cold action. A liquid which lacks fibrinogen penetrates the cell interspace, while in the blood vessel itself blood plasma rich in fibrinogen remains. The cell contents of the blood and also the viscosity increase. When the circulation slows down local clot formation can apparently easily occur.

In the majority of cases one finds around the demarcation line after cold damage the adventitia, the muscularis and the tunica elastica fairly unharmed, in fact well-preserved.

This led some pathologists to conclude that the damage must come from within the blood vessels. The muscular coat is always widely distributed within the specimens due to the high state of concentration. The arterial lumen is more or less filled by the colagenous germinal tissue rich in fibre, which is interspersed with fibroblasts. New capillary growth has sometimes been observed. There is a regular swelling of the intima, and also a tendency to further narrowing and finally to occlusion of the vascular lumen. One also finds protruding fungiform endothelial detachments (Fig. 65).

According to Staemmler the arterial vessels are never all changed to the same extent, some remain intact and well supplied with blood for a long time. This may be the explanation for the juxtaposition of well-preserved and damaged cells. Furthermore in the more remote circulatory areas vacuolisation can be observed in the endothelium, a spreading of the intima with complete preservation of the edges of the endothelial tissue.

Strangely enough Staemmler observed in his experiments few thrombuses in the outflowing veins.

As early as 1915 Smith et al. described endothelial swelling of the vascular intima including vacuolation in the muscle fibrills of the media and perivascular cell reproduction after the extremities had been exposed to ice-cold mud for 2 or 3 days, but no genuine thrombosis was observed, which may have something to do with the fibrinolysis. In 1945 Lange & Boyd did observe agglutination of the erythrocytes on 6-day-old cold injuries but no genuine clot formation.

The investigations of Greene in 1940 (a, b), 1943 and Kreyberg, 1946, 1949, are worth mentioning. The former already observed a clumping of the erythrocytes and a swelling of the intima 24 h after exposure to salt water (immersion). He subsequently saw the blood vessels then blocked by hyaline thrombuses. The term *honeycombed endophlebitis* was used, with preservation of the external layers of the vascular walls. The network in the lumen of the veins contains fibrolasts nad migratory cells, the origin of which is unknown (Staemmler).

Incidentally, in 1943 Reimers occasionally found fat droplets flowing out of the veins during amputations after cold injuries. We also observed this on many occasions. Günther (1940) and Reimers (1943) have even seen them spreading to the lungs. In a

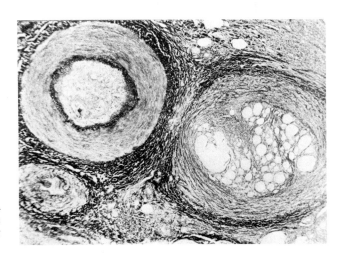

Fig. 65. Endarteritis and alveolated endophlebitis near the demarcation. (From Staemmler 1944)

histological specimen an enclosed fat droplet may show a typical fat staining colour and later settle, which explains the strange honycombed state of the thrombuses in the vascular lumina. Fat droplets were sometimes also phagocytised.

The lymphatic vessels were found to be either unchanged or dilated and then usually filled to an extreme with fibrins and cell accumulation. A change in the walls was not regularly observed.

Special Remarks on Vasotrophy, Significance and Nature of the Intima

According to the opinion of all important pathologists and clinicians the anatomical, nutritional condition of the vascular walls is of great significance for the etiology of obliterative, vascular diseases (Goecke 1942; Killian 1943; Hochrein and Schleicher 1959; Letterer 1962; Ratschow 1963).

It is a well-known fact that about two-thirds of the arterial vascular wall is fed from the inside by the bloodstream and only one-third from outside. To be more precise the intima and the inner two-thirds of the media are nourished by the blood and the outer third of the media and the adventitia by the vasae vasorum. A pathological influence on the vascular walls may, therefore, come either from the blood or be due to outside effects. Harmful chemico-toxic substances contained in the blood first affect the intima and the layers beneath, the basal substances. Bredt (1962) made the point that a disturbance of the composition of flowing blood can lead to a disease of the vascular wall, whereby in particular the inner layers are involved. Changes in the angioneurotic innervation, in the vasotonia, apparently are of influence here. In accordance with the anatomical conditions, it is assumed that there is a double lymph stream in the vascular wall, going namely from the adventitia to the endothelium and vice versa.

If one bears these circumstances in mind it becomes clear that in the *middle part of the vascular wall there is a critical area, where a nutritional deficiency might most easily occur.* Probably the alimentation of the central part varies according to the functional state and the strain. It may be assumed that hypoxaemic influence or a disturbed carbohydrate metabolism in the cells is most likely to be noticed in the area of the intima and of the inner part of the media.

According to the author the double feeding of the blood vessels is the reason why the free vascular transplantation first attempted by Lexer (1952) was a success and that the vein implanted in an arterial defect not only survived and settled but even adapted to the increased pressure and was converted into an artery substitute.

The endothelium of the intima constitutes a biological membrane of utmost importance as a blood tissue barrier. It is in a state of permanent functional fluctuation and is exposed to damage.

According to Bredt (1962) there is a definite possibility that blood changes may lead to a disturbance of the absorption and of the fluid exchanges in the vascular wall and damage to the intima occur long before clinical symptoms appear. The most varied assortment of noxa of physico-thermic, toxico-infectious und physiologico-chemical nature can, it is true, have an effect on the endothelial membrane, but the reaction of the vascular wall remains more or less the same, and in such a way namely that the term nosological unit has been used (Block 1943, 1951; Bredt 1962). In every case it is the processes which take place in the area of the intima itself and in the subendothelial area which are decisive, as well as of the basal substances, for which variety of names have been chosen and which is considered as the basic process in a reactive, inflammatory, obliterative vascular disease.

The Relationship Between Primary Cold Damage to the Nerves and the Blood Vessels (Thorban's Theory)

It is a well-known fact that Thorban in 1962 carried out extensive animal experiments to clarify the question of the relationship between the nerves and the corresponding vascular area, in order to find out whether delayed damage due to cold action could occasion obliterative arterial vascular diseases, such as endangiitis obliterans (cold endangiitis). His results favoured the presence of such a relationship since the nervous elements under all tissue substrata proved to be the most sensitive to cold. In order to check these ideas, and at the same time, however, to clarify the controversial question of vascular damage above an organic cold injury, demarcation and necrosis, Hager and Hofstedter (1977) performed histological investigations. They were provided with the opportunity of carrying out cellular investigations on a man with ankle fractures after 7 h exposure to cold and 2nd to 3rd degree frostbite on both sides of the upper and lower extremities after the subsequent amputation of both feet because of gangrene. The tissue sample did not originate from the demarcation area or the area surrounding it but from a much higher part around the middle of the lower leg. They found the epineurium to be fibrotic on the nervus tibialis, the perineurium and endoneural connective tissue covered, preserved nerve fibres alternated with areas of segmental degeneration. The usual investigation technique was complemented by the use of the new enzyme reaction according to Badycula and Hermann. The adenosine phosphatase is normally localised in the perineurium of the nerve. One observes deposits in the perineurium with fine septal processes towards the centre of a nerve cable. Thomas (1969) found after exposure to cold an increase in the adenosine phosphate activity with the formation of coarse grained precipitates. The authors then discovered in the arteria tibialis posterior in the middle of the lower leg fibrosis of the adventitia, a slight swelling of the intima resembling a sort of padding and a splitting of the elastica interna. There were, in addition, signs of thrombophlebitis, obviously secondary, of the tibial veins with perivenous, inflammatory infiltrates, an inflammatory impregnation of the vascular wall and accumulations of thrombuses in the lumen. Hager and Hofstedter (1977) also found changes to the skeletal muscles in the same area, namely widespread atrophy in the centre of swollen, hydropic muscle fibres, the sarcoplasm of which was inhomogeneous and had disintegrated into plaques, and contained giant cells with polimorphous nuclei, a sign of an over hasty regeneration. The changes were arranged in patches and resembled the clinical picture of neural muscular atrophy (Fig. 66).

Thorban had observed the development of vascular changes, which corresponded to the clinical picture of endangiitis obliterans, only in the case of partial nerve lesions and not with total lack of function. After total injury to the nerves he observed only an oedema of all the layers of the vascular walls and all signs of repair were absent. He emphasised the fact that the nerves and the corresponding vascular damage was never

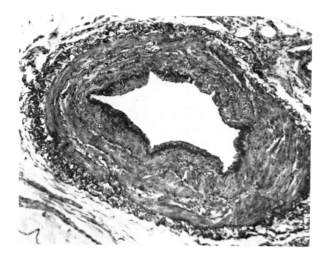

Fig. 66. Artery of the thigh 6 months after a 3-h exposure of the lower extremity in ice water at +2⁰ C. Intense, pad-like thickening of the intima with narrowing of the vascular lumen. (From Thorban)

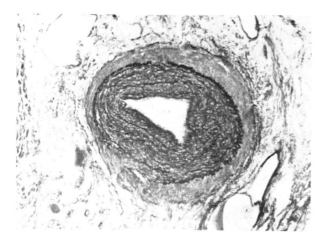

Fig. 67. Artery of the foot 3 months after isolated frost injury of the sciatic nerve. Well-advanced fibrosclerosis of the vascular wall with severe narrowing of the lumen. (Elastica-staining x 340) (From Thorban)

restricted to the spot where the intensive cold action had been felt but reached far into proximal, apparently healthy areas, i.e. to the regions without visible changes due to the effects of the cold, a fact which the author has repeatedly stressed (Fig. 67).

Hager and Hofstedter's (1977) more recent results indicate that Thorban's theory is right. Their pathological findings on nerves and blood vessels applied to areas way above the gangrenous region. An increased adenosine phosphate activity was observed. In these areas vacuolation of the adventitia cells, of the media and of the intima was also found, as is nearly always the case after nerve injuries. The muscle changes with fresh signs of regeneration presented the clinical picture of neural muscular atrophy. All this was found within an area where the skin surface was intact and without visible cold damage. These results are not only confirmation of Thorban's theory of the possibility of cold damage, but also abov a necrotic zone.

Hyperergic tissue reactions were sometimes referred to, sometimes one spoke of exudative serous inflammation (Rössle), sometimes of albuminuria in the tissue based on a primary disturbance of the permeability (Eppinger) or of dysoria (Schürmann). Klinge also called the symptoms a fibrinoid swelling and Meyer an interstitial fibrinous inflammation, whereas Selje refers within the framework of an adaptation syndrome to hyalinosis. Despite the varied terminology one and the same process is undoubtedly meant.

How a local or general vascular disease develops is dependent on several factors.

According to Rössle and Bredt for example, glucopolysaccharide is of utmost significance in metabolic vascular diseases of the fibrosclerosis type, other authors, on the other hand, consider a disturbance of the cholesteral metabolism to be decisive. In contrast, in all forms of reactive inflammatory vascular diseases, endangiitis obliterans and associated conditions, cellular and humoral influences should be present. It thus becomes possible to assume a certain damage to the cells, to the ferment activity and to the neurovascular relations of the accesoria (Bredt 1962), which precedes the clinical manifestation and is an assumption which does not go beyond a working hypothesis. It would not be justified at least to generalise these ideas and to refer them to more or less all relevant cases, as has unfortunately been done.

Inflammatory Processes in the Vascular Wall

In 1962 in his main lecture Ratschow gave a description of the nature of the basic processes in the region of the intima of the subendothelial area, of the basal substances and of the accesoria, which we will refer to reservedly as much of it is still very uncertain.

An endothelial disturbance of the permeability which allows protein containing liquid (plasma) to penetrate the subendothelial area is considered by all authors to be the decisive process.[1] Here it is assumed that there is a disturbance of the diffusion and filtration of the vascular wall itself which has an effect on the interaction between the vascular wall and its contents. The blood coagulation system obviously becomes disturbed too, and there is an increased tendency for thrombuses to form (Ratschow 1962). It may be assumed that according to the etiology individual differences in degree and extent are to be found. The substrata, which is critical for all forms of reactive vascular disease, is a focal swelling of the intima. Around the source of such swelling the elastica interna are found to be split up, from where the old name "arteriitis elastica" was obtained. It is, of course, clear that a splitting of the elastica of this kind leads to hydrostatic changes in the vascular wall itself. The latter were investigated more closely by Linzbach (see vol. I, p. 140).

This strange splitting of the elastica interna has been the cause of many different attempted explanations of a mechanical and also of a chemical nature. Many authors assumed that the amorphous basal substance could be dissolved by depolimerisation. It is certain that the damage to the elastica leads to a disturbance of the inner structure of the vascular wall and to a decrease in its stability. Whether or not this causes an increase

---

1 This change is generally found independent of the etiology. It is accompanied by changes in the basal substance.

in the filtration pressure and encourages transsudation, as many claim, is as far as we can see still unknown.

It is assumed that the increase in the thickness of the vascular wall due to the swelling prevents the possibility of diffusion for liquids and gases, which is of great importance in as far as the inner two-thirds of the media and all the intima are dependent on being fed from the bloodstream.

Oxygen deficiency in the vascular wall is apparently also due to substances deposited in or on the walls. Furthermore, it is assumed that there is damage to the normal fibrin film which covers the endothelium, as a result of toxis substances from the blood. Sealing substances deposited on the endothelium have been considered, which apparently inhibit the diffusion of liquids and gases, such as, for example, plasmalipoids, cholesterol, or fatty acids according to their nature and the amount. In all these cases, in the opinion of Hueper (1945), on oxygen deficiency of the vascular cells is the main cause of the damage (anoxia theory). That may be so in the case of normal temperature tissue, it is not, however, in the cooled state.

This encouraged discussion of the significance of *mast cells,* which were present in large numbers in the swelling focus of the intima. Mast cells provide the body with heparin and in this way have considerable influence on the coagulation of the blood. Heparin deficiency, which can occur as the result of hypoxaemia increases the coaguability and leads to thrombophilia due to a decrease in the zeta potential. As besides, every form of tissue damage encourages thrombocinase, the clot formation is apparently encouraged in the area of the intima foci.

As a result of Hahn's observations of 1943 that alimentary lipaemia can be overcome in vivo in a matter of minutes with heparin, the idea was conceived that a special *clearing factor* must be released from the lipoid protein, lipase in the tissue itself which splits the triglyceride into glycerine and free fatty acids. This clearing reaction is apparently dependent on age, and subsides with increasing age.

In the opinion of the authors this is the reason why in time hypoxaemic and anoxic damage to the vascular wall occurs more easily. According to Hueper (!945) the deposita-tion of cholesterol or fibrin makes not only the gas metabolism in the vascular wall more difficult and the diffusion of oxygen but also the passage of energy giving dextrose via the epithelial cells. Furthermore anoxia of the vascular wall apparently leads to a disturbance of the breaking down of the muscle polisaccharide and to a release of Hall's elastase and so prepare the way for a splitting of the elastica interna.

We would like to refer to a more detailed description of these interesting although by no means final theories, which Ratschow gave in 1964 in his last work in the Medizinische Wochenschrift.

Thanks to more recent scanning electron microscopic investigations carried out by Forst and Hess in 1970 not only has Siegmund's view of the vascular wall and its contents as a pathological unit received support but also quite new aspects have been introduced to help clarify the question of the biological processes in the vascular wall and in particular in the inside wall. The effects of these investigations are still unknown. Both authors were able to observe adhesions on the intima within a short space of time as the result of cold action (and due to other effects), i.e. deposits of thrombocytes, endothelial cells and fibrin in the form of a network, which may be considered as an initial symptom of vascular wall changes of an obliterative character. These adhesions certainly do not appear as the only cause of obliterative processes but they do seem to encourage the development of such pathogenic occurrences. The cholesterol level in the blood would therefore appear to be of the utmost significance.

The significance of blood platelets and their change after exposure to cold. Hess (1977) confirmed Siegmund's opinion that cold has an influence on the whole functional unity: blood vessels and blood-stream, and that the lasting pathophysiological changes which follow also affect both. Both the vascular wall structure and the plasma with its blood cells are sensitive to the cold. Due to an increase in viscosity and suppression of the fluidity of the blood the circulation slows down and finally comes to a standstill. In the terminal vessels stasis can be observed. The reaction of the thrombocytes to cold is here of considerable significance.

Hess stresses the particular sensitivity of the blood platelets and from his scanning electron microscopic observations describes how they are stimulated by the cold. They lose their disc shape, and after low temperature stimulus not only do they assume a spherical shape but they also develop pseudopodia, which stick to the surfaces, whereas thrombocytes which have not been stimulated in normal circulation with an intact endothelium never stick. As is well known the blood platelets cover within seconds any endothelial defect. The film is later fully integrated and leaves behind no traces.

According to Hess local cold action to the arteria femoralis caused the thrombocytes which pass through the lumen to be stimulated so that they changed their form and became deposited on the endothelium. Hess questions whether the changes are the direct result of cold action or whether the stimulus perhaps originates from the vascular wall. The speed of the blood flow proved to have a critical influence on the formation of adhesions, for if the circulation slows down the thrombocytes become separated and deposited on the inner walls with clotting processes and the formation of partial microthrombuses, which can lead to obturation and stenosis. A restriction of the blood patelet aggregation is no longer effective in the case of a fully developed cold injury. It is, however, to be recommended as a prophylactic measure. After preliminary treatment with 0.5 g of acetylsalicylic acid the thrombocytic adhesions were no longer to be seen on the tin walls of the coronary arteries. Whether this kind of prophylactic administration of aspirin after cold injuries is effective is still not absolutely clear. If thrombosis of the terminal vessels and a blocking of the draining veins is already present, experience has shown that attempts to prevent or restrict sludging and the aggregation of the blood cells unfortunately come to late.

Hess hoped that an increase in the flow velocity would have a favourable effect. Simple haemodilution or isovolaemic haemodilution combined with the administration of streptokinase is apparently of service in this respect, the latter causing the fibrin deposits to be dissolved and the vascular system thus cleared. The proportion of fibrinogen, which is mostly increased, is also decreased during this process. The effect of the streptokinase lasts for about 24 h, compensation follows and the viscosity increases again.

A new form of treatment has apparently been introduced in the form of the snake poison, *Arwin,* with which it is possible, after subcutaneous application, to create and maintain for a longer period, for several weeks, a controllable form of fibrinaemia. Maximum effectiveness is apparently around 70—80 mg % fibrinogen without danger of haemorrhage. It is also hoped that an increase in the flexibility of the red corpuscles with the use of Oxypentifylline *(Trental)* will produce favourable results.

147

Incidentally in 1974 Schmid and Schönbein were able to show that the erythrocyte aggregates also changed when they moved from an area of fast blood flow into an area of more slow blood flow or stasis. A fine network then forms which hold the cell elements together (cf. also the report of Zink et al. 1977).

Cold Endangiitis and Its Relationship to Endangiitis Obliterans

All the vascular changes which have been described are not specific to cold effects. They represent rather more a "basic pathological reaction" (Siegmund 1943a, b; Block 1951; Ratschow 1962; Killian 1962), which applies more or less to all reactive vascular diseases involving a serous inflammation. These include genuine endangiitis obliterans, according to Billroth et al. Raynaud's disease, cold endangiitis and related forms of disease. There are simply not many biological ways in which the blood vessels can react to noxa. The course is just about always the same and this is ultimately the reason, especially in the more advanced stages, for the difficulties concerning differential diagnosis. Between 1941 and 1945 and thereafter a distinction had not yet been made between arteritis or endangiitis after cold injury and genuine Buerger's disease. They were still grouped under the collective name "endangiitis obliterans". I then intentionally coined and introduced the term *"cold endangiitis"*, to clearly classify this form of vascular damage as an *acquired, regional condition* and to point out a few of its peculiarities. Constitutional factors are only occasionally of significance here. The effects of the cold are very extreme and can, like the effects of heat, harm any healthy organism. In only 10%–12% of all cold damage cases is it possible to diagnose a disposition to cold injury. It became all the more necessary to define cold endangiities, as Ratschow declared Buerger's disease, i.e. endangiitis obliterans, despite its reactive, inflammatory character, to be a constitutional disease and this was then considered to apply to the sequelae of cold injuries too (Fig. 68).

It is advisable, within the discussion on the relationship between endangiitis obliterans and cold endangiitis to bear in mind the historical development of the subject as it has

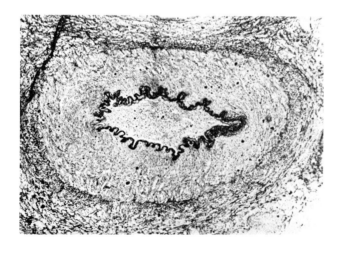

Fig. 68. Endarteritis obliterans of the posterior tibial artery well above frost injury. (See also Fig. 63 according to Block)

been presented, for example, by Lassmann and Fuchsig (1956), by Asang and Mittelburger (1957), or by Gänsslein (1940), as in these works mistakes which have crept in become evident. We cannot go into this more closely in this monograph.

Cold endangiitis is an acquired disease of an inflammatory character. It can occur after 2nd or 3rd degree frostbite, if larger arteries have been affected by the cold. In the majority of cases, however, there is first of all an interval of weeks, months or even years, with hardly any symptoms, before objective and subjective circulatory disturbances, delayed damage resembling endangiitis obliterans become apparent. This is partly due to the formation of sufficient collateral vessels. Direct cold damage to the sensitive blood vessels, as is mostly likely to occur with immersion foot, is assumed (Fig. 69).

Even though the changes to the blood vessels in all reactive, inflammatory vascular diseases greatly resemble each other some *distinctions between cold endangiitis and Buerger's disease* can, however, be made. The most important difference is that *Buerger's disease is basically a generalised condition, in other words a systemic disease, whereas cold endangiitis is only ever restricted to the larger or smaller area which was affected by the cold, never becoming generalised with sympathetic affection of other parts of the body.* Exceptions to this rule mostly apply to complications of an inflammatory nature in the frostbitten area.

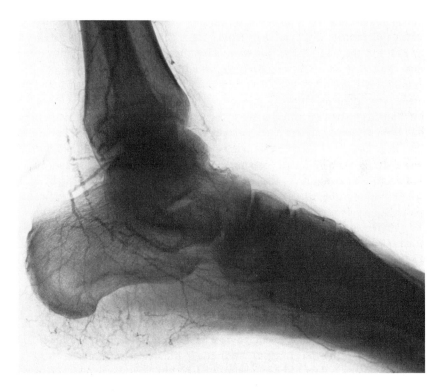

Fig. 69. Arteriography; posterior tibia broken in the middle, anterior tibia and inter ossa broken. Collateral formation, winding small arteries. Circumscribed endangiitis, caused by cold. (Darmstadt collection)

Primary sympathetic affection of the veins and their paralyses and thrombosis is a regular finding and a characteristic of cold injuries, whereas primary implications of the veins does not occur so frequently in endangiitis obliterans, namely only in 50% of all cases, as many authors have maintained (Allan et al. 1955; Ratschow 1959). In sclerosis involvement of the veins is only a secondary development and is restricted to the large body veins (cava, venae pulmonalis etc.).

Furthermore, a *honeycombed phlebitis with fatty inclusions* and the appearance of pseudoxanthoma cells according to Staemmler is characteristic of cold endangiitis.

As we know today, cold damage may be caused indirectly as the result of a disturbance in the neurovascular series of reactions, i.e. of the autonomous accompanying fibres of the peripheral nerves, which can cause serous inflammation of the corresponding arterial region. Permanent damage to the vascular walls may still develop months or years later and lead to loss of limb. That such damage to the autonomous nerve fibres of the blood vessels is of great significance especially with regard to the delayed effects of the cold was already assumed by Leriche (1940, 1941, 1945), by Sunder-Plassmann (1943) and by Block (1951) as the result of histopathological findings after investigations probably made on the ganglions, but it was not proved until more recently after the experimental studies of Thorban (1962).

He carried out immersion experiments on rabbits at relatively mild temperatures below and above $0°$ C. In his first series of experiments the nervus ischiadicus was exposed under anaesthesia and subjected to varying degrees of cold for varying lengths of time. When the animals woke up their labyrinthine reflexes and their sensibility were checked, in addition the clinical changes were subsequently observed, namely with regard to oedemas, muscular atrophy, contractures and the appearance of trophic ulcers. An aortography was carried out each time before death (by aero-embolism), and the nerve specimens were then investigated macroscopically and histologically with a series of dyeing methods. Similar experiments were carried out after the sympathetic nerve in the neck had been exposed and damaged by an ethyl chloride spray until frost formed (freezing).

In a further series of experiments on 30 animals, after preliminary tests cold damage was induced via a standard freezing method according to degree and duration at average temperatures of minus $5°$ C and plus $4°$ C on depilated animals partly under anaesthesia, partly without anaesthesia. The anaesthesia proved to be of no significance as far as the pathological changes were concerned.

Unlike all other experimenters Thorban carried out histological investigations from then on not only immediately after exposure but also at intervals of up to months. The first result obtained revealed that of the substrata the nerves are by far the most sensitive part to the cold.

In an immersion experiment on an animal marked, progressive changes to the nerves could be observed not only in the actual chilled area but also far above it after only 1 hour's exposure to cold water at $+4°$ C to $+2°$ C. In a lower leg affected by a cold injury Thorban found even in the thigh area partial nerve damage, i.e. to the ischiadicus, so that the histological picture always showed intact and degenerate cables.

As early as 8 days after exposure the first histological changes and also arteriographic changes to the corresponding, subordinate part of the vascular system could be observed, namely the classic, clinical picture of an acquired endangiitis obliterans of the cold endangiitis type. Thorban also discovered occlusion in the area of the arteria femoralis. He succeeded in administering the icy water (+2° C to +4° C) in such doses that no cold damage to the skin became visible after exposure of up to 5 h. None of the animals died, and there were no cases in which the labyrinthine reflexes and sensitivity were no longer present.

Only under the microscope could slight damage to the epidermis be seen. It was relaxed and had in parts an alveolar appearance with slight blisters. In the subcutaneous fatty tissue an oedematous softening could be observed, especially of the perivascular and the perifollicular areas. In more advanced cases in the course of time atrophy of the epidermis, basal pigmentation, a wasting of collagen and acute loss of the elastic fibres occurred, as has also been found by other authors.

The changes to the peripheral nerves were absolutely regular and also the most pronounced even at around +2° C after exposure of 1 h. The nerve damage was intermittent. The majority of the cables were preserved. In animals whose skin was macroscopically fully intact, similar partial nerve damage was observed. After a whole limb had been exposed to the cold, changes to the lumbar part of the cord and to the sympathetic ganglia occurred, in that even a loss of the Nissl substance was observed. The most important result was the discovery that only partial cold damage to the nerves, and not total paralysis, is capable of causing the peripheral development of organic damage to the vascular wall, part of cold endangiitis.

We quote here, word for word, because of their importance, points 4, 5 and 6 of the summary of his results: "In the case of local, limited cold damage the condition of the skin is not a reliable guide for assessing the degree of actual cold damage to more deepseated and sensitive tissues. It is therefore possible, even with skin that was macroscopically intact, to show regressive changes to the peripheral nerves. In these cases the local blood vessels reveal after some months the same organic damage to the vascular walls as we have found in the peripheral nerves after direct damage caused by the cold. The changes to the nerves described are not only found in the area where the cold effects are visible (e.g. the lower leg) but they also reach far into the proximal area."

Corresponding to the extent of the changes to the nerves beyond the region of visible cold influence organic vascular changes can also occur in the parts of the extremities, which were not directly exposed to the cold.

The investigations of Schönbach (Schönbach and Thorban 1959) who discovered that disturbances in the permeability and the barrier function are a typical result of innervation disturbances of the blood vessels, so that a serous inflammation with albuminuria in the tissue can follow, link up with the results of other authors and together they help to form the clinical picture of obliterative organic vascular disease (Fig. 70 and 71).

In his summary the question put at the beginning concerning the existence of invisible cold damage is affirmed and the question of the relationship between local cold injuries and local obliterative vascular changes, at least in animals and under the conditions mentioned, is also acknowledged. On this subject Thorban (1962) writes:

"These observations are naturally only completely valid in the experimental field, where they have their origin, but we may in human pathology consider them as a support for the assumption that there is a causal link between a locally restricted cold injury and the formation of an obliterative vascular process outside the actual frozen area."

In addition we would like to quote the following from the summary of his work: "The vascular changes described of the endangiitis obliterans type were caused by the

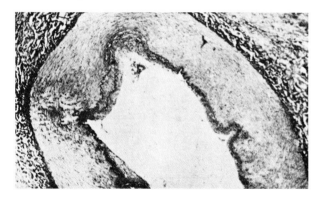

Fig. 70. Posterior tibial artery from the middle part of the lower leg after gangrene of the forefoot (amputation). (Unterdörfer and Umbach 1976)

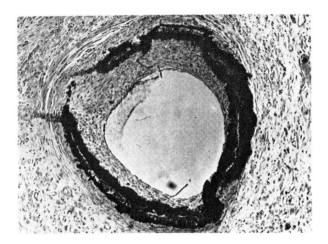

Fig. 71. Arterial calcification in the internal membrana elastica (Hahn et al. 1976)

effects of exogenous factors. In earlier work we have together with Schönbach repeatedly referred to the fact that the so-called endogenous active components such as constitution, disposition, sensitisation etc. could not convincingly explain endangiitis obliterans. The pathogenetic significance of the morphological changes to the different tissues after cold injuries seems to us by comparison all the more important. From the results of our investigations it is difficult to imagine that endogenous factors are involved in the development of organic changes to the vascular walls after cold damage."

There is no doubt about the fact that these experimental investigations conducted by Thorban have made a considerable contribution to the understanding of the whole cold problem.

References

Abrammson DJ (1944) Monograph. University of Chicago Press, Chicago
Allan EV, Barker NW, Hines LA (1947) Periphere Gefäßerkrankungen. Saunders, Philadelphia
Allan EV, Barker NW, Hines LA (1955) Periphere Durchblutungsstörungen, 2nd end. Saunders, Philadelphia
Ariev TV (1939a) Vestn Khir 57:527
Ariev TV (1939b) Sov Krad Zhur 43:391
Bader ME, Mead J (1949) Fed Proc Bull 6
Beecher HK (1936) Skand Arch Physiol 73:123
Block W (1942) Arch Lin Chir 1:64
Block W (1943) Zentralbl Chir 70:1691
Block W (1951) Durchblutungsstörungen. Berlin
Boettcher H (1944) Virchows Arch Pathol Anat 312:46
Bredt (1962) Report. Sachverständigentagung des Arbeitsministeriums
Breitner B (1932) Munch Med Wochenschr 1:573
Breitner B (1943) Klin Wochenschr 22:220
Breitner B (1944a) Dtsch Z Chir 259:273
Breitner B (1944b) Chirurg 16
Brown RB, Hill (1923) Proc R Soc 94:297
Bruns A, König F (1920) Z Phys Ther 24:1
Büchner F (1943a) Klin Wochenschr 80
Büchner F (1943b) Mitt Geb Luftfahrtmed 7
Burch G, Ray T, Ochsner (1947) Ann Surg 126:850
Burton AC, Taylor RM (1946) Am J Physiol 129:565
Ceelen E (1932) Arch Klin Chir 173:742
Craigh HK (1945) J Nerv Ment Dis 101:272
Crismon HJ, Fuhrmann FA (1947) J Clin Invest 259, 268, 286
Ducuing J, Harcourt J, Folch H, Bofold J (1940) J Chir (Paris) 55:385
Fontaine R, Bollack C (1960) Wien Med Wochenschr 110:509
Forst H, Hess H (1970) Report. 7. Tagung der deutschen Gesellschaft für Angiologie, Berlin
Fuerst E (1897) Medical dissertation, Königsberg
Fuhrmann FA, Crismon HJ (1947) J Clin Invest 26:229, 236, 245, 476
Geiger A (1933) Klin Wochenschr 1313
Goecke CA (1942) Munch Med Wochenschr 89:542
Gracey L, Ingram D (1968) Br J Surg 50:302
Greene R (1940a) Zentralbl Chir 695
Greene R (1940b) Lancet 303
Greene R (1943) J Pathol Bacteriol 55:259
Grosse-Brockhoff F (1950) In: Handbuch der inneren Medizin, vol 6/2, p 46
Günther H (1940) Mitt Biochem 47:18
Häussler H (1943) Munch Med Wochenschr 90:301
Hager J, Hofstedter F (1977) Aerztl Prax (Suppl) 41
Hahn PF (1943) Science 98:19
Hellmuth W (1930a) Medical dissertation, Cologne
Hellmuth W (1930b) Arch Klin Chir 158:702
Hess H (1977) Aerztl Prax (Suppl) 47
Hochrein M, Schleicher J (1959) Herz- und Kreislaufkrankheiten, 2nd edn. Steinkopff, Darmstadt
Hodara H (1896a) Munch Med Wochenschr 14:341
Hodara H (1896b) Z Dermatol 22:445
Hueper WC (1945) Biochem Symp 11:1
Ipsen A (1936) Wärmetopographie. Thieme, Leipzig
Jarisch A (1943) Mitt Geb Luftfahrtmed 7
Judmaier F (1949) Wien Klin Wochenschr 61:85
Judmaier F (1950) Schweiz Med Wochenschr 44
Judmaier F (1952a) Munch Med Wochenschr 94:255
Judmaier F (1952b) Wien Klin Wochenschr 64:100
Jung A, Fell H (1942a) Dtsch Z Chir 285:244
Jung A, Fell H (1942b) Bull War Med 3:219
Kappert, Rupp, Rudelli (1948) Helv Med Acta (A) 15:404
Killian H (1942a) Zentralbl Chir 1763

Killian H (1942b) Arbeitstagung beratender Chirurgen, Berlin
Killian H (1943) Zentralbl Chir 70:50
Killian H (1962) Sachverständigentagung, Bonn (Report of Ministry of Labour)
Killian H (1966) Der Kälteunfall: Allgemeine Unterkühlung. Dustri
Killian H, Doenhardt A (1955) Wiederbelebung. Thieme, Stuttgart
Koch (1892) Biol Zentralbl 12
Kramer K, Schulze W (1944) Klin Wochenschr 23:192, 201
Kramer K, Schulze W (1948) Pflügers Arch 250:141
Krauspe C (1943) Osttagung beratender Ärzte, Berlin
Kreyberg L (1946) Lancet 1:338
Kreyberg L (1949) Physiol Rev 29:156
Krieger H (1889) Virchows Arch Pathol Anat 116:64
Laewen A (1942a) Dtsch Mil Arzt 7:479
Laewen A (1942b) Zentralbl Chir 69:1253
Lange K, Boyd L (1944) Science 102:151
Larrey JD (1817) Memoires du chirurgie militaire et de campagne, vol 4. Paris
Leriche R (1940) Presse Med 48:75
Leriche R (1941) In: Handbuch der inneren Medizin. Springer, Berlin
Leriche R (1945) In: Physiologie pathologique et traitement chirurgical des maladies artérielles de la
    vasomotricité. Masson, Paris, p 65
Leriche R, Kunlin J (1940) Mem Acad Chir 66:14, 196
Lewis RB (1927) Blutgefäße der menschlichen Haut und ihre Reaktion. London
Lewis RB (1928) Blutgefäße der Haut. Berlin
Lewis RB (1938) Gefäßstörungen der Glieder. Thieme, Stuttgart
Lexer EW (1952) Dtsch Med Wochenschr 920
Lindemann H (1942) Erkrankungen der Arterien durch Kälteeinwirkungen. Lecture 25 March 1942
Mantscheff Z (1943) Bruns Beitr Klin Chir 174:357
Marchand F (1908) Handbuch der allgemeinen Pathologie, vol 1
Marx H, Schoop W, Zapata C (1956) Z Kreislaufforsch 45:658
Meiners H (1952) Pflügers Arch 254:557
Moser H (1942) Dtsch Med Wochenschr 68:549
Müller O (1918) Dtsch Arch Klin Med 82:547
Nägelsbach E (1919) Munch Med Wochenschr 353
Nägelsbach E (1920) Dtsch Z Chir 160:2051
Natus (1910) Virchows Arch Pathol Anat 199:1
Piroszinski WJ, Webster DR (1953) Clin Am Coll Surg 4:204
Quintanilla R, Krusen FH, Essex HE (1947) Am J Physiol 149:149
Ranke OF (1943) Klin Wochenschr 22:113
Ratschow M (1933) Klin Wochenschr 1:860
Ratschow M (1936) Verh Dtsch Ges Kreislaufforsch 220
Ratschow M (1953) Periphere Durchblutungsstörungen, 5th edn. Steinkopff, Berlin
Ratschow M (1959) Angiologie. Thieme, Stuttgart
Ratschow M (1963) Med Klin 9:344
Recklinghausen F von (1883a) Dtsch Z Chir 213
Recklinghausen F von (1883b) In: Handbuch der allgemeinen Pathologie des Kreislaufes. Stuttgart
Reimers TC (1943) Zentralbl Chir 44:1573
Rein H (1931) Ergeb Physiol 32:28
Rein H (1943) Lehrbuch der Physiologie. Springer, Berlin
Ricker G (1924) Pathologie als Naturwissenschaft. Springer, Berlin
Ricker G (1927) Sklerose der inneren Arterien. Berlin
Rischpler A (1900) Beitr Pathol Anat 28:541
Rosenhain FR, Penrod EK (1951) Am J Physiol 166:55
Rudnitzki TJ (1900) Zentralbl Chir 9:237
Sapin-Jaloustre J (1956) Enquêtes sur les gélures. Herman, Paris
Schade H (1920) Munch Med Wochenschr 449
Schneider M (1941) Arch Klin Chir 201:109
Schneider M (1952) Nauheimer Fortbildungslehrgänge 18:15
Schneider M (1953) Langenbecks Arch Klin Chir 276:25
Schneider M (1954) Lehrbuch der Physiologie
Schönbach G, Thorban W (1959) Langenbecks Arch Klin Chir 291:217
Schulze W (1942) Klin Wochenschr 646

Schwerner K (1944) Medical dissertation, Breslau
Shumaker HB, Lempke RE (1951) Surgery 30:873
Shumaker HB, White BH, Wrenn EL (1947) Surgery 22:900
Siegmund H (1942a) Munch Med Wochenschr 827
Siegmund H (1942b) Arbeitstagung beratender Ärzte, Berlin
Siegmund H (1943a) Zentralbl Chir 1558
Siegmund H (1943b) Mitt Geb Luftfahrtmed 7:43
Siegmund H (1950) Dept Air Force 2:858
Smith JL, Ritchie J, Dawson J (1915) J Pathol Bacteriol 20:159
Staemmler M (1933) Beitr Pathol Anat 91:30
Staemmler M (1942) Zentralbl Chir 45:1757
Staemmler M (1943) Erfrierungen. Thieme, Leipzig
Staemmler M (1944) Virchows Arch Pathol Anat 312:437, 501
Stray K (1943) Oslo I Kommisjon hos dybwad 216, Report
Sunder-Plassman P (1943) Durchblutungsschäden. Encke, Stuttgart (Neue deutsche Chirurgie, vol 65)
Thomas E (1969) Veröffentlichungen aus der mophologischen Pathologie, vol 80. Fischer, Stuttgart
Thorban W (1962) Bruns Beitr Clin Chir 207:87
Tittel S (1944) Z Exp Med 113:698
Veghelyi P (1960) Die künstliche Hibernation. Ungarische Akademie der Medizin, Budapest
Volkmann R (1893) Beitr Pathol Anat 12:233
Webster JW, Eckmann CH, Douglas WM (1955) US Armed Forces Med J 6:171
Weiss E (1921) Wien Klin Wochenschr 1981:1
Weisswange (1944) Medical dissertation, Innsbruck
Zink RA, Schaffer W, Lutz M, Bernett P, Messmer K (1977) Report. Angiologische Tagung, September 1977
Zoege von Manteuffel J (1902a) Mitt Grenzgeb. Med Chir 10:343
Zoege von Manteuffel J (1902b) Zentralbl Chir 63
Zoege von Manteuffel J, Rudnitzki TJ (1902) Mitt Grenzgeb Med Chir 10:373

Eye Disorders Due to Cold

Michel (1882) and Jarisch (1921 a, b, 1943) noticed during their cold experiments on animals a cloudiness of the cornea. It sometimes acquired a porcellanous appearance. Defective vision apparently also occurred. The turbidity is reversible and disappears automatically during the rewarming process. This is why it is assumed, probably rightly so, that a change in the colloidal protein state in the refractory media is responsible for the cloudiness due to cold.

It may, however, also be the case that anoxia triggers off the protein changes, for Krogh (1924) and Killian (1925) were repeatedly able to observe reversible cloudiness of the tissue after adrenaline with its vasoconstrictive effect had been applied to frog tongues.

The investigations of Rein (1931), König (1943a, b) have revealed the enormous importance of a regulation of the supply of blood to the mucous membrane of the paranasal sinus for the thermal protection of the orbital cavity, and especially the importance of keeping the temperature of the eyeball and of the nervus opticus constant. They are protected from the cold because the sinuses provide good insulation. It has been proved that the latter are capable of astonishing adaptability to different outside temperatures. The rewarming process as a reaction to cold outside air is completed in a matter of seconds and the whole area of the orbital cavity is thus maintained at a normal temperature. Only under these optimal conditions does the vision function properly. We do not, in fact, experience impaired vision even in very heavy frost. It does not occur until the whole body has begun to cool down, as this then extends to the nervus opticus, the retina and the optical tracts.

It is well known that during cooling the pupils react more slowly and finally cease to move altogether. In 1940 Sudo carried out comparative checks of the temperature of the thigh, the breast, the eye-lid in the conjunctival sac and also in the anterior aqueous chamber and the vitreous body, the ventral aorta and of the rectum of rabbits with the help of thermo-elements. When cold was applied to remote parts of the body the eye temperature only changed in accordance with the cooling of the circulating blood. In contrast to these observations Goven maintained that there were direct vasomotorial influences on the eye temperature. When cold was applied directly to the eye the eye temperature dropped in accordance with the general laws of heat conduction. The conjunctival sac reached the lowest temperature, then the anterior chamber, then the vitreous body.

The conjunctiva and the cornea only possess cold receptors, no thermo-receptors. We are indebted to Fritz (1939) for his studies of the reaction of eye pressure to the cold.

The effects of ice on closed eye-lids was to produce a drop of $5 - 10$ mmHg in the eye pressure in normal eyes as well as in eyes affected by glaucoma.

It even has the effect of counteracting myotics. The changes seem to arise as a result of a general change in the circulatory state under the influence of vasomotor nerves and are perhaps associated with a decrease in the production of vitreous humour.

156

Changes to the rotary nystagmus before and after cooling have also been investigated by Niko. It was shown that under the influence of cold the nystagmus time decreased considerably, namely from the normal 12 — 13s to 8.5 — 10.5 s after cooling. Delayed damage was not observed.

In the surgical literature on the cold problem there are no reports of conjunctivitis due to the cold. It does, however, occur. Between 1914 and 1918, nubecula due to the cold was sometimes observed in pilots. For details of this clinical picture the special ophthalmic literature must be consulted. The symptoms are usually mild and recede in the warmth.

Changes to the Lungs

Many authors have declared the respiratory system of warm-blooded animals to be particularly sensitive to the cold. (Krueger and Blümel 1977a, b). All measurable values of respiration and gaseous interchange undergo changes during exposure. Apart from a considerable slowing down of breathing due to depression of the respiratory centres (until they reach a standstill) there is a secondary disturbance of the gas interchange caused by atelectasis, congestion and oedemas.

If the blood gas is checked during exposure respiratory acidosis is always diagnosed as the result of a disturbance of the acid-base balance, which additionally increases the acidosis of metabolic origin. Due to impaired diffusion the PO_2 in the blood and in the tissue drops. The CO_2 threshold, on the other hand, is not influenced to any appreciable extent. A consequence of "cold" acidosis is a move to the left of the O_2 dissociation curve, which still does not mean that the oxygen supply to the tissue is harmed, specially since the requirement becomes less.

Vital cold injuries to the lung have been affirmed and described in the literature. Epithelial damage to the mucous membrane of the respiratory tracts apparently occurs which have led to the formation of focal bronchopneumonia with subpleural haemorrhages.

Neither Unterdorfer and Umbach (1977) nor myself, ever observed such genuine pulmonary cold damage during the cold periods of the Second World War. A relationship between such bronchopneumonia and cold effects seems doubtful. The idea was conceived that such cold damage to the lung tissue during heavy frost and strong winds might be the result of strained breathing through an open mouth. We are rather more inclined to believe that these inflammatory symptoms came into existence with the flaring up of old infections in the respiratory tracts (cf. Killian 1966, p. 153).

Nevertheless, in his scanning electron microscopic investigations after exposure to cold Hess (1970, 1977) found an increase in the atelectasis, a swelling of the alveolar septa to four times the normal size, caused by an interstitial oedema and intra-alveolar haemorrhages, in addition, within the pulmonary capillaries changes to the erythrocytes and the blood platelets (see above).

References

Hess H (1970) Report. 7. Deutsche Angiologentagung, Berlin
Hess H (1977) Ärztl Prax (Suppl) 47
Jarisch A (1921 a) Pflügers Arch 192:255
Jarisch A (1921 b) Pflügers Arch 186:192
Jarisch A (1943) Mitt Geb Luftfahrtmed 7
Killian H (1966) Der Kälteunfall: Allgemeine Unterkühlung. Dustri
König FH (1943 a) Klin Wochenschr 22:45
König FH (1943 b) Klin Wochenschr 3:46
Krueger P, Blümel G (1977 a) Ärztl Prax 39:516
Krueger P, Blümel G (1977 b) V. Internationale Tagung der Bergrettungsärzte. Werk, p 11
Rein H (1931) Ergeb Pzysiol 32:28
Unterdorfer H, Umbach P (1977) Ärztl Prax (Suppl) 41

Causes of Cold Necrosis

Hypoxia and Rewarming Damage

Towards the end of 1945 the opinion prevailed amongst almost all pathologists, physiologists, surgeons and specialists in internal medicine that cold damage, and especially necrosis, was ultimately the result of oxygen deficiency or asphyxiation (e.g. Lutz 1942, 1949, 1951; Werz 1951; Judmaier 1952 a, b; Benitte 1950; see Rosenstiel's summary of 1946). Most of them denied any direct effect of cold action.

In his monograph in 1956 Sapin-Jaloustre devoted much attention to a presentation of the causes of cold necrosis. It resembles a lecture on all the different theories on cold gangrene, which have been postulated over the years, such as, for example, the vascular theory, the anoxia theory, the belief that thrombosis or freezing were responsible for the necrosis and many others. Even complex ideas in which it was claimed that a number of causal factors led to necrosis, are discussed. German authors were rarely mentioned here.

Our information on death from exposure (white death) revealed clearly that it is never a case of death due to cold damage to the cells and tissue, since the tissue temperature at the time of death is much too high, on an average around 26° to 27°. The white death is not, therefore, the result of local cell damage but solely to a failure of vital organic functions during exposure, in particular to the termination of the function of vital centres and the failure of nerve conduction. There must, therefore, be different causes of death according to the viability of the different organs, in particular of the heart (see Killian 1966).

It is different with local cold injuries since here the peripheral parts of the body and the tissue reaches low temperatures above 0°C or even below it. From minus 3°C downwards they can freeze, which raises special problems in as far as the nature and duration of the freezing process are of the utmost importance. As the freezing of tissue, however, is in practice not often found as the reason for necrosis, other causes of cold gangrene must instead be considered, including firstly the question of tissue anoxia due to ischaemia, which can be of primary or secondary nature. In this respect our views changed considerably soon after 1945.

The regular observation of a primary cold spasm of the arteries with peripheral oligohaemia or ischaemia actually led to the adoption of the hypoxia theory of necrosis, particularly as the blood supply to the limb or area affected is restricted in two ways:
1) By a local blockage, apparently predominantly of chemical origin, of the blood supply and vasoconstriction of the terminal vessels, which becomes quite extensive.
2) By a spastic contraction of the main supply arteries, the small arteries and the arterioles and a cutting off of the frozen area. It occurs via the autonomous nervous system and reduces the backward fow of large amounts of cooled blood to the centre of the body in the interests of thermo-regulation and the maintainance of a positive heat balance.

Both processes are combined and co-ordinated. The cold damage was taken to be a kind of asphyxiation due to the impression of defective circulation, created as the result of the primary arterial spasm. This is why in nearly all studies dating from this time one finds mention of "asphyxiation metabolism". Incomplete metabolic processes, the formation of amines and H substances, such as histamine, with the effects of which one associated the severe disturbances in the vascular permeability and the development of serous inflammations with all their consequences, all these were thought to be caused by a lack of O_2. The author considered all these ideas to be absolutely unsatisfactory since the success of our treatment, even when we had managed to get rid of the arterial spasm, was often extremely limited. Necrosis occurred nevertheless.

At that time the question "when" was raised, i.e. when hypoxia and asphyxia due to the effects of cold were at all possible. In 1942 Schürer, Killian (1942 a, b) and some other surgeons observed that after application of Esmarch's rubber bandage ischaemia could be tolerated, still in an exposed state during transport, not only for 4 h as at room temperature, but for 12 – 24 h without any harm being caused. This proved that the tissue metabolism, i.e. the oxygen requirement, of the area cut off was reduced to such an extent by the cold that it was able to survive. At around +6°C the metabolism comes to a standstill and the oxygen requirement drops to almost zero.

In 1939 Allen studied the consequences of putting a tourniquet on a limb at different temperatures. A rubber tube, placed round the bottom of a rat thigh for 5 h, produced at 38°C, after it had been loosened, a highly oedematous swelling and reddening of the extremity. Nearly all the animals died. If, on the other hand, this extremity was placed in water at +2°C to +4°C neither a severe oedema, nor hyperaemia, nor a general state of shock were to be observed after the ligature had been removed. The extremity which had been tied off recovered. The animals survived the state of ischaemia. Even more impressive were the experiments of Brooks and Duncan (1940),who exposed rat tails to an increased pressure of 135 mm of quicksilver, and thus produced necroses. The relationship between the temperatures of the ischaemic areas and the degree of the necroses were then registered.

At + 40°C necrosis was already observed after 2 h, at +35°C after 7 h, at +15°C after 26 h, at +5°C after 72 h and at + 1°C after 97 h.

It was shown that the development of necrosis is definitely dependent on the tissue temperature during the rewarming process. The higher it is, the more quickly and easily can necrosis occur. Exudation, the formation of oedemas and toxins, the development of bacterial infections was sometimes reduced and sometimes even prevented and thus the shock state often avoided.

According to Bergmann and Friedländer it is possible to produce a skin temperature of +4°C using ice bags, so that in layers 5 cm deep temperatures between +6° and +10°C are reached. After 1.5–2 h the area becomes anaesthetised. In many cases it was possible to keep the tissue cooled for days without any damage. The American authors succeeded in cooling the limbs to +4°C in a state of bloodlessness. One could then leave a rubber bandage on for up to 90 h, operate under refrigeration anaesthesia, without any cold damage occurring after careful thawing out.

In 1944 Schaar et al. tied up rat tails, cooled the tissue and were able to preserve it for 4 days, whereas without cooling total necrosis could be observed after only 4 h ischaemia. Lewis and his colleagues (Lewis and Moen 1952 a, b; Lewis and Freymag

1951) compared not only the physical effects of cold with the effects of heat (about +52°C) but also the effects of heat and cold on ischaemia. If ischaemia was created artificially for the time of cooling by ligature fortis, no necrosis occurred, whereas in the controls which were not cooled necrosis was observed. All these observations clearly indicated that cold alone does not necessarily cause any damage, that on living matter it has the effect of preserving tissue, a view also held by Bigelow (1942), White (1943), Krey-berg (1946a, 1948a, 1949a, 1950), Shumaker (1952), Shumaker and Lempke (1951), Shumaker and Kunkler (1952), and Allen (1945). *For this reason we doubted the existence of an "asphyxiation metabolism" during cooling.*

In 1942/44 Schwiegk et al. tried to prove the existence of an asphyxiation metabolism, which most authors assumed to be a prerequisite for serous damage and necrosis. The results were, however, completely *negative*. They were unable to find it since during the cooling period the tissue does not suffer from an oxygen deficiency. On the contrary the oxygen requirement decreases parallel to the drop in tissue temperature and the decrease in the tissue metabolism.

The only evidence that asphyxial processes do nevertheless occur and amines form in the cold damaged area was provided by Loos (1939, 1941 a, b, 1943, 1953) who, in a pharmacological test, found large amounts of H substances (histamine) in the exudate of fully formed cold blisters on the unstriped muscles. This was later confirmed. Oxygen deficiency of the tissue must at some time or other have been apparent, but when?

On evaluating the apparently conflicting observations, the author came to the conclusion in 1944 (Killian 1944) that *so-called cold damage must be understood in the main to be rewarming damage,* since it is not until the thawing out phase that a critical disproportion between oxygen supply and requirement leading to asphyxiation of the cells occurs. This is the result, on the one hand, of arterial spasms, on the other of a blockage of the venous bloodstream, after the tissue metabolism has begun to function again, around +4° to +6°C. When this view was expressed for the first time, at a South West German conference of surgeons in Freiburg in October 1948, it was met with great surprise. It was, nevertheless, soon accepted and has become common knowledge. Cold damage is, therefore, more likely to be rewarming damage than be actually caused by physical cooling, (the only exception is freezing). Schwiegk came to a similar conclusion.

If oxygen deficiency is maintained for a long time the preserving effect is gradually lost. During the discussion after my lecture in 1948 Druckrey expressed the view, based on older experiments with salivary gland tissue at the Kaiser Wilhelm Institute in Berlin, that cold alone does not damage the tissue before 0°C (probably not before 2° or 4°C), but that it enables it to bear an acute oxygen deficiency (which would kill the cells at 37°C) without any detectable damage being caused. If however, the oxygen deficiency persists, the preserving effect gradually disappears. The damage, Druckrey specified, was not actually the result of exposure to cold itself, but of oxygen deficiency during the recovery period, which totally confirms our ideas about *rewarming damage.* In 1949, in his work which was later published, Druckrey wrote on this subject: "There is therefore no such thing as cold damage, only rewarming damage due to acute lack of oxygen."

Similar views have incidentally been expressed by some botanists. All this brings us much nearer to an explanation of the whole subject. It must, however, be mentioned (from Druckrey's experiments) that in the case of long-term cooling even without freezing after 2 to 3 days signs of metabolic disturbances appear on the tissue cells, which finally become irreversible and can ultimately cause cytolysis. This limitation must be applied to the clinical situation.

Our understanding of rewarming damage is not altered by the fact that according to Barcroft's dissociation curves for oxyhaemoglobin oxygen is more strongly bound to the haemoglobin and it is, therefore, more difficult for it to be released to the tissue. Some authors believed in a reduction in the activity of the respiratory enzymes and explained in this way the inadequate use of the oxygen since bright red blood containing oxygen was fact supplied to the vessels as could be dearly seen in the disappearance of the arterio-venous difference (Crismon and Fuhrmann 1946). As far as we know, however, this theory has not been confirmed. Most ferment systems are resistent to the cold.

As is well known, in 1943 Werz (a, b) concluded that an "oxygen scissor effect" and state of asphyxiation developed, as the oxygen was more strongly fixed when increased oxygen was required, a theory which led to heated discussions but which has today been rejected.

As far back as 1917 Lake held the view that anoxia was the cause of cold necrosis. He maintained that anabolism ceased in tissue cultures around 25°C, catabolism, on the other hand, continued until below 10°C. Between 10° and 25°C he believed there to be a particular danger of metabolic products from the cells accumulating. This apparently explained the development of a "pied de trenchée". This theory has never been checked or acknowledged.

In 1950 the Russian authors Ariev and Seneckow (quoted according to Ariev 1950) claimed that cold damage was the result of anoxia of the tissue because the balance between oxygen supply and demand was lost mainly during the rewarming process. They believed asphyxiation to be the result. Sapin-Jaloustre (1956) added to this that the success of rapid rewarming could be seen as evidence of the fact that the lack of oxygen can easily be overcome. In our opinion, however, the apparent success of rapid rewarming is not a reliable enough premise to be used as the basis for the anoxia theory — the more so since most experiments involving ultra rapid cooling were carried out with cold mixtures apparently favouring ultra rapid thawing, in order to prevent the development of coarse ice-crystals, which takes time.

Sapin-Jaloustre's experiments, quoted in this connection, on golden hamsters, which after freezing were not harmed by rapid rewarming, but after slow thawing out suffered severe cold injuries, are not acknowledged or proved, since the hamster is a genuine hibernator with a tissue which possesses an increased resistance to cold and to a lack of oxygen. In our view anoxia cannot be considered as the only cause of cytolysis after exposure to cold.

Most authors, including Laborit (1962), Vagliano (1948) and ourselves, tend towards the view that there is a combined cause, normally direkt damage to the tissue due to the cold, and at the same time vascular damage, which can lead to a state of hypoxaemia or anoxia. This theory applies, however, in particular, in our opinion, to primary cold necrosis.

Necrosis Due to Direct Exposure to Cold

From Allen's first attempts in 1937/38 (Allen 1939) to develop refrigeration anaesthesia and observations made in Russia in 1941, 1942, one had gained the impression that cold only then caused direct damage to the tissue, when the tissue had been frozen at around minus 3°C. Only in such cases did one assume that direkt cold damage had been caused. It was supposed to arise on the one hand as the result of a decomposition of the protoplasm (Schade 1919, 1920, 1923, 1949; Gehenio and Luyet 1937–1952), on the other because of a freezing of the free cell water, which has a destructive effect on the structure.

This claim cannot be upheld anymore today either, in such a form, since as is well known the freezing of a group of tissues does not necessarily lead to necrosis or the loss of a limb. The very contradictory and confusing data on the direct effects of cold have today been clarified a step further, since a distinction has now been made between gradual cooling to a low temperature below 0°C and ultra rapid cooling, which alone is capable of maintaining the tissue in an amorphous state and of fixing the metabolism, producing a preserving effect, so that rapid rewarming causes no appreciable damage.

One critical error of ultra rapid cooling was discovered, namely the possibility of *vitrification of the tissue,* i.e. a skipping of the crystallisation phase or the formation of crystallisation nuclei, which are the basis of the growth of *coarse ice crystals, which destroy the structure.* When this stage of numbness has been reached (vitrification), the affected tissues can be further cooled to the lowest temperature without any damage being caused, provided that there is an appropriate rewarming technique to ensure that during the thawing out phase no structural damage is caused by coarse ice needles.[1] Unfortunately this information plays a relatively small part in clinical treatment, since ultra rapid cooling occurs relatively seldom in practice. It occurs most often to the limbs via contact with metal, in high mountains in heavy frost accompanied by strong air movement. It was observed by Davis et al. in 1943 among pilots.

Unfortunately for experimental purpose techniques of *ultra rapid cooling* with ethyl chloride spray, cold mixtures or carbon dioxide snow were used to produce frostbite without these technical procedures being taken into consideration in the conclusions. Many errors were made and wrong conclusions drawn as a result of this.

In the biological part of the "Kälteunfall" (Killian 1966) we drew attention to the numerous freezing experiments carried out by Koch (1892), Sturdza, Aulor-Klinge, Gehenio and Luyet (1937–1952). Since these experiments there can be no more doubt about the fact that with a relative shortage of water in the cells, freezing to as low as minus 25°C can be reached and endured using the ultra rapid cooling technique without the viability or the ability to reproduce and propagate being affected. It seems particularly surprising that it was possible to cool a large number of tumor cells, e.g. the Brown-Perce tumour and the Jensen sarcoma, to minus 253°C without all the cells being destroyed. After careful rewarming the tumour cells could be further cultured.

It was also possible in many cases to freeze small living creatures, poikilothermal fish, frogs and other animals, so that ice crystals formed in their bodies. They could then

---

1 The expansion of the extracellular and intracellular water on freezing with its explosive effects certainly plays an important part here too.

carefully be thawed out without any damage being caused. The latter, however, possess protoplasm, which is different to that of warm-blooded animals. It is not at all astonishing that Kreyberg (1946, 1948, 1949, 1950) and Adams (1941, 1940 a, b, 1944, 1952, 1956) were not able to save Raverdin's skin graft in situ from necrosis by cooling whereas skin grafts which had been ultra rapidly cooled healed smoothly after transplantation. The same applied to blood vessels, bones and similar tissue substrata, which can be transplanted without difficulty after preservation by ultra rapid cooling. It is also well known that it was possible to ultra rapidly freeze the beating heart of a chicken embryo to 195°C in liquid nitrogen, then to rapidly defreeze it at 42°C. It went on beating for hours after. Genuine hibernators could be cooled to such a point that ice crystals appeared in the tissue and yet they still survived. These are, however, special cases, which cannot be applied to human conditions.

It is not, therefore, the absolute degree of cold which causes damage but the manner and duration of the cold action which are decisive, as they determine the chances and the nature of the crystallisation of the cell and tissue water and thus the fate of the cells and tissue. Lewis and Moen (1952 a, b) as well as Piroszinski and Webster (1952 a, b) belong to the group of authors who consider the physical effects of the cold to be the main damaging factor as a result of their experiments and who attempt to show that anoxia of the tissue is of relatively little importance in the development of necrosis.

To sum up, it may be said that the direct effects of cold can and may only then be held responsible as a damaging factor when certain physical conditions are met. Otherwise the tissue will be preserved by the cold. How direct cold damage to the tissue ultimately occurs, is still today not yet completely clear.

Role of Catecholamines

According to Monsaignon (1940), Hunter apparently knew that wounds on a cooled limb hardly bleed at all as the blood vessels contract. The arterial vasoconstriction which is the basis of this manifestation has been proved by the most varied methods, such as skin thermometry, oscillography, arteriography and other biological methods, and also histologically. (See here Shumaker et al. 1948; Leriche and Kunlin 1940; Breitner 1944 a, b). It is based on cold reflexes and an increase in the tonus of the sympathetic nervous system, caused by the secretion of adrenaline and noradrenaline.

Some authors have attempted to explain the development of necrosis on the grounds of this increase in the sympathetic tone and the arterial spasms alone. In 1940 Leriche and Kunlin considered cold injuries to be a vasomotorial form of disease with a tendency to thrombosis. Their success with the blocking of the sympathetic nerve had an essential influence on this view. In 1948 Vagliano, after acute frostbite on the 3rd day, and Leriche and Kunlin in 1940, on the 5th day, registered a pronounced spasm of the afferent arteries arteriographically. Their results were confirmed again more recently, in 1953 during the Korean campaign, by Canty and Sharf. Both authors used arteriography systematically in order to discover the necessary position for an amputation. It soon became evident that clinically it was not the narrowing of the afferent arteries but their pathological condition which was of critical significance, for the blocking by thrombuses was the result of primary and secondary damage to the vascular walls. It was discovered that the arterial walls also suffered from the serous inflammation of cold damaged areas and that this later led to "cold arteriitis" and obliterative cold endangiitis, which could cause necrosis, if an adequate collateral circulation did not develop.

Many authors did not observe arterial thrombosis with fresh cold injuries, e.g. Grezillier (1919), Killian (1942 a, b, 1943), Vagliano (1948), Webster (1952, 1953) and Lewis (1952). Mallet-Guy and Lieffring (1940) did not find any arterial thrombosis either in over 100 cases of fresh cold injury.

In high mountains Davis et al. (1943) observed capillaroscopically a spasm of the small arteries in the fingers causing a circulatory standstill and finally secondary thrombosis of the terminal vessels. When necrosis developed on a large scale, he also found thrombuses in the arterioles and small arteries. Arteriovenous thromboses did not develop according to Leriche's observations in 1945, in total agreement with our later observations, until days after exposure during the inflammatory, reactive phase of hyperaemia and mainly affected the veins and also large and small arteries where the cold penetrated more deeply (immersion). Leriche refers to acute dystrophy of the arterial vascular walls.

According to clinical experience it seems to be possible in the case of Raynaud's disease that an excessive reaction to the cold may lead, despite a relatively warm environment, to oxygen deficiency in the affected area due to an arterial spasm of too long duration. This can cause necrosis. As a rule *a cold spasm alone is not sufficient to destroy the tissue.* Adrenaline damage and necroses, e.g. local anaesthesia is unfortunately not common. (See Killian et al. 1973.)

Occlusion of the Venous Pathway and Microcirculation

Many authors have held the slowing down of the circulation in the paralysed veins responsible for a further cause of the development of necrosis after exposure. This leads to congestion of the blood, circulatory failure and finally to thrombosis or irreparable occlusion of the drainage pathways.

This is contradicted by the fact that in other forms of blocking of the veins and thrombosis of the venous drainage pathways (even of the vena femoralis) generally no necrosis occurs, only a marked oedema and a postthrombotic condition. In his experiments Lewis observed no thrombosis in the blood vessels before the 24th h of exposure, Piroszinski and Webster (1952 a, b) before the 36th h. It occurred after 48 h with the development of necrosis. The authors considered this blockage of the veins to be a secondary sequela and concomitant affection, but by no means as a cause of the necrosis.

It is therefore not possible to treat this maximum dilation and paralysis of the veins and venous plexuses so typical of cold injuries as the sole cause of necrosis. In our opinion a blockage of the venous side is, however, of significance in necrosis, if the rewarming process takes place too rapidly and signs of asphyxiation appear. The arterial intake and pressure can only then be effective and contribute to an improvement in the oxygen supply to the tissue, if the outflow is more or less secure and free. If it begins to function early enough the clumps of erythrocytes are released again. The sludging and the agglutination disappear and no irreparable damage remains. This is unfortunately not the case with most severe cold injuries. During the healing process of localised cold damage the venous drainage may be diverted or rechanneled via dilated collateral vessels. If the drainage remains inadequate, a chronic oedema remains for a longer time in the frostbitten area. Postthrombotic symptoms only occur if the deeper lying veins are permanently blocked.

The Marked Cold Oedema

The cold oedema also poses problems with regard to necrosis. It is of primary origin and develops gradually after long exposure, and is not, in our opinion, the result of abnormal permeability of the damage vascular walls, but of a physical change in the salt concentration and of the osmotic pressure in the tissue and in the extracellular fluids. Of decisive importance is the tissue acidosis which certainly develops during exposure. This acidosis was partly regarded as the result of electrolyte disturbances, partly, however, also as their cause. Water accumulates in large amounts in the acid tissue. Albuminuria in the tissue is not yet found.

It takes time for a cold oedema to develop. After days of exposure to a mild degree of cold (e.g. immersion in water at +4°C) the feet become ice cold and swell acutely before they are rewarmed. *The rapid development of a primary cold oedema within a few hours is only observed in the case of recurring cold injuries, which makes it possible to draw conclusions about previous tissue damage.*

The actual marked oedema in fully developed cold injuries does not form until the rewarming phase, when warm blood has flown into the frostbitten areas. This *secondary* oedema of the hyperaemic stage is therefore definitely the result of disturbances in the permeability and damage to the vascular walls, the latter being partly due to direct exposure, partly, however, also to the effect of amines (H substances) which owe their existence to a lack of oxygen in the tissue.

Sapin-Jaloustre (1956). Lange and Boyd (1944) and others found evidence of the involvement of H substances in cold necrosis in the apparent success of treatment with antihistamine preparations. According to the experiments of Cier and Froment in 1954, the tendency of the blood vessels to dilate is apparently reduced and permeability disturbances partly counteracted after such treatment. There is no clinical confirmation of such success, which remains doubtful. And yet the opinion generally prevails that H substances are in fact associated with secondary vascular dilation during the inflammatory phase of the cold injury.

In 1947 Fuhrmann and Crismon investigated the oedema fluid in biological intestinal tests but there were no H substances present, presumably because the samples were taken during the cooling phase and not afterwards.

The development of the marked, secondary oedema is rapid and can, in the area of the limbs, which are firmly enclosed by fascial sheaths, (e.g. in the area of the lower leg) reduce the arterial blood flow mechanically to such a degree that ischaemia occurs, which necessarily leads to asphyxiation and necrosis, if the period of 4 h at normal temperature is exceeded. The simultaneous obstruction of the venous drainage vessels must also be remembered.

This fact prompted Sauerbruch et al. (1944) in the case of marked oedemas of the lower extremities (lower leg and foot) to insist on the area being relieved as quickly as possible by multiple incisions being made and the skin, the subcutaneous fatty tissue and in particular the fascial sheaths opened. Those who kept to this procedure were able to save a number of limbs.

Electrolyte Disturbances

Not until recently was attention drawn to the intensive, progressive changes which the electrolyte and water distribution undergoes during exposure. Considerable changes in the concentration of the blood salts in the intracellular and extracellular areas were observed. It is considered possible, it is true, that the cause of the necrocytosis during exposure may be the too high concentration of salts, especially of Na and Ca with a simultaneous loss of potassium. The information on such changes in the electrolyte concentrations, about which there is actually no doubt, varies, however, to such an extent in the literature that it is first necessary to wait for further results before changes in the internal environment can be included among the causes of necrosis after exposure.

References

Adams RJ (1941) Acta Chir Scand 85:1
Adams RJ (1942a) Nord Med 915
Adams RJ (1942b) Bull Var Med 915
Adams RJ (1944) Acta Chir Scand 89:527
Adams RJ (1952) 2nd Conference on Cold Injuries. Josuah Macy Jr Foundation
Adams RJ (1956) Nord Med 56:1581
Allen FM (1939) Am J Surg 45:495
Allen FM (1941) Am J Surg 52:225
Allen FM (1942) Am J Surg 55:451
Allen FM (1945) Am J Surg 68:170
Ariev TV (1950) Klin Med (Mosk) 28:3,15
Benitte AC (1950) Rev Corps Santé Mil 4:347
Bigelow GW (1942) Can Med Assoc J 47:529
Breitner B (1944a) Dtsch Z Chir 259:273
Breitner B (1944b) Chirurg 16:8
Brooks B, Duncan GW (1940) Am Surg 112:130
Canty J, Sharf AG (1953) Ann Surg 138:65
Crismon HJ, Fuhrmann FA (1946) Science 104:408
Davis L, Scarff JE, Rogers N, Dickinson M (1943) Surg Gynecol Obstet 77:561
Fuhrmann FA, Crismon HJ (1947) J Clin Invest 26:229, 236, 245, 476
Gehenio PM, Luyet BJ *1937–1952) Les accidents dûs au froid
Grezillier A (1919) Medical dissertation, Paris
Judmaier F (1952a) Munch Med Wochenschr 94:255
Judmaier F (1952b) Wien Klin Wochenschr 64:100
Killian H (1942a) Zentralbl Chir 1763
Killian H (1942b) Arbeitstagung beratender Chirurgen, Berlin
Killian H (1943) Zentralbl Chir 70:50
Killian H (1944) Forsch Fortschr 2
Killian H (1966) Der Kälteunfall: Allgemeine Unterkühlung. Dustri, Deisenhofen
Killian H, et al. (1973) Local anaesthesia and local anaesthetics, 2nd edn
Koch (1892) Biol Zentralbl 12
Kreyberg L (1946) Lancet 1:338
Kreyberg L (1948) Arch Pathol 45:707
Kreyberg L (1949) Physiol Rev 29:156
Kreyberg L (1950) Acta Pathol Microbiol Scand (Suppl) 91:40
Laborit H (1962) Presse Med 60:1256
Lake NC (1917) Lancet 2:557
Lange K, Boyd L (1944) Science 102:151
Leriche R (1945) In: Physiologie pathologique et traitement chirurgical des maladies arteriélles de la vasomotricité. Masson, Paris, p 65
Leriche R, Kunlin J (1940) Mem Acad Chir 66:14, 196

Lewis RB (1952) Mil Surg 110:25
Lewis RB, Freytag F (1951) Proc Soc Exp Biol Med 77:816
Lewis RB, Moen PW (1952a) J Med Sci 224:529
Lewis RB, Moen PW (1952b) Surg Gynecol Obstet 95:543
Loos HO (1939) Dermatol Wochenschr 1017
Loos HO (1941a) Zentralbl Chir 10:449
Loos HO (1941b) Med Klin 37:54, 84
Loos HO (1943) Mitt Geb Luftfahrtmed 7
Loos HO (1953) Munch Med Wochenschr 90:155
Mallet-Guy P, Lieffring JJ (1940) Mem Acad Chir 14:136
Monseignon A (1940) Presse Med 48:166
Piroszinski WJ, Webster J (1952a) Ann Surg 136:993
Piroszinski WJ, Webster J (1952b) Proc Soc Exp Biol Med 80:306
Rosenstiel M (1946) PM 18:257
Sapin-Jaloustre J (1956) Enquêtes sur les gélures. Herman, Paris
Sauerbruch F, Jung H, Klapp R (1944) Dtsch Z Chir 258:319
Schaar, Jones, Lehan (1944) Surg Clin North Am 1326
Schade H (1919) Munch Med Wochenschr 1:1021
Schade H (1920) Munch Med Wochenschr 449
Schade H (1923) Physiologie und Chemie der inneren Medizin. Steinkopff, Dresden
Schade H (1949) Z Exp Med 7:275
Schürer F von (1942) Zentralbl Chir 69:486, 1797
Shumaker HB (1952) Report. 1st and 2nd Conferences on Cold Injuries. Josuah Macy Jr Foundation
Shumaker HB, Kunkler AW (1952) Surg Gynecol Obstet 94:475
Shumaker HB, Lempke RE (1951) Surgery 30:873
Shumaker HB, White BH, Wrenn EL (1948) Yale J Biol Med 20:519
Vagliano M (1948) Erfrierungen. Masson, Paris
Werz R von (1943a) Arch Exp Pathol Pharmacol 211:561
Werz R von (1943b) Mitt Geb Luftfahrmed 7
White JC (1943) N Engl J Med 228:211

Complications of Cold Injuries

Non-specific Complications

There is an acute danger of infection with every 2nd—4th degree cold injury. Experience has shown that it is far greater in the area of the lower extremities than in other parts of the body. Inflammation does not stem from the infected rhagades, from open cold injury vesicles or cold injury ulcers, but from the permanently infected line of demarcation.

Not only clinicians but above all pathologists (Siegmund 1942 a—c, 1943 a—c; Schulze 1947) have confirmed this fact. General septic infections can emanate from the line of demarcation. Schulze pointed out that it is often not possible to tell from the external state of a cold injury that beneath the apparently dry scab a dangerous focus has formed. From personal experience I can only confirm this. Small areas of frostbite on the limbs, especially on the tips of the toes, have been sufficient to produce most serious symptoms and systemic infections with a fatal outcome.

As a rule the healing process of a 2nd degree cold injury or even the dried mummification of 3rd degree damage does not involve any fever worth mentioning. We have, however, unfortunately experienced exceptions. Severe frostbite of a more extensive kind on the lower extremities, sometimes even on all four limbs, results as a rule after the 2nd or the 3rd day in high septic temperatures and signs of severe intoxication, even though the further development did not always involve wet gangrene. It may be assumed that due to the generally weak condition high fever occurs as the result of the resorption of highly toxic and pyrogenic substances from the frostbitten area. However, the remittent rise in temperature is normally caused by the development of purulent or putrid multi-infections, which are mostly accompanied by concomitant germs of the proteus-pyoceaneus group and anaerobes. The information in the literature on the frequency of such septic infections varies considerably. According to Riehl (1915), unlike large area burns, with frostbite there is at first no great danger to life. We can confirm this, since the total rate of deaths from the septic sequelae of local cold injuries is nowhere near comparable to that from burns. If, however, more serious septic processes occur with thrombophlebitic symptoms or an anaerobic infection sets in, the mortality of these cases is then known to be very high.

This is made clear in a dissertation by Grezillier (1919), who reports on 6 deaths from 78 cases of cold injury to the feet. The remark of Vagliano (1948), that a serious infection after frostbite was a certain case for early amputation, has been confirmed by all experienced surgeons, including Russian authors (Guerasimenko 1950).

Apart from the signs of systemic infection the appearance of local lymphangitis and lymphadenitis is nearly always observed. The inflammatory swelling in the frostbitten area increases considerably, and usually also spreads in the direction of the healthy tissue. The areas become hot and dark red and show all the symptoms of an acute, severe cellulitis phlegmon. The skin is often as smooth as silk and taut. Ulcers or perforations often occur.

All variations of phlegmonous processes are found in the subcutaneous epifascial and subfascial area. Furthermore we have often observed the development of chronic tendon sheath suppuration, tubular abscesses, osteomyelitic processes and empyema of the joints. Sometimes toxic erysipelas formed, emanating from the line of demarcation. Occasionally even stomatonoma has been described.

These are, however, non-specific forms of purulent complication, which could occur with more or less any wound. We have, on the other hand, experienced inflammatory complications which must be considered simply as characteristic of cold damage.

These include firstly purulent, progressive thrombophlebitis, which Larrey had already observed after cold injuries. It occurs much more often to the lower extremities than to the upper and is by no means restricted to the gangrenous area but according to the pathological findings of Riehl in 1915 and 1938, also Siegmund (1943 a-c) and Schulz in 1943, extends far beyond this area frequently as far as the groin or even as far as the vena iliaca. We sometimes found in apparently healthy parts above the amputation area an infected vein, from the stump of which liquid pus or a purulent, pulpy, thrombotic substance appeared. In 1943 Biebl (personal communication) observed in such a case the vena saphena magna full of pus from one end to the other. The veins are not always continually filled with clots, but contain here and there smaller or larger thrombophlebitic foci, over which the skin is red and swollen. In 1943 Siegmund (a-c) also referred in a lecture to most severe phlebitic purulation, sometimes reaching up as far as the hollow of the knee or even the groin. He thereby confirmed the above findings and also described the too narrow yellow tubes, the changed veins, which resemble maccaroni. In the course of the development of purulent lymphangitis and thrombophlebitis *septic systemic infections* occur in some cases. In view of this fact in cases where there was danger of this happening the vena saphena magna was partly removed as early as possible and the stumps tied up. The transition from a common purulent infection to a systemic infection is not always accompanied by severe symptoms but can also occur, as we know from experience, first slowly, then suddenly become evident via high septic temperatures with shivering.

As far as one can tell from the data, it is normally a systemic infection of thrombogen origin with metastasis. The lymph tract seems to be of less importance in cold injuries. According to my table of systemic infections, (see Handloser 1944, p. 199) it is mainly the pulmonary type which occurs, in other words a coarse embolic form of dispersion of septically infected clots via the bloodstream with the typical formation of metastases in the lung filter. In the past Siegmund described two cases of this kind. Both died of pulmonary abscesses. Sometimes small embolisms develop, are filtered through the lungs and then dispersed in a very fine, infected form all over the main circulation. Then metastases occur in the area of all organs, e.g. in the muscles, in the subcutaneous tissue, in the liver, the spleen, the kidneys and in the heart. Even metastatic empyemata and metastatic pericarditis have been observed after cold injuries. Of the main joints the hip joint, the knee·joint, the shoulder joint and the sternoclavicular joint are most often affected, the elbow joint seldom. In the majority of cases haemolytic, highly toxic streptococci and staphylococci were observed in the bacteriological investigations.

Further septic complications after cold injuries include the development of a fresh form of *endocarditis,* namely the verrucous, ulcerous form which likewise must have emanated from the infected line of demarcation. In our experience acute endocarditis occurs far less often with other wound infections. It has been confirmed by many pathologists after cold injuries. It may serve as a second focus of dissemination and from here metastases can form in the most varied organs.

In 1943 Boehnig described changes to the muscle fibrils in the heart and the clinical picture of interstitial myocarditis after cold injury similar to that found after diphtera. In some cases septic processes with changes to the kidneys have been observed after frost-bite. In addition to heavy protein secretion during the infectious and necrotic development epithelial damage and swelling of the glomerular coils and the renal tubules have also been found. Occasionally a granular degeneration of the larger organs has been observed, e.g. the liver, which occurred in the course of the septic systemic infection and led to the organ gaining a considerable amount in weight.

All these septic complications have become much less common since the discovery of antibiotics. This includes the cases of osteomyelitis and severe, progressive, phleg-monous processes.

Specific Complications

Wound Diphtheria

Cases of wound diphtheria after cold injuries have occurred more often. During the years 1941/43 our bacteriologists discovered that in almost 40% of the cases of 3rd degree frostbite diphtheroid rod-shaped bacilli were to be found around the demarcation area. These include all forms of paradiphtheritic and pseudodiphtheritic bacilli and here and there also genuine diphtheria bacilli. The vast majority of these bacilli are of a saprophytic character. Their presence here is not, however, without importance, since they, too, have an unfavourable effect on the wound. The transition from the atoxic to the toxic form in the diphtheria bacilli has been described and confirmed in experiments (Killian 1943). Positive bacteriological findings can only be acknowledged if the results of Römer's toxin experiment or even of more recent tests are positive and the clinical symptoms support them. If such a super-infection with diphtheroid rods or genuine diphtheria bacilli develops the granulation becomes soft, there is heavy purulation which is difficult to curb and the healing process is delayed. In most of the cases the infections do not yet have the chronic necrotising effect, which is characteristic of genuine wound diphtheria. Only in exceptional cases do tissue necrosis, a typical undermining of the edges or the formation of a pseudomembrane occur. In isolated cases toxic paralysis or an injured myocardium were observed, which were sometimes fatal. We have not experienced any of those acutely dangerous cases of torpid surgical diphtheria from the point of view of necrotising erysipelas, which does occasionally develop after a wound (pure culture of genuine Di bacilli in the slide preparation).

Cases of wound diphtheria have been observed by a large number of authors, for example, Wagner, as early as 1915, Klages (1942), Kingrin (1943, personal communication), Killian (1943), Starlinger (1942). In the past wound diphtheria was one of the most dreaded complications, today it has become extremely rare thanks to the effects of the antibiotics, which can be used to treat the diphtheria bacilli. Diphtheritic anti-toxins must be administered if the culture and toxin tests prove positive. If the patient has been actively vaccinated against diphtheria, the protective titre must be increased

171

with a follow-up dose of the toxoid. We refer to the more recent literature on diphtheria bacilli and their sensitivity to certain antibiotics (Walter-Heilmeyer).

Tetanus

As early as 1817 Larrey observed and described lock jaw after cold injury. A whole series of surgeons have since confirmed his observations (Lagorce 1814; Desmoulins 1815; Bienoust et al. 1817; Vernoun and Sonnenburg 1876).

In the Crimean War six such cases were observed among the French, and three among the English troops. During the Russian-Turkish war, of 42 cases of lock jaw, two were accompanied by cold injuries; both were fatal.

Furthermore Middeldorf (1883), Wagner (1886), Boehler (1917), Hecht (1915), Lumiere and Astier (1917), Mayer and Kohlschütter (1914), Buzello (1923) and Stricker (1940), all confirmed the occurence of tetanus after cold injuries.

Almost all army pathologists have reported on this subject and individual cases were described by Heller (1908), Killian (1943), M. Madlehner (1943, personal communication), Kingrin (1943, personal communication). After Wagner's list was compiled in 1915 the total number of cases had probably by far exceeded 100. In 1939 Glagolef observed 34 cases of lock jaw, 7 after cold injuries and he makes special mention of the fact that all developed very rapidly and that none of the patients could be saved. Of all the tetanus cases in the Leipzig University Hospital 3.4% occurred after local frostbite. In 1923 and 1930 Fuss also reported that the cases of tetanus after cold injury tended to take an extraoridnarily serious and dramatic course and that the mortality rate increased from an average of 34% to 95%.

In all monographs on cold injuries emphasis is laid on tetanus (Floerken 1917, 1920 a, b; Sonnenburg and Tschmarke 1915; Redwitz 1940; Lucke 1941; von Brandis 1943; Starlinger and Frisch 1944; Whayne and Coats 1958).

Our views on tetanus infections have changed in the recent past in as far as the belief that the effective toxin is propagated via the nerves, which was assumed for a long time (Buzello 1923; Abel 1934, 1936; Doerr 1935, 1936; Bromeis 1937; Schmidt 1940), must be considered outdated. Today, on the other hand, it is assumed that, as with most other infections, the effective toxin is spread by diffusion via the lymph or the blood throughout the body. The lymphatic channels of the nerves are also involved. The incubation period is therefore only a question of the time of the enrichment of effective amounts of toxins in the site of action, and the toxin found in the nerves corresponds to the difference and migration in the lymph current as in all other tissue (c.f. here my section on tetanus in Handloser 1944, and our diagram of the effects of the toxin, Killian 1951).

If effective tetanus toxin is quickly produced in high concentrations and distributed via the blood, this becomes clinically evident because of the short incubation period with unfavourable prognosis. The early cases are very often fatal.

By comparison to this we have seen in Russia, where the soil is poor in tetanus bacilli, some *late cases* after cold injury of purely *ascending,* in other words, *tetanus* caused by the lymph nodes, the prognosis of which is rather more favourable (Madlehner, personal communication; Killian 1943). It is very often difficult to make a sufficiently early diagnosis because of the slow course of the disease and its inadequate, sometimes quite vague, misleading symptoms. Complaints from the patients of acute and painful feelings of tension in the affected extremity and the occurrence of *rigid postures, strange contracture positions, as well as hardness of the local muscles,* may all be signs of the onset of the disease. Lock jaw is not normally diagnosed until after the development of the typical emprosthotonos of the trismus, and then it is often already too late.

See the description of a case like this in my book: "Im Schatten der Siege" (Killian 1964, pp. 67, 73).

For decades it has been compulsory after 1st to 3rd degree frostbite to administer tetanus antitoxins. Today tetanus immunisation has become generally accepted.

For a long time little could be done therapeutically about tetanus. In the meantime the possibilities have improved considerably thanks to long-term artifical respiration, relaxants, the methods of hypothermia (hibernation) and also the introduction of very powerful antibiotics.

Penicillin G in heavy doses (10–20 mill IE/die) is recommended as being therapeutically effective after the dressing of very dirty wounds. Tetracyline and cephalosporine may also be used in treatment. It is more important to keep the wound open while it is being dressed, so that the tissue is well supplied with oxygen, a condition which is very difficult to keep to in the case of 3rd and 4th degree frostbite. Once tetanus has broken out, treatment in an intensive care unit is strongly recommended according to the experience of anaesthetists.

Gas Gangrene, Gas Phlegmon, Malignant Gangrene

It is not surprising that after local cold damage a genuine anaerobic infection of the gas phlegmon or malignant gangrene type may develop in the region of tissue decay. The whole demarcation area lacks oxygen, is anoxic, a condition which greatly favours the formation of the bacilli of the gas gangrene group and anaerobic, haemolytic streptococci and staphylococci.

As far as I know, in the literature throughout the world cases of gas gangrene have only been reported after cold injuries to the lower limbs, and not to the upper limbs or other parts. None of the four clinically defined forms of gas gangrene was predominant. The cases which we saw were mostly the brown form.

Brown gas gangrene should not be confused with the very similar malignant gangrene (Killian) where there is no formation of gas due to anaerobic, highly toxic, haemolytic streptococci, or with an infection which simulates gas gangrene due to aerogenic strains of the coli imperfectum, which were described in 1913 by Schönberg and in 1947 by Killian et al.

Infections of the demarcation area with Coli bacteria have often been described (e.g. Vagliano 1948).

Mixed infections with fungus, such as were mentioned by Raymond and Parisot in 1930 as being essential for wet-type damage (pied de trenchée, trench foot and Flanders' foot) may occur. We were not, however, able to find any documents with more detailed information on the subject.

In 1943 Sigl observed a peculiar greenish blue discoloration of the whole area in two cases of gas gangrene after cold injury. It is sometimes extremely difficult to tell the difference between the frostbitten gangrenous areas and those affected by clostridium, especially if a malignant oedema is involved. Cases of gas gangrene after cold injuries have been reported by Partsch (1943), Orator (1943, with metastases), Killian (1942 a, b, 1943), Laewen (1942 a, b, 1944), Hofheinz (1943), Schulze (1943, 1947) and Siegmund (1943 a–c). The on-coming danger can be recognised by the rapidly developing symptoms of gangrene which has suddenly become malignant, whereby it is not the septic fever (which is not always present) which is the most important sign, but the rapidly increasing general decay and the toxic depression of the circulation accompanied by a relaxation collapse.

One normally also finds the formation of gas in decaying areas and should not be misled by this fact. It is not found with malignant oedemas and not with Welch's infection either. If, on the other hand, a rapidly developing pneumatisation of the tissue is observed and the fast formation of gaseous emphysema with the typical signs of cracking and tympanism in the direction of the thigh, then there is no longer any doubt of the presence of a gas phlegmon caused by organisms of the gas gangrene group (Welch-Fränkel: Bacillus perfringens, of the Clostridium hovyi or Cl. septicum; Koch and Pasteur) or the bacillus hystoliticus and Cl. sordelli bifermentans groups). If need be, an X-ray picture will clarify the situation, since with these specific infections the ubiquitous formation of gas causes the muscle fibrills to split, which becomes a characteristic sign (see Killian 1939). Pure infections of the gangrenous type hardly ever occur after cold injuries. It is always a question of putrid, anaerobic multi-infections with rapid tissue decay and an unpleasant smell.

For all these cases the method of making copious incisions, which has often been successfully applied, may be considered, also treatment in an oxygen tent, and more recently the increased oxygen pressure method. Amputations have become less common, since the introduction of a large number of antibiotics: penicillin G (in heavy doses), tetracycline, amphicillin, chloramphenicol and cephalosporin (Walter-Heilmeyer), which are effective against clostridia and which, in our opinion, have become considerably more effective. Anti-gas gangrene serum was a disappointment. (See Killian and Denk 1943.)

References

Boehler L (1917) Med Klin 11
Brandis HJ von (1943) Vorträge aus der praktischen Chirurgie, vol 27. Encke, Stuttgart
Buzello A (1923) "Habilitation" thesis, Greifswald
Floerken H (1917) Bruns Beitr Klin Chir 106:4
Floerken H (1920a) Zentralbl Chir 47:1651
Floerken H (1920b) Die Kälteschäden im Krieg. Springer, Berlin (Ergebnisse der Chirurgie und Orthopädie)
Glagolef (1939) Zentralbl Chir 404
Grezillier A (1919) Medical dissertation, Paris
Guerasimenko NJ (1950) Klinika i letchneie otmorogeniy, vol 1. Moscow
Handloser (1944) Innere Wehrmedizin. Steinkopff, Darmstadt
Hecht K (1915) Wien Klin Wochenschr 65:1487
Heller E (1908) Dermatol Z 630

Hofheinz S (1943) Berichte der beratenden Chirurgen
Killian H (1939) Pneumopathien. Encke, Stuttgart
Killian H (1942a) Zentralbl Chir 1763
Killian H (1942b) Arbeitstagung beratender Chirurgen, Berlin
Killian H (1943) Zentralbl Chir 70:50
Killian H (1951) Dtsch Med Wochenschr 408
Killian H (1964) Im Schatten der Siege. Ehrenwirth, Munich
Killian H, Denk W (1943) Lectures. Military Medical Academy, Berlin
Killian H, Meyer O, Sigl O (1947) Bruns Beitr Klin Chir 176:538
Klages F (1942) Zentralbl Chir 1242
Laewen A (1942a) Dtsch Mil Arzt 7:479
Laewen A (1942b) Zentralbl Chir 69:1253
Laewen A (1944) Dtsch Med Wochenschr 70:141
Lucke (1941) In: Handbuch der inneren Medizin. Springer, Berlin
Larrey JD (1817) Memoires du chirurgie militaire et de campagne, vol 4. Paris
Lumiere A, Astier E (1917) Munch Med Wochenschr 64:223
Mayer AW, Kohlschütter R (1914) Dtsch Z Chir 127:518
Orator (1943) Erfahrungsberichte der beratenden Chirurgen
Partsch F (1943) Erfahrungsberichte der beratenden Chirurgen
Riehl (1915) Wien Klin Wochenschr 11
Schulze W (1943) Arch Dermatol 184:61
Schulze W (1947) Klin Wochenschr 646
Siegmund H (1942a) Munch Med Wochenschr 827
Siegmund H (1942b) Arbeitstagung beratender Ärzte, Berlin
Siegmund H (1942c) Arch Dermatol 184:84
Siegmund H (1943a) Zentralbl Chir 1558
Siegmund H (1943b) Mitt Geb Luftfahrtmed 7:43
Siegmund H (1943c) Jahreskurse Aerztl Fortbild 34:9
Sonnenburg E, Tschmarke P (1915) (Neue deutsche Chirurgie. Encke, Stuttgart
Starlinger F (1942) Zentralbl Chir 69:1179
Starlinger F, Frisch OW (1944) Die Erfrierungen. Steinkopff, Berlin
Vagliano M (1948) Erfrierungen. Masson, Paris
Wagner K (1915) Wien Klin Wochenschr 28:1385
Whayne TF, Coats (1958) Cold injuries groundtype. USA General Surgeon of the Army

Prophylaxis and Treatment of Localised Cold Damage

Prophylaxis of Localised Cold Damage

General Information

Apart from the avoidance of a general loss of temperature, which greatly increases the risk of the development of peripheral, localised frostbite, a number of special preventive measures, learnt from experience, must be observed.

Every group leader bears the full responsibility for the avoidance of cold damage during exposure to cold. It is also the duty of every single member, however, to observe his comrades and to report any sudden paling with a danger of freezing, especially in the area of the face, of the nose, the cheeks, the ears and the hands, since the person affected very often notices nothing of this. After an initial burning pain, the area too quickly becomes insensitive, all sensitive qualities are lost.

Some practical rules should be observed:
1) Maintain a good circulation (movement).
2) Avoid every kind of obstruction of the local blood circulation during exposure, either from shoe-laces, bandages or from forced positions with the joints maximally bent with angulation or possibly closing of the arteries, in the shoulder region the art. axillaris, in the elbow region the art. cubitalis, to the leg in the hip region the art. femoralis, in the knee the art. poplitea.
3) Avoid poisons which would cause the peripheral arteries to contract, such as nicotine and sympathicometica (as opposed to moderate amounts of alcohol).
4) Avoid contact with metal.
5) Check the limbs after exposure: Take off wet gloves, shoes, every kind of wet clothing: shirt, socks, trousers etc. Here a few additional remarks should be made: shoes which fit well are essential. The fact that leather contracts when wet must be taken into account. Three pairs of dry socks should fit easily into winter shoes without pressure. It should be possible to move the toes freely. Leather shoes afford poor insulation at very low temperatures and should, therefore, if possible, be replaced by felt shoes or felt overshoes, when the weather is extremely cold and dry. In wet weather, on the other hand, felt shoes present a great danger. Fur shoes ware worse than felt ones as far as protection from the cold is concerned, since its hair and hair layer becomes flattened. Fur worn on the outside offers more protection than fur on the inside. In an emergency felt insoles or paper insoles, straw overshoes or wrapping leather shoes in straw is sufficient, to achieve better insulation.

The floors of military stations, as well as the floors of aircraft, tents, sledges etc., must be adequately insulated.

There is a particular danger during exposure if socks becomes wet as the result of the wearing of high rubber shoes. Rubber shoes do not allow ventilation, inside dampness accumulates, which greatly increases the conductivity and danger of cooling.

176

In the same way hyperhidrosis of the extremities has an unfavourable effect (clammy hands and feet). Treatment with dry powder, frequent washing or bathing in lightly astringent solutions are necessary to prevent cold injuries occurring.

From the practical side it is important to insist strictly on the prevention of snow getting into the upper edges of the shoes. They must be made leakproof. Third and fourth degree frostbite often resulted when snow penetrated the army boots, melted, and then froze hard, so that the whole foot became totally frozen. Often the frozen feet had to be knocked out of a solid block of ice, once the army boots had been sawn open.

One should never rest or sleep in severe cold with damp clothing, wet shoes or wet gloves or socks. The transport of the wounded or injured with wet bandages, or fresh plaster casts, which are still wet, has had disastrous consequences in heavy frost and should be avoided. All these preventive measures should be followed, although the peripheral limbs, the fingers, the hands and also the toes and the forefoot are naturally protected from too acute a loss of temperature by periodic phases of warming up (Aschoff-Lewis reaction, Hunting phenomenon). The main danger arises when the Aschoff-Lewis reaction stops and the limbs begin to loose heat like a physical body.

Frank carried out experiments on human beings with the sphygmomanometer cuff in order to measure the drop in skin temperature parallel to the decrease in the blood flow — this at a room temperature of $-26°C$. The following diagram shows the results (Fig. 72).

It can be seen that the changes in the blood flow on the back and the palm of the hand make relatively little difference but that the finger temperature is very much affected. The temperature drops as a result of the circulation stopping much more quickly here than in other areas. The spot in most danger is the tip of the finger. At $-40°C$ air temperature it already reaches a skin temperature of $10°C$ within 6 min and of $0°C$ after 10 min (Fig. 73).

An effective form of protection of the hand and fingers against the cold is gloves and a woollen wristlet to warm the pulse. Corresponding results can be achieved in the same way in the area of the feet and the toes.

Attempts at thermic protection by using anti-frost ointments and the same experimental techniques resulted in no changes in reaction being observed after the application of ointments to which histamines, adenyl-phosphoric-acid, acetylcholine or hormones had been added. The main value of anti-frost protection lies, in our opinion, in an avoidance of the top dermal layer becoming wet through. Apart from this, sensitive parts of the skin and parts where the mucous membrane begins, such as the lips, should be kept smooth and be protected from cracks, rhagades and brittleness.

The prevention of the skin freezing to metals: It is particularly dangerous if the skin freezes onto metal. This happens suddenly, if the skin of the hand, the fingers, the toes or the soles of the feet, which are always slightly moist, come into contact with the smooth surface of cold metals at $-15°C$. The skin becomes frozen to the metals so quickly that it is, in most cases, no longer possible to free it and in most attempts to do so the epithelium sticks to the metal, so that unpleasant superficial injuries result. Completely dry and well oiled skin does not freeze onto metal.

As the process is dependent on the heat conductivity of the metal in question there are considerable differences between the individual metals. The greater the conductivity, the smaller the risk of the skin freezing to the metal. The hand does not usually freeze

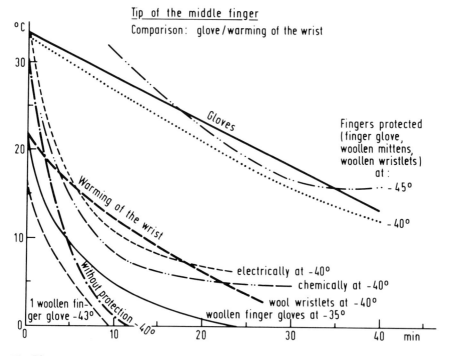

Fig. 72. Comparison of the protective effects of gloves and wristlets. (From Frank)

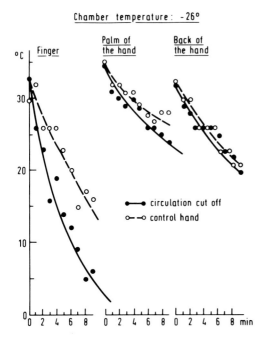

Fig. 73. Rewarming trials after circulatory cut off with exposure to cold (comparative measures in the finger, palm of the hand and back of the hand). (From Frank)

onto silver or shiny copper, whereas it does to aluminium, which is a poor conductor and to iron in different forms. It can occur on window glass, but not, however, on perspex or on wood. Metals with a satin finish or burnished metal surfaces prevent it occuring.

To eliminate the danger of freezing, it is sufficient to lay an insulating layer between the metal and the skin. This can be a material such as wool.

Prophylactic Thinning of the Blood by Infusion or Isovolaemic Haemodilation

During the last two Himalayan expeditions, in 1975 to the 25,314 ft high Kanchenjunga mountain and in 1977 to the 25,533 ft high Lhotse mountain for the first time artificial blood thinning was planned as a preparatory measure before the ascent (Zink et al. 1977). The reason for this was the recognition of the fact that during longer periods at high altitudes, due to the beginning of an increase in the erythropoiesis, slight increases in the haematocrit values to 0.55 — 0.60 Vol. % and more can be observed, which causes a further thickening to 0.80 %, resulting from an additional change in the water distribution in the organism, a migration of the water to the tissue. The water balance is gradually negatively affected, of course, during exposure. This means that due to an increase in the viscosity of the blood the circulatory conditions deteriorate in particular in the periphery, and there is, therefore, also an increase in peripheral resistance and an added strain on the heart. In order to overcome this 14 members of the group were pretreated with infusions of 500—750 ml of Biseko, a further 9 via isovolaemic haemodilution, i.e. blood was taken in two or three steps and immediately topped up with a colloidal blood replacement fluid (5% human albumin, dextran etc.) As reported by Zink et al. (1977), not only was a remarkable improvement in the performance of the mountaineers observed afterwards — of 21 men 19 reached the 8500 m high summit, a unique achievement — but no signs of a retina haemorrhage or any other cold injury to the limbs was registered after their return, whereas untreated members suffered from such injuries. One group member was even able to stand these heights for the first time without oxygen and came back down to the valley unharmed (with haematocrit 0.47 Vol.%). The haematocrit value was always taken as the criterion for the thinning of the blood. Before the final ascent but after preliminary treatment, values of 0.58 and 0.56 Vol.% were registered and after the return from the summit of Mt. Kantsch 0.59 Vol.% (n=10), and from the summit of Mt. Lhotse 0.56 Vol.% (n=4). Those men who had been subjected to isovolaemic haemodilution showed haemodilution values of 0.59, 0.51 or 0.53 Vol.% after the return (normal = o 42.6, o 40.6 Vol.%).

This observation indicates, in our opinion, what significance must be attached to increased viscosity of the blood with a slowing down of the circulation, the sludging phenomenon, the accumulation of erythrocytes and finally the formation of stasis and agglutination thrombosis in low pressure areas for the development of localised cold injuries. The region of the precapillaries and post-capillaries, the miscrocirculation, which can cease to function, and also the venoles and the veins are particularly affected. It must not be forgotten that during exposure the afferent arteries are narrow and considerably restricted as the result of a reflectorial impulse of the sympathetic nervous system, and that a blockage of the venous drainage vessels has an inhibiting effect on the afferent arteries which may even bring the circulation to a standstill. The affected areas inevitably suffer from asphyxiation during the rewarming phase unless the blockage of the microcirculation and the venous drainage vessels is stopped before the oxygen requirement of the tissue increases critically, when the tissue metabolism begins to function again at above around 6°C. It was not possible to risk using haemodilution in the Himalayas until Klövekorn had begun his experiments in Boston with Moore (Klövekorn et al. 1973) and a team under Messmer in Munich at the Institute of Surgical Research had discovered the biological effects of hae-modilution on animals. From the numerous publications of this group of authors we ob-tained the most important data to be able to give an impression in particular of the changes in the haemodynamics and the oxygen supply to the tissue.

According to Klövekorn et al. (1975), neither the arterial mean pressure nor the central venous pressure changed in animals to any appreciable degree due to isovolaemic dilution. The heart rate remained constant and as can be seen on many diagrams the blood pressure amplitudes stayed at about the same height. PCO_2 and the pH values hardly changed at all (Figs. 74 and 75). As early as 1970 Sunder-Plassmann et al. had registered an increase in the cardiac output and the stroke volume and minute volume in animals due to haemo-dilution with volume replacement (dextran 60), if the viscosity of the blood had been artificially lowered parallel to the haematocrit value. These observations were later cli-nically confirmed on a larger number of patients. The decrease in the oxygen binding power of the blood caused by the removal of erythrocytes was fully compensated by the relief and the increase in the supply of blood to the tissue and organs. The extraction of oxygen from the red blood corpuscles was not thereby increased since the arteriovenous

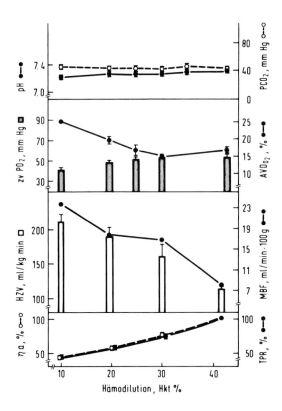

Fig. 74. Behaviour of haemodynamic and blood chemistry parameters during isovolaemic haemodilution with dextran 60 (mean values ± SEM)

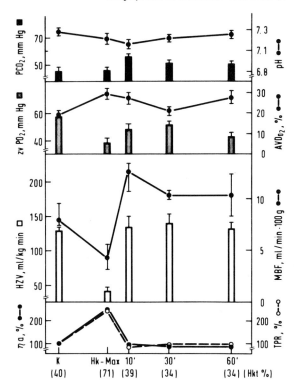

Fig. 75. Behaviour of haemodynamic and blood chemistry parameters during acute haemoconcentration and subsequent haemodilution with dextran 40 (mean values ± SEM; K: control value; max: maximum haemoconcentracion)

difference proved to be almost constant. The venous oxygen pressure and content also remained high enough so that there was no danger of hypoxia. The authors were able to establish that isovolaemic haemodilution to haemocrit values of 25–30 Vol.% could be endured without any danger occurring provided that no cardiac insufficiency was present (which must be considered as a contra-indication) (Fig. 74).

The blood viscosity as well as the colloidosmotic pressure are clearly decreased by haemodilution (Klövekorn et al. 1975; Peter and Lutz 1975). Inspite of a reduction in the oxygen capacity and a lowering of the haemoglobin values, there is no significant drop in the oxygen supply to the tissue (Lake et al. 1972). Via special investigations on the O_2 diffusion – the oxygen pressure with haematocrit values of 20–45 Vol% – this reaction was confirmed in the muscles, the liver, the kidneys, the pancreas and the small intestine (Messmer 1972, 1975). The most favourable effect lies around 30% haematocrit, (corresponds to 10 gr % hgb), the lowest clinically tolerable value is about 25%. Below 20% the oxygen supply to the capillaries deteriorates critically (Messmer and Sunder-Plassmann 1973). If the flow velocity in the terminal vessels drops below a certain critical level, there is actually a prestatic increase in viscosity (Sunder-Plassmann, Messmer). As early as 1969 Weatherley and White et al. (1969) associated the "sludging phenomenon" of the erythrocytes with an increase in the viscosity of the whole bloodstream accompanied by a decrease in the plasma viscosity. A thinning of the blood should therefore counteract the sludging, the clot formation and the infarction. Within the framework of cold action it is above all of importance to maintain the functioning of the microcirculation and of the venolum

181

veins, occasioned by a lowering of the haematocrit, as well as of the peripheral resistance in the endovascular system with an increase in the fluidity of the blood (Fig. 75).

In this way the blood can circulate more freely and quickly and the venous blood supply through and from the heart is encouraged. The clotting factor of the blood changes according to the degree of the thinning. The fibrinogen concentration is decreased. The proportion of blood platelets decreases in accordance with the withdrawal of blood. Prothrombin time and partial thromboplastin time are extended in the normal range. No signs of an increased tendency to haemorrhage were observed during operations after haemodilution.

The impressive part of the procedure is the improvement or maintenance of the microcirculation, which, after a haemorrhagic shock and also after exposure, is severely restricted or even interrupted (Chien 1967). It has even been established that, thanks to blood thinning of the nature of haemodilution, the number of cases of thrombo-embolisms dropped statistically (Messmer to be published).

The fact that it is possible to avoid a transfusion of blood from another person by reinfusing the patient's own blood is considered a favourable side-effect.

In 1977 Zink et al. referred to the special conditions which prevail in high mountains. From personal experience he confirmed that, thanks to haemodilution, the oxygen supply to the microcirculation is improved and the functional capacity of the organism preserved. The improved heat supply to the limbs has a favourable prophylactic effect on the development of cold damage to the extremities, quite apart from the fact that due to the reduction of the viscosity of the blood the heart is under considerably less strain.

At high altitudes one is always concerned with a combination of hypoxia, a reduced oxygen partial pressure and also with an unavoidable, abnormal loss of water, which leads to haemoconcentration. It has been shown that this loss of water can barely be made up by an intake of 3-4 litres of water per day. Oliguria also often occurs in high mountains, i.e. there is a considerable decrease in urination. The haematocrit values rise on an average to the high but still acceptable levels of 0.6–0.7. They are not only the result of high-altitude poliglobulism after acclimatisation but of an abnormal loss of water, which automatically leads to haemoconcentration and an increase in viscosity. Apart from the administration of large quantities of water, solutions containing proteins are also used at high altitudes in order to counteract the abnormal loss of water.

Treatment of Localised Cold Damage

The procedures for the treatment of localised cold damage comprise such an assortment of prescriptions, methods and processes that it is very difficult to obtain an accurate impression of the usefulness of the individual measures.

Sapin-Jaloustre (1956) refers, quite rightly, to a chaos of therapeutic data and lashes out at any enthiusiastic praise of a certain method. When one knows that the causes of cold damage are of varying kinds, one is forced to deduce that no one single medicament or method can ever be one hundred per cent successful (as has often been maintained). Apart from this fact, it is quite certain that those tissues, the fate of which has already been decided before the beginning of treatment, can no longer be saved by any therapeutic measure whatsoever.

As it is very important with cold injuries at what stage in their development the patient comes for treatment, it is necessary to make a fundamental distinction between the methods of early treatment and those for manifest cold damage and delayed damage. As is natural the initial emphasis is on the former. We understand here the thawing out of a cold damaged area and treatment within the first few hours or days after exposure. Fortunately it has been shown that many methods of early treatment have later proved to have beneficial effects.

Treatment of localised frostbite, which does not take account of the general condition of the body is inappropriate and misguided. A prerequisite for the success of local treatment is the warming of the whole body, so that the circulation can begin to function properly again. As long as the patient is still cold and his temperature is still too low, no lasting results can be expected from the application of heat to the extremities. On the contrary we strive to warm the centre of the body so that the peripheral blood vessels are reopened in the interests of physical heat regulation. The means which are available for this were out-lined in our monograph on cold injuries (Killian 1966).

Occasionally difficulties may arise if the patient has not only suffered localised frostbite, but at the same time another injury too, so that it is not possible, for example, to warm up the whole body in a hot bath. In such cases one must use other methods to quickly warm up the body, e.g. wrapping it in hot, wet cloths.

Shivering can incidentally be overcome by means of calming the autonomous nervous system, and also with endo-anaesthesia by blocking the cold receptors. Pierau et al. (1965) tried to achieve the same effects on animals with benzonatate (Tessalon). In animal experiments Pierau et al. attempted to eliminate shivering by calming the peripheral cold receptors via endo-anaesthesia with Tessalon (an ether). This can also be achieved with sedatives. In our opinion it does not seem advisable to use this method since shivering is a natural defence reaction against loss of heat through the creation of additional heat, which should not be counteracted.

Whereas in the past one only recommended warm baths at 39°C or in the case of the politraumatised used hot packs (in Russia in 1941/42 the author also used warm infusions of about 40°-41°C), today we have a whole series of other effective methods of rewarming frozen limbs at our disposal, which can work even in the case of unconsciousness and cardiac arrest due to cold. Besides short-wave therapy which can be applied locally (Hirsch et al. 1977; Leitner and Kronberger (1977), gastric lavages with hot solutions (Lee et al. 1959) and transperitoneal dialysis of the stomach, as well as artificial respiration with damp, warm air (Lloyd et al. 1972; Shanka 1975), were reported to be effective. Of particular importance, in our opinion, in the case of cardiac arrest due to exposure is the lavage of the pericardium with a warm, sterilised isotonic saline solution or with Ringer's solution.

An impressive incident reported by Höflin (1977) at the conference of alpine rescue physicians in Innsbruck in 1976 is proof of the extraordinary rescue work which can be achieved with this method (see p. 12).

The water- and windproof gold/silver aluminium foil, which was developed by W. Soehngen, has become indispensable for saving body-heat and protecting from coldness in various kinds of accidents and especially in cases of injured persons who were exposed to the cold. Electric blankets which are heated beforehand should not be used, not packs, however, are recommended (Neureuther-Flora). Both authors recommend the Hibler pack, which is similar to the old Priesnitz pack.

The technique: A five times folded linen cloth is soaked with hot water from a thermos bottle and is not put on the skin, but on the underwear which covers the breast and abdominal regions. Sweater, anorak are pulled over it. The whole body is wrapped in aluminium foil.

F.K. Pierau, K.O. Plesch and F.W. Klüssmann tried to eliminate the cold tremors by means of endo-anesthesia with tessalon (kind of ether) in experiments in order to sedate the peripheral receptors of coldness. This can also be produced by sedatives. Such a procedure, however, does not appear to be recommendable, because the cold tremors belong to the natural physical mechanisms of protection from coldness in order to produce additional body-heat, which should not be cut off if the glycogen reserves are not too much exhausted.

Attention has been drawn to the fact that when the body and the blood are cold the effect of well-known medicaments may be reserved and toxic, so that they should be avoided. The same applies in the early treatment of frostbite since all vasoconstrictive preparations of the adrenaline – effetonin ephedrine group which increase the tonus of the sympathetic nervous system must be strictly avoided. Lippros (1942) (Fig. 76) has shown their harmful effects. Stronger doses of painkillers, hypnotics or narcotics should not be administered since they in fact lead to a gradual centralisation of the circulation, to vasoconstriction and a decrease in blood pressure with a reduction of the oscillographic pressure amplitudes and thus to a noticeable deterioration in the peripheral circulation. This also includes opiates such as morphine and also barbiturates of the hexobarbital-sodium type.

Treatment of Early Cases

Thanks to our present-day knowledge of the development of cold injuries the aim of treatment must be to get the circulation in the threatened tissue areas working again as quickly as possible. This fulfills the dual aim of rewarming the affected limb via the blood and of carrying out this rewarming process without sensitive phases of oxygen deficiency of the tissue, i.e. without the development of a regional asphyxiation metabolism. This can be

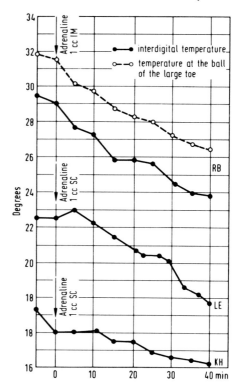

Fig. 76. Interdigital temperature changes and temperature changes at the ball of the large toes after adrenaline in various patients. *R B*, 60-year-old with pernicious anaemia; *L E*, 32-year-old girl with arterial spasms in the hands; *K H*, 18-year-old girl with acroasphyxia. (From Lippross 1942)

most easily achieved if the limb which has been exposed is still cold when it is submitted for treatment, so that the thawing process is under the control of the physician himself. In most cases the patients reach us too late, which makes it all the more important for the layman to be generally well informed. Several processes of rewarming have been developed for early treatment:

a) Cool treatment or the refrigeration technique.
b) So-called physiological rewarming at room temperature without additional, artificial means.
c) The recently suggested and frequently recommended artificial rapid rewarming of a fresh cold injury.

Cool Treatment and the Refrigeration Technique

The method so often practised in the last century of rubbing a cold limb with snow can be traced back to a recommendation of Larrey's during Napoleon's Russian campaign in 1813.

He believed that it was sufficient to rub the frozen limbs with snow to start the circulation moving again and achieve a gradual rewarming. He applied the cold snow with every

185

intention of avoiding too rapid a rewarming, since he had observed the most dreadful results from this. This method is considered obsolete today. It led not only in some cases to a deterioration of the cold injury but the helper himself often contracted frostbite too on his hands and fingers. This unfavourable experience is similar to that made by famous Polar explorers such as Scott, Byrd and Shackleton, who totally rejected such methods. A final attempt with this technique was apparently made by Greene during the British Himalaya expedition in 1941 and 1942 and by American surgeons, such as Edholm (1952), Heaton and Davis (1952), Canty and Sharf (1953) and Pratt (1953) during the Korean campaign in 1952/53. They all gave up this from of cool treatment at once in favour of a gradual rewarming.

Refrigeration treatment of manifest cold injuries at an advanced stage of development was recommended by Webster et al. (1942), and Greene in 1942, White and Scoville (1945) considered this method at that time even to mean great progress, since it alleviated the acute pain and still allowed regeneration. If airflow cooling, (which certainly has advantages) was not sufficient to stop the pain caused by oxygen starvation, cooling with icebags or in iceboxes (as for regional hibernation according to Allen) was even used. As a rule three to four icebags were enough, which were renewed every 3 to 4 h. This treatment was extended for up to 2 weeks and then the limb was gradually warmed, as with Bundschuh's method. Severe cold injuries were supposed to have been avoided in this way.

If a limb has been cooled in this manner the blood supply to the damaged area is sensitively reduced and disturbed for a long time and, according to experimental and clinical results, probably more harm than good is done, since the nerves and blood vessels are not able to stand cooling for a longer period, even though the drop in temperature makes them resistent to oxygen deficiency. This is why many authors such as Davis et al. (1943), Lange and Loewe (1946), Lange et al. (1947, 1950, 1955), Lempke and Shumaker (1949), Quintanilla (1947), Crismon and Fuhrmann (quoted according to Sapin-Jaloustre 1956), Ariev (1937, 1939a, b, 1950), Bellander (1940 a, b), Killian (1946, 1959, 1972) rejected the refrigeration technique in the treatment of cold injuries.

Although we have recommended keeping the peripheral frozen areas relatively cool while the centre of the body is being rewarmed, this has nothing to do with proper 'refrigeration'. It simply means that temperatures of $8°$ to $14°C$ are used, i.e. temperatures which enable the metabolism to start functioning again without the oxygen requirement of the tissue becoming too high. The aim of this is simply to keep the groups of tissues still relatively resistent to an oxygen deficiency during the thawing process and the time of the regeneration of the peripheral circulation.

Sudden changes in temperature from $+32°C$ to $-13°C$ room temperature always cause a rapid reduction in the supply of blood to the toes and fingers which is followed by a slow and almost linear drop in the skin temperature (cf. Abrammson's summary of 1944).

It was seen that the toes and fingers warmed up by far the most quickly and the best when the centre of the body was kept warm or was heated up which is of utmost importance from a practical point of view.

Physiological Method of Rewarming

For many mild cases of cold injury it is sufficient to rewarm the central part of the body and to leave the extremities at room temperature to warm themselves alone via the blood-stream. Then a slow, spontaneous rewarming of the limbs can be observed. This procedure was referred to in 1919 as the "physiological rewarming method" according to Grezellier, and in 1939 further developed by Fievez in as far as the latter made his patients practise active gymnastic exercises of the extremities at room temperature, to improve the circulation and to stimulate natural heat production in the muscles.

Slow Active Rewarming

During the second world war and the Korean campaign nearly all surgeons used exclusively a very guarded technique of rewarming. In general the technical practice involved the frozen limb being put as a whole into a luke-warm bath, the temperature of the limb was slowly brought up to 4°C by the addition of hot water. In Switzerland the technique of slowly thawing freshly frozen limbs by gradually heating a bath from about 10°C to 40°C is attri-buted to Campbell (1952, 1966, 1977). It was, however, already carried out between 1914–18 by most surgeons at the front on the German side. Campbell's vast experience (Pontresina) confirms the intense pain, which is caused by rapid rewarming, which should be avoided since it leads indirectly to renewed secretion of adrenaline and noradrenaline, thereby causing vasoconstriction. During the gradual thawing out process the skin slowly becomes red, softer and more elastic, so that the patient is more easily able to move his limbs by himself.

   If this commonly practised technique does not meet with our approval this is due to consideration of the fact that the peripheral frostbitten areas are often already rewarmed, before an adequate flow of blood is able to supply the oxygen requirement of the tissue. Those who practise this method create in the extremities the very conditions which lead to the development of a local asphyxiation metabolism of the tissue and increase the danger of necrosis. In order to avoid this we have insisted on a gradual rewarming of the limbs to be effected via the blood after the main part of the body has been rewarmed, furthermore on having the cooled limbs cold, in order to allow the organism to go on warming up milli-meter for millimeter in the direction of the periphery. A cool air flow from a ventilator is sufficient to keep the extremities cold.

   It seems in the meantime to have become generally accepted that it is of the utmost importance to warm the centre of the body before or during the thawing out of the extre-mities as suggested by us, since it is stressed repeatedly in relevant literature (Campbell et al. 1946; Guerasimenko 1950; Judmaier 1952 a, b; Douglas 1952).

Rapid Rewarming

As early as 1917 Lake attempted rapid rewarming experimentally and clinically on mild cold injuries without achieving any success. Later Ariev (1937, 1939 a, b) and Girgolaw (1943) carried out primitive animal experiments by freezing rabbit ears with an ethyl chloride spray and made comparisons between a spontaneous rewarming and a rapid re-warming in a hot bath. There were reports of amazing success.

Although after general loss of temperature as the result of a cold accident (e.g. a fall into icy water) rapid rewarming of the whole body is the only correct procedure, on is forced to take into account the dangers of a rewarming collapse (Brendel), since the rescue collapse presents a far greater danger, and such treatment, in the case of peripheral cold damage, gives cause for concern.

Naturally everybody strives to rewarm the organism and improve the circulation as quickly as is appropiate, but it has been observed time and again that the tenet, too rapid rewarming of cooled areas causes harm, is right, and not incorrect as Sapin-Jaloustre claimed. The rapid rewarming of cooled or even frozen groups of tissues, accompanied by a lack of oxygen, has the effect that chemical transformation due to this oxygen deficiency occurs prematurely, which can cause general decay and tissue decay as has been proved by numerous clinical observations since Larrey's (1817) day (e.g. Lewis and Loewe 1926). In this respect we share the view of Paunesco-Podeanu and Tzurai (see their monograph, 1946), who re-jected rapid rewarming on the grounds that it destroyed the tissues.

In the experiments of Brooks and Duncan (1940) the harmful effects of rapid rewarm-ing with ischaemia were made particularly clear. They reported that *the oedema is sub-sequently much more pronounced, the tissue pressure increased, the inflammation and the pain considerably worse and gangrene of the tissue sets in and develops more rapidly.*

It must be admitted that contradictory claims have been made as far as we know by Kreyberg in 1949. We would like to mention here Sapin-Jaloustre who went to great lengths to compile from the whole world literature until 1956 the relevant experimental results on rapid rewarming in animals and in man.

The main error of all these experiments therefore seems to have been that the method of cooling (technique) and its influence on the possibilities of treatment were ignored and the interval between exposure and the beginning of treatment was also disregarded. To test the efficiency of rapid rewarming ultra rapid cooling was used almost exclusively, partly with an ethyl chloride spray, partly with carbon dioxide snow at $-22°C$, partly with cryogen mixtures of up to $-55°C$. Vitrification occurs in these cases, i.e. a fixation of the tissue in an amorphous state without the formation of any harmful, coarse crystals, which is fairly certain to allow recovery at least for a certain time with relatively little damage. If under such experimental conditions rapid rewarming then appears to be successful, this still does not prove anything. On the contrary, the success is deceptive. The tissue is not seriously damaged by the short-term ultra rapid cooling. Therefore rapid rewarming can be tolerated and no damage of an appreciable degree is caused. Unfortunately these factors escaped Sapin-Jaloustre, which accounts for his relatively optimistic assessment of the animal experiments (Harkins and Harmon 1937; Ariev 1939 a, b; Crismon and Fuhrmann 1947; Finneran and Shumaker 1950; Shumaker et al. 1951; Pichotka et al. 1949, 1951 a, b; Entin et al. 1954) — despite very varying results.

In 1977 Höflin, Rahn et al., Perren and Ziegler reported on a new series of experi-ments on the problem of the rapid or slow warming of freshly frozen limbs. The experi-ments were carried out on the anaesthetised ears of rabbits after rapid cooling with alcohol to $-55°C$ and the damaged area thawed according to various methods of rewarm-ing, for example at $-15°C$ for 15 min at $+22°C$ in the open air and by rapid rewarming either from $10°-40°C$ within 10 min or immediately in a warm bath ($+40°-42°C$). In a second series the experiments were repeated using the backs of mice. The authors reported that after 3 weeks' observations the results were better after rapid than after slow rewarming and therefore recommended rapid rewarming for human cold damage, although the unbearable pain which this causes is well known.

The same authors made at the same time histological and radiological studies of the changes to the rabbit's ear after artificially induced cold damage and came to the same conclusion, namely the superiority of rapid rewarming (after rapid cooling with alcohol to $-55°C$). They claim to have observed less necrosis after rewarming. The damage was evidently correlated to the arterial vascular supply and very noticeable calcification of the ear cartilage was observed histologically.

Very few reasonably comparable experiments have been carried out on human beings, e.g. Davis et al. (1943), Adams and Falconer (1951), and Lange et al. (1947). Unfortunately here, too, artificial cooling methods with ethyl chloride spray or carbon dioxide snow, in other words ultra rapid cooling, were mostly used, so that the results remain questionable.

In 1940, at the time of the sea disaster involving the British cruiser "Glorius" before Narvik, Ungley had the opportunity to treat the frozen limbs of the rescued according to the technique of rapid rewarming in a hot bath. He observed *a considerable deterioration of the oedemas and an intensification of the pain,* which at times became unbearable. He apparently did not observe any deterioration in the cold damage but appropriate checks were not made. Furthermore, in 1942, in a case of frostbite on hands and feet Glenn et al. rapidly rewarmed the limbs in a hot bath at $43°-48°C$ without any loss of limb resulting. It is not possible to use such reports since no comparisons exist.

Apparently as early as the Finnish — Russian war Russian doctors attempted rapid rewarming under the influence of Ariev in 1940 and of Girgolaw in 1943, but no reliable reports of success are available. In 1947 Lange et al. created localised cold damage on the thighs of volunteers but did not observe any significant differences afterwards between rapid and slow thawing. Simon and Filhoulaud (1940, 1941) did not achieve better results from rapid thawing either in his experiments compared with the controls, *on the contrary, after rapid thawing the results were worse.* De Bakey came to a similar conclusion in 1947. He confirmed that rapid thawing out can at the most be useful within an hour immediately after exposure.

If one overlooks all these experimental and clinical data one will not be able to help regarding rapid rewarming with great scepsis and only then allow its application in the case of ultra rapid cooling and when treatment can begin within the first hour after exposure.

Vasodilators and Spasmolysants

It was natural to use vasodilating, sympathicolytic, adrenolytic and spasmolytic medicaments in the treatment of arterial cold spasms. It was not until 1941/42 that they were systematically tested. It was hoped in this way not only to improve the circulation and to save areas in danger, but also to counteract thrombosis and secondary necrosis. If the blood vessels are blocked, our medicaments do not reach the required spot irrespective of the manner of application and the effect is therefore questionable in every case.

189

The oral application of preparations which dilate effectively has the advantage that they can be taken at an early stage by the patient himself (e.g. by pilots in action). The number of preparations[1] which were used for this purpose, is very large. An increase in the skin temperature was usually used as a criterion for the effectiveness. A direct improvement in the state of the circulation was sometimes observed too, and the recovery of functioning registered.

Papaverine, Eupaco, Eupaverin, Aminophylline (Euphyllin)

Numerous surgeons including the author started in the disastrous winter of 1941/42 to try to relax arterial spasms by administering papaverine and eupaco suppositories. The results were not satisfactory however. See, here, the reports made by Starlinger (1942) von Brandis (1943 a, b), Wagner (1915), Gerlach (1943), Killian (1946, 1959, 1972), Adams (1941, 1942 a, b, 1944, 1952, 1956) and many others. It was not until 1947 that Quintanilla et al. tried to influence cold injuries by using papaverine on rabbit ears. He was not successful.

The effectiveness of the derivates of papaverine, eupaverin and euphyllin (administered in a glucose solution) was somewhat better, but still left a lot to be desired, which may be connected with the fact that the reactions of cooled blood vessels are very poor and the required effect does not appear until after thawing out (as opposed to the effect of adrenaline which is resistent to cold). Nevertheless in 1942 v. Schürer and Starlinger appear to have achieved relatively good results with the intra-arterial administration of a eupaverin-glucose solution. The pain in the frostbitten area is said to have disappeared quickly and the circulation to have improved.

Priscol

Attempts were also made to treat early cases of cold injury with Priscol. We were not, however, able to achieve any definite success with it. This preparation mainly affects the arterioles and the arterial capillaries. This is the reason why Priscol has proved to be of service in the treatment of frost damage, chilblains and delayed damage. In 1951 Fishman treated cold damage with 25 mg of Priscol per day over a period of six months and was apparently successful. Adams and Falconer also claimed in 1951 to have been successful in treating the severe frostbite of a skier with Priscol (Figs. 77 and 78).

Padutin

Padutin has also been disappointing in the early treatment of cold injuries. The depot Padutin was frequently used in the treatment of the remaining damage to the blood vessels.

---

1 In the following section only those medicaments are listed which were really tried out on a large scale in the treatment of cold injuries!

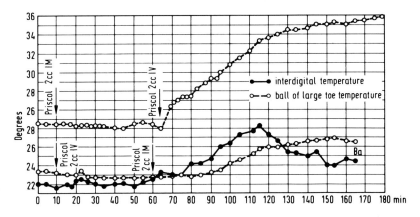

Fig. 77. Effect of *Priscol* injections (I V and I M) in a 48-year-old man with varicous vein complaints (Bu), and also in a 55-year-old diabetic patient with paraesthesias of the feet (Ba). The first injection was not responsive, the second had an effect on the vessels. Measurements taken at the finger tips and balls of the toes. (From Lippross 1942)

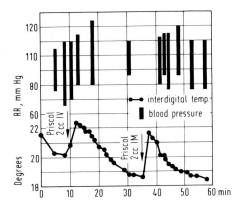

Fig. 78. Comparison of the Priscol effect on the interdigital temperature and blood pressure in a 26-year-old patient with acrocyanosis of the hands. (From Lippross 1942)

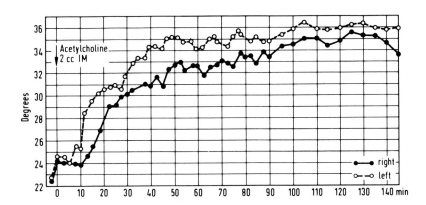

Fig. 79. Interdigital temperature after injection of 2 ml *acetylcholine* intramuscularly in a 57-year-old woman with a spastic circulatory disturbance owing to scleroderma of the finger. (From Lippross 1942)

Histamine and Acetylcholine

Quintanilla et al. in 1947 and also Meiding and Kolsky in 1953 tried in experiments on rabbit ears to relax the cold spasm and dilate the blood vessels in cold injuries produced by using an ethyl chloride spray by applying histamine. Their results, however, were not favourable. Gill found acetylcholine to be totally ineffective on 2nd and 3rd degree cold injuries, sometimes even harmful. The reports of Ullarthet (1931), Saltner (1940), Bohnstedt (1932) and Adams (1944) on the use of acetylcholine are equally doubtful. No clear improvements were observed. These negative reports are in accordance with the findings of Monsaignon (1940 a, b). In 1943 Kutschera—Aichen and Bergen ventured to administer acetycholine intravenously without being able to improve the results to any appreciable degree. Despite these, on the whole, negative results acetylcholine is still used occasionally on cold spasms and circulatory disturbances (Figs. 79 and 80).

Ergot Alkaloids

These derivatives of ergot are of importance in the relaxation of arterial cold spasms because of their marked sympathomimetic effect, as has been shown partly experimentally, partly clinically *Hydergine* was mostly used. It must be remembered that Hydergine or droperiodol cause a decrease in the blood pressure and in particular in the body temperature. The effectiveness of Hydergine is supported by the experience of Tiel and Schneider (1949), who were able to show in cold experiments on rabbit ears that it relaxes arterial cold spasms and improves the blood circulation. The disadvantage of this method is an increased development of oedemas in the affected areas, which generally does not occur if the arterial spasms relax spontaneously.

In 1951 Hurley et al. carried out cold experiments on rat tails (anaesthetised using Nembutal). The artificially induced frostbite was treated with a mixture of ergot alkaloids, partly orally, partly by injection (with intervals of 6 h). An improvement was apparently observed or a decrease in the loss of tissue. In the controls necrosis of 4.8 cm diameter usually developed, in the animals under treatment of only 1.35 cm.

In 1952 Hurley et al. repeated these experiments on rats under high altitude conditions, i.e. with a lower O_2 tension and at low temperatures. After freezing they administered Hydergine (orally or by injection). They achieved the best results when the Hydergine had already been administered before the development of the frostbite. In these cases

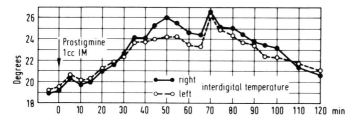

Fig. 80. Effect of intramuscular injection of *Prostigmine* on the interdigital temperature in a 21-year-old girl with acrocyanosis. (From Lippross 1942)

the loss of tissue in the animals under treatment was only 64% (until the 30th day of treatment) compared with 84% in the controls. As a side—effect, however, a considerable increase in the death-rate of the experiment animals was observed, apparently due to a disturbance in the heat balance or damage to the hypothalamus.

The effectiveness of the ergot alkaloids was checked by Lewis and Moen in 1953 in experiments on rabbit paws, but it was not confirmed. An increase in the death rate of the animals was once again observed.

In 1953 Meiding and Kolsky tested two sympathicolytic experiment preparations in comparison with anti-histamines by producing artificial cold injuries on rabbit ears using an ethyl chloride spray. The oedemas became worse but the scabbing formation was apparently less.

Chalinot et al. reported in 1954 having been successful with the administration of Hydergine in two cases of cold injury.

Ganglionic Blocking Agents

Very few surgeons have so far used endo-anaesthesia with procaine i.v. (given to tone down the whole autonomous nervous system and in particular for vasoconstriction) in the treatment of cold injuries. It was known that American surgeons used as an infusion the Osaka anti-frost solution, which contains a procaine additive. Its composition: 12 ccm alcohol, 250 mg procaine, 250 ml 5% glucose and heparine additive. As this solution also contains alcohol and heparine, it is not possible to exactly assess the effectiveness of procaine or other local anaesthetics which are suitable for endo-anaesthesia.

In 1950 Finneran and Shumaker tested ammonium on rats and rabbits and were said to have been successful. They began treatment after cold damage set in and apparently obtained 97.3% very good results without necrosis or with only slight necrosis (of 1.4 cm diameter), compared with only 8.8% good results without necrosis (diameter of 3.6 cm) in the controls. The time factor is of importance; within the 1st h there was an increase in the successful cases, after the 1st h no further favourable effects could be registered.

The experiments of Entin and Baxter of 1952, who used hexamethonium on dogs and rats are also worth mentioning. Only a slight decrease in the loss of tissue of 42.8% in the animals under treatment was observed compared with 50% in the controls. In a second series of experiments using hexamethonium bromide and pentamenthonium bromide starting 24 h earlier) the loss of tissue in rats was 42% compared with 51% in the controls and in animals, which had not been anaesthetised, 22.3% compared with 24.4% in the controls.

As early as 1948 Holmes reported on a case of 3rd degree frostbite which he had successfully treated with tetraethylammonium. It was said to have healed quickly.

The experience gained during the Korean war is of decisive importance for the assessment of the value of vasodilators in the early treatment of cold injuries, especially that of Talbott, Movrey and Farago, Orr and Fainer, all from 1952.

Movrey and Farago (1952) used the Osaka anti-frost solution in 593 cases of frostbite for the treatment of early cases without having any convincing success. During the third hypoxaemic phase with disturbed circulation besides procaine they also used ronicol and priscol, furthermore moderate amounts of whisky (56 − 113 g daily). The authors observed, with a decrease in the arterial blood pressure, an increase in the skin temperature. Their optimistic reports contradict, however, the findings of other surgeons. In 1952, for example, in 1.880 cases of cold injury in Korea Orr and Fainer applied vasodilators between the 2nd and the 15th day after exposure, but observed no success in comparison with their control cases.

Talbott (1952), who administered alcohol (IV) and hexamethonium, priscol and niacine came to the same negative conclusions, as did Heaton and Davis, also in 1952.

As early as 1950 Avena et al. had reached the opinion that in the acute stage of a cold injury vasodilators do more harm than good. In 1951 Blain went even further: he claimed that tetraethylammonium was of more harm than of good service as a blocking agent.

In 1951 in a summary Shumaker and Lempke objected to the use of this group of medicaments. Vagliano (1948) had already passed the same negative judgement when he expressed the belief that Padutin, Acetylcholine, Papaverine, Priscol, Acrotherm, Euphyllin and Amynitrite are of no use in the early treatment of frostbite.

After all this it must be admitted that neither in experiments nor on human beings has it so far been possible to produce exact evidence of the favourable therapeutic influence of vasodilators in the early treatment of cold damage. They do, on the other hand, undoubtedly possess a certain therapeutic value in the treatment of the circulatory disturbances which occur later.

Porter and Wäsche recently attempted to block the sympathetic nervous system intra-arterially with 0.25 − 0.5 mg of Reserpine in five cases of fresh cold damage to the hands. The fact that the peripheral arteriospasm had been relaxed was proved after a preliminary check by means of an arteriogram. In 1975 Porter and Reiney had already studied the effects of small doses of Reserpine on the Norefedrin content of the vascular wall. See also the data provided by de Jong and Golding and Sawyer (1962) on local sympathectomies after cold injuries.

Fever Treatment

The disappointment which we experienced with vasodilators in the early treatment of frostbite, forced us to look for new methods. Thus my idea was conceived to warm the body and the limbs internally via the blood by artificially creating a fever. In 1941 − 43 this at first seemed absurd. When the blood was heated the body was naturally forced to emit heat, i.e. the physical heat regulation started to function, the peripheral arteries including the terminal vessels opened, and there was an increase in infrared radiation and a moistening of the skin. At first no one knew, however, whether it would be possible, by intentionally regulating the heat balance with pyrogenic substances, to relax the cold spasm in the arteries. Fortunately we were not mistaken in believing it might be possible. This method of vasodilation even proved to be much more effective than vasodilating medicaments. The concern of specialists in internal medicine, who feared collapse symptoms as the result of peripheral vasodilation, proved to be unfounded. Besides, with centrally induced fever there is an increase in the chemical heat production, so that subsequently, by way of adjustment, the physical heat regulation started to function. Here the danger of an acute decrease in blood pressure with collapse symptoms was far smaller.

The fact that regulating reactions are able to withstand different kinds of resistance was already known to Rein (1943). He considered them to be of a dominating character. Rein had observed such reactions during the relaxation of an arterial adrenaline spasm. In the past Häusler (1943) was able to provide evidence of the fact that in cold injury experiments no positive results worthy of mention could be achieved by localised rewarming, whereas a rewarming of the whole body or a centrally induced rewarming by means of fever preparations proved to be effective and successful.

During the search for an appropriate preparation for the artificial creation of fever we selected the weakest dose of Pyrifer, a pyrogenic substance from the coli bacterium instead of milk (Caputo 1941; Cianotti 1942; Nowack 1942). v. Schürer (1942) undertook similar experiments with typhoid vaccine.

Pyrifer was only used when the patient showed no signs of a high temperature caused by the cold damage itself. The Pyrifer 1 was injected in intervals of 2 − 3 days, beginning as early as possible. As the rise in the blood and the body temperature does not occur until 4 − 6 h after the intravenous administration of Pyrifer the interim period must be bridged with other thawing methods. Pyrifer usually takes 2 days to take effect. Subsequently it is possible to give further injections. The rise in temperature of the limbs is greater than that in the centre of the body. In the damaged areas, for example, one finds a rise in temperature $3° − 9.3°$ C, whereas in the centre of the body it is only $2° − 3°$ C.

The lower the initial temperature of the limb is, the poorer the circulation, the greater the changes are. As a rule the cold oedemas are seen to disappear quickly, the tissue pressure to become reduced, and the local blood supply to improve.
Furthermore, progressive rewarming with a rapid return of feeling is observed. In the case of marked oedemas it is possible to avoid incisions. The demarcation lines move towards the periphery and show a fresh redness. The healing process is speeded up. Unpleasant pain and sensations of various kinds quickly recede. An improvement in the patient's circulation is noticed subjectively at an early stage by a tingling sensation, itching and a feeling of thawing. Some areas which had initially lost all feeling become sensitised again. A delayed rise in the body and blood temperatures after the administration of Pyrifer is always a bad sign and indicates danger.

Not only do the oedemas rapidly disappear, the vesicles dry up and the swellings disappear, but as a rule rapid epithelialisation of the open spots is observed. In addition, dry mummification, in tissue areas which were already bound to become necrotic before the beginning of treatment, occurs more quickly. With this method we never saw a case of wet-type gangrene. The time of treatment was also shortened.

Comparative experiments carried out by Gerlach have proved that fever treatment with Pyrifer is far superior to the administration of vasodilating preparations such as eupaverin and Euphyllin and corresponds approximately to periarterial anaesthesia or to the blocking of the sympathetic nervous system.

In 1943/44 Killian, Vogt, Hemmer and Koch investigated the effects of fever treatment on the circulation via the sphygmographic method according to Brömser and discovered that fever action is the counterpart of cold action (Killian et al. 1946). It leads to a rapid movement of the extracellular water from the tissue back into the blood vessels and the state of the whole circulation is thus improved.

At the same time a rapid compensation of the disturbances in the mineral metabolism, the water distribution and the osmotic state takes place.

195

Similar conclusions were reached by Reigber (1945), who discovered that the rise in temperature due to the induction of artificial fever after cold damage is as a rule much greater than in cases of manifest endangiitis obliterans, Raynaud's gangrene or vascular sclerosis, which shows to what extent the arteriospasm is due to poor circulation. In the past Lewis (1951, 1952) found out that the lower extremities possess a greatly increased vasomotorial tonus. He did not succeed, in the hot—box, in counteracting this tonus. We, on the other hand, had no difficulty with centrally induced fever in overcoming and relaxing the spasm of the arterial blood vessel. See also the experiments of Killian et al. (1946).

It has been known for some time that during fever a decrease in the blood pressure occurs. According to Schleicher and Gligore (1946) it affects the systolic as well as the diastolic blood pressure. After the fever has gone down this is compensated. In our own series of experiments the mean blood pressure also dropped as the temperature rose. The highest point of the fever curve usually coincides with the lowest blood pressure values, only in exceptional cases are the reactions delayed. The blood pressure amplitudes increase as the temperature rises, which indicates that the amount of blood flowing is greater. This fact was not noticed by Schleicher and Gligore (1946).

The elastic resistance in the wind kessel blood vessel, particularly in the aorta, increases. The total peripheral resistance, on the other hand, decreases regularly. The reaction of the cardiac output varies according to the initial state. The minute volume increases regularly during fever. This corresponds to a general mobilisation of the circulation in the interests of heat regulation, which, in Kirsch's and Bruns' investigations too, is expressed in an increase in the basal metabolic rate. In our experiments the heart action and output varied to such an extent that no conclusions could be drawn.

Parallel to the sphygmographic method according to Brömser we also applied the carbon monoxide method in some cases to determine the amount of blood flowing and also found an increase in the amount of blood circulating during fever. At the same time the number of erythrocytys in cm^3 of blood usually increased, as did the value for the haemoglobin in the blood. On the other hand the plasma protein content dropped slightly during the fever period, which corresponds to the afflux of a larger quantity of fluid from the extracellular areas.

The development of hydraemia of the blood during fever, a movement of the fluid into the blood vessels, is well known. By many it is considered as a pre—requisite for the increased release of water through the skin in the interests of physical heat regulation. We may consider hydraemia of the blood caused by artificial fever, not only as an expression of the mobilisation of quantities of blood which had been immobile, or of the releasing of blood depots, but we are also forced to explain it as the result of the migration of water from the tissue, a factor which is of particular service during the fever treatment of cold damage. *Whereas the cold has the effect of causing anhydraemia and an increase in the water content of the tissue, the fever treatment forces a reversal and the compensation of this disorder.* The increase in the erythrocyte content and the haemoglobin values often observed despite the thinning of the blood, are, in our opinion, to be understood as the release of the body's erythrocyte depot, in particular from the spleen.

Reduction of Viscosity by Artificial Thinning of Blood

After the Swiss surgeon, Kronecker, in 1886 in Berne, had successfully attempted for the first time to give animals an infusion of isotonic saline solution in the treatment of depression of the circulation, shock and acute loss of blood, this method was commonly used in the mastering of circulatory conditions in which there was a danger to life and in general life saving. Even in the First World War one had no other choice. It was still not possible then to make up the blood volume with colloidal solutions, since these did not then exist. At that time only a few physicians ventured to carry out direct blood transfusions for fear of serious complications due to incompatibility. In the Second World War colloidal blood substitutes, such as 6% − 7% glucose solutions and Polyvinylpyrrolidone (Periston, Weese), were introduced. We were also able to give blood transfusions according to blood groups. Banked blood was available and later also human serum or dried human plasma.

The search for possibilities of reducing the viscosity of the whole bloodstream and thereby of increasing the fluidity of the blood, in order to avoid a critical slowing down of the circulation during exposure, sludging of the erythrocytes, congestion and finally stasis and agglutination thrombosis, so that the microcirculation is maintained, appears to be fully justified, especially as hopes cherished in connection with the use of anticoagulants were shattered. From the impression that one gains today it, in fact seems to be more important to facilitate and encourage the reduction of viscosity during exposure than to reduce the clotting properties of the blood. This treatment usually comes too late. Although haemodilution has so far only been used as a prophylactic measure on expeditions at high altitudes, before special kinds of operations or after a loss of blood of 1000 − 2000 ml, there is a chance that positive results may also be achieved with it within the framework of the early treatment of cold injuries, in other words, during the thawing out period, and that one may be able to limit the danger of loss of tissue. Rieger et al. (quoted according to Messmer) have also noticed advantages to haemodilution in the treatment of arterial occlusion.

As early as 1964 Mundt et al. tried to thin the blood using dextran in the treatment of fresh cold injuries to the limbs and reported good results. In 1971 Gödecke tried the same during the rewarming of the whole body with simultaneous alkalisation of the organism and administration of noradrenaline, artificial respiration and fibrinolytic treatment.

In 1974 Kyösola and Trasima also used low−molecular dextran solution to prevent a failure of the microcirculation and the beginning of stasis. He only obtained positive results, however, during early treatment. After 24 h, i.e. after the completion of thrombosis in the terminal vessels, no further favourable effect could be achieved. The intravascular obstruction could no longer be removed.

Today we have quite a number of different colloidal solutions at our disposal for the artificial thinning of the blood, leading to a subsequent decrease in viscosity, improvement in the fluidity and maintenance of the microcirculation during exposure. Apart from dextran (40 and 60) as was used from 1971 by Sunder−Plassmann et al. and Messmer et al., and Macrodex and Rheo−macrodex, today we also have Emagel, Gelfundel, Neo−Plasmagel and Physiogel, in addition, Haemaccel (with a gelatine base (Muscha-

197

weck) and 5% human albumin, as well as Bisko from the Biotest Int. Frankfurt. A 6% solution of hydroxyl-ethyl starch (HES) was also tried (Kettler et al. 1976).

Genuine isovolumetric haemodilution should be more effective than a pure infusion, i.e. a blood sample of 500 – 750 ml (erythrocyte sample) with subsequent retransfusion of the patient's own blood, provided that there is no injury or wound causing heavy loss of blood.

If cold damage has occurred after an injury the anaesthetist or surgeon will have to decide in each individual case whether a simple infusion to thin the blood can or must suffice or whether, on the other hand, one can attempt haemodilution. No large scale control experiments have yet been carried out to provide information on the usefulness of the method for such purposes.

All colloidal blood substitutes can cause anaphylactoid reactions. These must be taken into account, if there are advantages to carrying out haemodilution. They are in fact very unusual and for all preparations the number is about the same. In 1977, for example, Ring and Messmer quoted the following values: for protein plasma solution: 0.003%, for hydroxy-ethyl starch: 0.005% and for dextran: 0.008%.

A greater danger is a blocking of the kidneys. Corticoids can be of service in the case of severe allergic reactions.

Anticoagulants and Fibrinolytics

In 1942 Siegmund (a-c), Behrens (unpublished data) and Bigelow carried out experiments on cold injuries using heparin. This treatment is based on the assumption that congestion of the blood and thrombosis of the total venous drainage vessels in the frostbitten area is the main or a partial cause of the damage, and that one can expect to see an improvement in the healing process if clotting is prevented. Actually an error in reasoning has slipped in here, since at the beginning of treatment the arteriospasm is usually still present, the blockage of the veins and the venous plexuses already completed, so that the heparin will have difficulty reaching the area where it could be effective. This must be the explanation for some of the failures with this kind of treatment.

In 1956 Sapin—Jaloustre made the great effort of compiling all the available information on such experiments.

It is mainly the experiments and reports of success of Lange et al. (1947, 1950) and other colleagues which attracted considerable attention, since they claimed to have achieved 96% to 100% successfully healed cases compared with the controls. Other authors also reported favourable results after treatment with heparin, e.g. Shumaker in 1947, Shumaker et al., and Wrenn and Sandford in 1947, Finneran and Shumaker in 1950, Lempke and Shumaker in 1949 and Shumaker and Lempke in 1951, although to a far more modest extent.

In comparison with this a large number of animal experiments showed no favourable effects at all after treatment with heparin or bishydroxycoumarin (Dicumarol), Quintanilla et al. (1947), Pichotka et al. (1949), Fuhrmann and Crismon (1947). In particular Lewis's comprehensive control experiments of 1952 and those of Lewis and Moen of 1953 refuted Lange's claims (Lange et al. 1947, 1950). They maintained that no advantages of this method had been observed. On the contrary, the death rate of the animals treated with heparin increased considerably, which may perhaps have been something to do with damage to the adrenal cortex caused by the heparin, which has already been referred to earlier (Hoellscher in 1923 and Partoux 1953, quoted according to Sapin—Jaloustre 1956). This was confirmed, too, in follow-up investigations carried out by Lewis and Moen in 1953 on 468 rabbits, in whom standard 2nd degree cold injuries had been artificially induced (in part muscle necrosis without skin necrosis). Beside 154 controls, 314 animals were treated with heparin. The muscle necrosis was not affected, the main damage deteriorated noticeably and the death rate of the animals increased.

The questionable or even bad results with heparin could also be extended to other anticoagulants, e.g. to Parathrodyn, used in 1944 by Mantscheff and Locker (which is inferior to heparin according to Kaula) and Dicumarol and Thromexan (Brambel and Locker 1944), Fuhrmann and Crismon (1947), Pratt (1953) and Sapin—Jaloustre (1956).

More important than animal experiments is the experience with human beings. In 1946 Lange and Loewe (repetition in 1947) induced frostbite (2 to 5 cms) on the forearms of eight volunteers with carbon dioxide snow ($-22°$ to $-30°C$, for 30 min.) and then treated them with heparin, checking the coagulation times. Vesicles were observed on the treated subjects, but no necrosis.

The frostbite was produced by means of the *ultra rapid cooling* method ($-22°$ to $-30°C$ for 3 min), which is naturally of great importance for the evaluation of the results of the treatment. It was reported that no or hardly any gangrene was observed after administration of heparin, not even when the treatment did not begin until 24 h after exposure. These experiments should certainly not be taken into consideration, since the administration of heparin naturally has an influence on the controls of the other side as well and ultra rapid freezing does not produce any particular damage.

Theiss's data (Theiss et al. 1951) is important, since he reported that a severe retroperitoneal haemorrhage developed during treatment with heparin and simultaneous blocking of the sympathetic trunk and that the outcome was fatal. This case corresponds to a report made by Graven (quotated according to Bonika 1953), who referred to three deaths from retroperitoneal bleeding with ileus after a combined blocking of the sympathetic trunk and administration of anticoagulants (see Killian 1972).

The disapproving attitude towards treatment of fresh cold damage with anticoagulants derives mainly from bad experience with them in Korea (Talbott 1952).

In 1952 Orr and Fainer carried out heparin treatment for up to 10 days on 1880 cases of cold injury in the military hospitals of theAmerican units in Korea and Japan and reported the results to be somewhat more favourable than for the control cases. In 1952 Movrey and Farago reported on 593 cases of cold injury in Korea, of which 38 were treated with heparin after the 36th without any marked improvement being observed. Laufmann reached the same result in 1951. Heaton and Davis (1952) used the Osaka mixture with heparin (s. p. 201) on men with cold injuries (but without wounds), one 500 cm^3 ampoule every 6 h. No special advantages of this kind of heparin treatment were to be found.

The hopes raised in Siegmund (1942a-c), Behrens (unpublished data), Bigelow (1942), Lange et. al. (1947, 1950) by their animal experiments were therefore unfortunately not fulfilled as far as cold damage was concerned. It was not possible to free the already blocked venous capillaries, venoles or veins of clots and congestion and to allow the blood to flow again. On most cases such attempts are made too late. If the use of anticoagulants has become normal practice in the case of frostbite, (see, for example, the reports of Mundt et al. of 1964), this is due to the fact that it was thus hoped at least to prevent the development of thrombosis or even of an embolism.

In our opinion early treatment with anticoagulants is nevertheless of importance, if acute thrombophlebitis develops during the course of localised infection in the frostbitten area. In this particular case, as is common, treatment with *anticoagulants, fibrinolytics,* thrombolytics, streptokinase and plasmin is not to be disregarded.

For some time fibrinolytics and thrombolytics in the form of the enzyme strepto-kinase have been used in the early treatment of cold damage, since the latter is usually contained in the englobulin fraction of the blood. In general about 2 million streptokinse units are used daily in Ringer's solution or Ringer's lactate solution and regular checks made of the fibrinogen factor and of the fibrinogen generation products (Jeretin et al. 1976). The development of oedemas was considered to be a sign of the start of perfusion and thrombolysis. Heparin and Aspirin have also been used instead of streptokinase. It has been reported that urokinase is more effective than streptokinase when Trental is used streptokinase cannot be administered. The latter seems more important, however, since with falling temperature blood viscosity increases.

Anticoagulants such as heparin and Liquemin are administered parenterally in order to stop clotting medicinally (antidote; protamine chloride), the cumarin derivates are for short or long-term treatment, administered, however, orally, (antidote: vitamin K, Konakion). Here not only must the contraindications be strictly observed but also the effects must be constantly checked by means of the Quick test (prothrombin clotting time) or by determining the thromboplastin time.

Alcohol

Alcohol, taken internally in small quantities, is of unquestionable significance in the prophylaxis and treatment of localised cold injuries. The stimulating effect on the whole circulation and the peripheral vasodilation encourage and improve the supply of blood to the extremities. The vasodilating effect is revealed by a redenning of the superficial capillary region and an increase in the skin temperature. This is the basis of the fact, learnt from experience, that small amounts of alcohol, taken before or during exposure, give increased protection against frostbite and delay noticeably the onset of the cooling of the limbs. (Sullivan and Masterson 1953). Taken after and during exposure alcoholic beverages can stimulate a periodic restoring of the warmth the limbs have lost (Aschoff – Lewis reaction). In the monographs on cold damage of Paunesco – Podeanu and Tzurai (1946) and Vagliano (1948), the consumption of moderate amounts of alcohol is recommended as a valuable means of supporting the rewarming process and peripheral vasodilation. The dangers of alcohol lie only in its abuse, particularly in a state of exhaustion. Due to its narcotic effect alcohol makes the person drinking it tired, heavy, sluggish, and sometimes slow in his movements, and therefore encourages general loss of temperature. An urgent warning against the consumption of alcohol, as was common in our country, is not valid.

Daily doses of 50 g of alcohol have been given for medicinal purposes. Russian authors, such as Kiyaschev (1944) and others, have increased these doses up to 100 g daily, Bowery and Varhago allowed a daily consumption of 56 to 113 g of whisky. The Osaka anti-frost solution contains small amounts of alcohol. It was only used when there were no wounds. Talbott administered small doses of alcohol intravenously, which we do not support.

Vitamins

Two vitamins are evidently of particular significance in the treatment of frostbite, namely vitamin E and vitamin K. Information on this subject is extremely scanty and covers almost exclusively the treatment of chilblains.

Whitelaw and Woodman (1950), for example, administered 20 mg of vitamin K three times daily, then later 35 mg of vitamin K two to three times daily. In 90 % of the cases this apparently led to freedom from discomfort and a healing of the chilblains within 5 to 7 days. As a disadvantage they reported that it had been necessary to go on administering vitamin K throughout the year otherwise there had been relapses.

Schaalf's (1951), experience was similar, during the treatment of chilblains. He administered vitamin K in order to counteract the poor circulation and the increased permeability of the capillaries. He too reported apparently positive results with vitamin K. The consumption of vitamin E evidently affords the Eskimos particular resistance to cold. Its administration after cold damage has also been recommended recently by dermatologists. Vitamin A and Vitamin C, as well as the vitamin B complex, may be of use after extreme physical exhaustion.

Rutin and Calcium

In order to counteract the cold oedema the idea of artificially sealing the blood vessels with rutin and calcium was considered. Infusion solutions were added to these chemicals. It was not, however, possible to decrease the permeability of the capillaries by means of rutin, nor was it possible to achieve a marked reduction of prevention of the oedemas.

The corresponding animal experiments on rats and rabbits carried out by Fuhrmann and Crismon (1947) did not produce any satisfactory results either. They were, it is true, able to observe capillaroscopically a delay in the development of stases in the blood vessels and apparently also a limitation of the gangrene development on the paws, but there was no reduction of the necrosis on the rabbit ears. The experiments of Shumaker et al. in 1951 produced no positive results either. They administered up to 100 mg of rutin per kg of body weight for 4 days (cf. the negative results of Lewis and Moen in 1953).

The clinical experience from about 5,000 cases of cold injury in Korea was all negative.

Early Treatment With Oxygen and CO_2

Due to our knowledge of the fact that the circulation is disturbed to a large extent in the peripheral, cold-damaged areas and that hypoxaemia is especially likely to develop during the thawing out phase, we made use of oxygen treatment by inhalation at an early stage and in particular on patients suffering from shock, after loss of blood accompanied by acute loss of temperature.

In 1977 Haydukievicz made an interesting observation on this subject on himself. After good acclimatisation at a high altitude his legs became ice-cold and stiff and did not warm up or recover despite rubbing. After breathing in oxygen he immediately felt a sensation of warmth and relief in his legs. The smoking of one cigarette, and a dose of Palfium to a greater extent made the condition at once worse. The cold stiffness returned. The condition improved notably 15 min after two Ronicol tablets had been taken. The circulation was stimulated and the success of this effect lasted considerably longer than that of the breathing of oxygen.

The intravenous administration of oxygen has been successfully used for some time for every kind of circulatory disturbance (Moser 1942; Judmaier 1953). Since Eppinger, even before 1930, provided evidence of the fact that chemically cleaned oxygen, given intravenously, is immediately taken up by the blood and does not do any harm. In 1953 Judmaier carried out a total of 2000 oxygen insufflations on 160 cases of disturbed circulation with 15 % success and 25 % failures. This included not only cases of endangiitis obliterans but also cases of damage remaining after cold injuries. As far as we know this method has not yet been used in the early treatment of cold injuries but it is promising. In our opinion oxygen treatment, with the oxygen above atmospheric pressure, might also be considered.

In 1955 Leussner recommended carbon dioxide treatment for cold injuries. He introduced carbon dioxide into a hot bath and found an optimal analeptic effect of the gas at $20° - 22°C$. In this way it was possible to induce hyperaemia of the skin with a pleasant warm sensation. The flow velocity in the capillaries increased. The subcapillary venous plexuses should dilate and open branches which were previously closed. The carbon dioxide will, of course, have the effect of stimulating the peripheral circulation. It was in this connection that Leussner already observed after two carbon dioxide baths of $10 - 15$ min a rapid disappearance of the oedemas and a reduction in the secretion in cases of frostbite. Acute serous secerning spots were transformed into dry gangrene, the healing process was encouraged. Carbon dioxide baths of this kind apparently have a favourable effect on the spasms of the afferent arteries and arterioles accompanied by peristaltic symptoms in the peripheral vascular system. Schliepbach and Smerts (1955) have reported similar observations. It is still not clear whether these CO_2 baths are suitable for the early treatment of cold injuries. They have so far only been used in later treatment. Attempts have also been made to administer small quantities of the gas intraaterially.

Cortin and ACTH

Adrenal products of the cortin and cortisone type have been widely used in the treatment of severe burns and have apparently been effective (Götze 1944; Grassweller and Farmer 1950; Whitelaw and Woodman 1950). It was natural to carry out similar experiments on cold injuries. (Riml et al., quoted according to Killian 1942), especially as the adrenocorticotrophic hormone (ACTH), functioning together with the adenohypophysis, has a considerable effect on the phosphorylation process of the carbohydrate metabolism (Verzar quoted according to Killian 1942), the permeability and the functions of the limiting membranes. (See also the work of Tonutti 1940, Selje etc.) It became known that after severe intoxication, oxygen deficiency, over-exertion and inundation of the body with protein degradation products a state of exhaustion of the adrenal cortex may occur. As Riml points out, to these symptoms must be added the general loss of temperature and acute frostbite. An ACTH deficiency leads to acute disturbances of the circulatory condition and heat regulation. After this we had every reason to try an adrenal product of the Cortin and precortine type, although the results of animal experiments carried out by Entin and Baxter in 1952, Glenn et al. in 1952, and Lewis in 1951 with cortisone were disappointing.

We were never able to observe clinically definite improvements in cold damage as the result of the use of adrenocortical extracts. In 1952 Glenn treated 2 cases, Dickinson 18 cases, also in Korea, without success. It was the same with Higgins et al., Talbott (1952), and Movrey and Farago (1952), who treated comparable cases of frostbite with cortisone and ACTH. There were no advantages compared with their control cases.

It therefore seems completely pointless to try and use these hormone preparations in the early treatment of cold injuries.

Antihistamines

Assuming that capillary damage and disturbances in the permeability in cases of cold injury are partly associated with the formation of amines in the tissue (H substances) experiments were carried out using antihistamines (antistine, antergan, avil etc.). In 1946 Frommel and Piequet used such products and reported achieving more rapid healing and more favourable scars. After inducing artificial frostbite on volunteers Macht et al. (1949) used pribenzamin and benadryl (iontophoresis) and reported moderately favourable effects.

Shumaker's animal experiments on rat and rabbit ears using benadryl produced a moderate improvement. Other anti-histamines, such as neo-antergan, atosil, phenergan and multergan, were used on animals by Meiding and Kolsky (1953) with slight, positive results. According to these results a certain importance must be attached to anti-histamines in the treatment of cold damage.

Combating Pain and the Sedation of the Autonomous Nervous System

Local cold damage often causes considerable pain, which makes the general condition worse and the patient suffer sleepless nights. One is therefore often obliged to give anagelsics. During the disastrous winter of 1941 and 1942 in Russia we used morphine and oxycodone (Eucodal) reservedly since they can lead to vasoconstrictive side-effects (centralisation of the circulation), which are unwelcome. Meperidine (Dolantin Pethidine) was often used and occasionally hydromorphone (Dilaudid), Retobemidone (Cliradon), and after the war dextromoramide (Palfium), Diazepam (Valium) Chlordiazepoxide (Librium), 3-hydroxy-N-methylmorphinan (Dromoran) etc.

It is not yet clear to what extent the use of psychopharmacological agents, neuroleptic drugs and tranquillisers, in particular during mass cold catastrophes (e.g. earthquakes during frost periods) can be of service for their soothing influence in the treatment of additional cold damage after burial in avalanches and injuries with shock symptoms. The phenothiazine derivates: promazine, promethazine, chlorpromazine, mepazine etc. could probably be used, also promethazine (Atosil, Phenergan) fluo-promazine (Psyquil), Largaktil, Megaphen and Fentanyl, possibly Kentamine too.

Early Massage and Exercise

The rubbing of freshly frozen extremities is a common habit of laymen. Many a limb has been saved in this way, since there is no doubt that it does encourage the peripheral circulation. A careful massage with stroking movements seems to work well, if the cold stiffness of the muscles has been overcome and the circulation is functioning properly again. Block's (1942) warning against premature massaging of the limb in an ice-cold state, i.e. against rapid actions, is justified. In addition, there seems to be little point in massaging toxic substances (H substances) from cold damaged areas into the circulation in the direction of the heart. Krogh and Kohler recommend only gentle and careful massaging with stroking and kneading movements, but no exaggerated measures. Besides, it seems to be better, not to massage the actual frostbitten area, but instead the proximal area above it. Massages should not be entrusted to untrained nor to incapable personnel.

Similar cautiousness is also recommended with regard to passive movements of the limbs, since the cooled muscles are often still in a frozen state. Jerky flexions can easily lead to damage to the joints, and to the joint capsules, to laceration of the muscles and to bleeding. It is a different matter if one allows the patient to carry out active movements himself during the rewarming phase in order to stimulate the circulation and to encourage the local production of heat.

Measures of Dealing With the Marked Oedema

The best way of treating a marked cold oedema is definitely to quickly warm up the main part of the body. American surgeons, however, were not content with this, but went on to apply compression bandages in order to keep the severe secondary oedema, which occurs in the hyperaemic phase, under control, (plaster casts and pressure dressings). As this treatment is the consequence of false premises it is useless. As Lempke and Shumaker (1949) have already pointed out, the development of an oedema can be influenced in its cause but it cannot be mechanically restricted, so that the tissue pressure increases and the blood supply deteriorates.

An uncomplicated cold oedema is usually not all that pronounced. If, however, it is accompanied by an acute secondary oedema, the hydrostatic pressure within the fascial area, especially in the area of the lower leg, can increase to such an extent that ischaemic states develop as the result of compression of the arteries (as in the lacerations of the art. tibialis ant. and post.) In view of this fact, in the past Nösske (1910), Bundschuh (1918) and Witteck (1915) began to make 20 – 30 small 2 cm long incisions in the area of the marked oedema on the foot, the lower leg, the hands and the backs of the fingers, more precisely on the extensor surfaces, and on the forearm and lower leg also on the flexor sides, not only through the skin but also through the hard fascial sheaths. If the limb is still completely cold and without feeling, no additional anaesthesia is necessary before such an incision in the frostbitten area is made. This old method was revived in 1944 by Sauerbruch et al. and has certainly contributed to preventing the loss of many a limb. When the small wounds begin to bleed, this may be considered as a good sign of the recovery of the circulation (Floerken 1914, 1915). After Sauerbruch et al. (1944), Hempel (1930, 1931, 1933), Pernato (1941) Matais (1942) and others made positive reports on this method. It must be carried out under strictly aseptic conditions. Sauerbruch et al. (1944) made these relief-bringing incisions up as far as the thigh area and claimed that the effect was similar to that of a blocking of the sympathetic nervous system. The vascular spasm apparently relaxes. It is a fact that the circulation improves as a result of this decompression and that the oscillatory deflections are greater.

Further measures can help to dehydrate the oedema area. These include the prescribing of diets containing little salt during the time of treatment, the administration of hypertonic glucose solutions and diuretics (caffeine, Saliorgan, Novasurol, (Esidriex or Lasix). At the same time the water intake should be limited and any continuous intravenous drip necessary should be reduced to a minimum. Sudorifics have also been used in order to promote loss of water. As far as we know hyaloronidase (kinetine) has not so far been tried to alleviate full oedemas and to speed up absorption.

If the presence of a marked oedema jeopardizes the survival of a limb, one must try to dehydrate and decompress with a diuretic. Not all diuretic stimulants are appropriate. In the case of acute cerebral and pulmonary oedemas Lasix has proved to be good.

Blocking of the Sympathetic Nervous System

General

Beginning with the assumption that a primary arterial spasm is involved in the cause of the development of cold injuries, Lake (1917) had already carried out experiments to try and tone down the sympathetic nervous system. His reports, however, like Osipovski's studies on this subject made later in 1935, have been forgotten. It was not until 1940, at the time of the development of the surgery of the sympathetic nervous system and the recognition of a neuro-vascular relationship, that Lériche and Kunlin (1940) tested clinically the possibility of blocking the sympathetic cable and ganglia in the treatment of cold injuries and experienced favourable results.

Their method consisted of blocking the lumbar sympathetic chain with anaesthetic substances (Novocaine) after cold damage to the lower extremities and the stellate ganglion Th. 2 and 3, after fresh cold injuries to the hands and fingers. Of the first 39 patients treated in this way they found that with 1st and 2nd degree cold injuries infiltrations of this kind on 3 consecutive days were sufficient to overcome the arterial spasm and to prevent gangrene developing. The cold oedema and the pains disappeared quickly (Fig. 81).

Since that time the blocking of the sympathetic nervous system has been considered the most important measure in the early treatment of cold damage, as also of other kinds of circulatory disturbance.

Whereas on the German side attention was at once drawn to this method and it was used extensively in 1941 and 1942, American surgeons apparently only ventured very hesitantly to use it, as it was considered to be harmful or dangerous (1943). See the data provided by Telford (1943a, b) and Adams and Clemenson (1944). It was believed that the cold oedema became worse as the result of blocking the sympathetic nervous system, and that it could even be the cause of some gangrene. In addition to this some cold experiments on rabbit ears produced negative results. See the data provided by Crismon and Fuhrmann (1946, 1947), Shumaker and Lempke (1951).

Inspite of some technical difficulties the conclusion was reached that the blocking of the sympathetic nervous system in animals leads to an improvement in the condition of the cold oedema, relieves pain and even reduces the danger of necrosis, as Lériche had already maintained (1945). The healing process of local cold damage was encouraged.

More important than comparative animal experiments are those carried out on human beings, of which we unfortunately know very little. Only those cases are of decisive importance in which a double-sided cold injury of the feet and hands of the same kind on both sides occurred and the surgeons only blocked on side for control purposes.

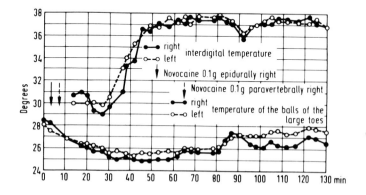

Fig. 81. Example of the effect of blockade of the lumbar sympathetic chain. Behaviour of the inter-digital – and ball of the large toe – temperatures in a 46-year-old woman with chronic rightsided sciatica, after epidural and paravertebral injection with novocaine (LI – LIII): comparison of both sides. (From Lippross 1942)

One of these cases was a very impressive blocking of the stellate ganglion carried out on double-sided frostbite of the hands by v. Schürer (1942). The comparative photographs are reproduced here (Fig. 82). Whereas on the control side necrosis formed and the limbs had to be amputated, the limbs on the side under treatment were saved. It can clearly be seen to what extent the condition of the hand, which had been treated with the blockage, is better than that of the untreated control.

Similar positive results were obtained by Mallet – Guy and Lieffring (1940) and Jung and Fell (1942a, b), Block (1943), Breitner (1944a, b), Tantini and Baggio (1941a-c), Isaacson and Harrell (1953), v. Schürer (1942), Killian (1942), von Brandis (1943a, b), Starlinger and Frisch (1944), Paunesco-Podeanu and Tzurai (1946) and Vagliano (1948); more recently also by Martinez et al. (1966).

Jung and Fell (1942), Breitner (1944a, b) and Mallet – Guy and Lieffring (1940) checked the results of the effectiveness of the blocking of the sympathetic nervous system using *arteriograms* and *oscillograms*. At the same time other test methods were also applied.

It was always observed that in the frozen section of the limb together with a moderate drop in blood pressure considerably increased oscillation occurred, which was regarded as a sign of arterial vasodilation and improved circulation. Series of arteriographs produced the same results. The arterial pathways were found to be fuller and more dilated on the blocked side, which was proof of an alleviation or a complete relaxation of the cold spasm. With fresh cases the reactions were clearer and more pronounced than with old cold injuries in which irreparable damage to the vascular wall of the cold endangiitis type had already set in. Jung and Fell pointed out that long after the cold injury occurs positive results can be obtained from the blocking of the sympathetic nervous system.

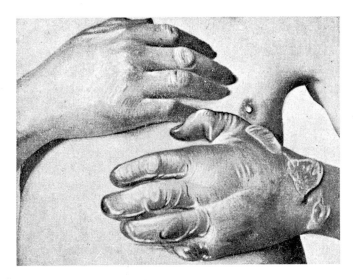

Fig. 82. Comparison of the effect of sympathectomy in severe frostbite in both hands; 4 days after the operation good reversal of the cold injuries can be seen on the operated side, only the distal phalanges of the 2nd, 3rd and 4th fingers are mummified. On the left side, however, there is extensive blistering with underlying necroses. The entire hand is lost. (According to v. Schürer 1942)

Similarly successful results were also achieved when reproduced by many other authors. In 36 cases of double-sided frostbite, all more or less equally severe, Tantini and Baggio (1941a-c) apparently found a 90 % improvement of the blocked side compared with the controls – whereby in 9 % of the cases the attempt at blocking failed. In 61 % of the cases his oscillograms produced favourable values, which was recognised by a sharp increase in the pressure amplitudes. In a comparison between periarterial infiltration in the region of the arteria femoralis (beneath the inguinal ligament) and a blocking of the lumbar ganglion the latter proved on an average to be considerably better.

In 1952 Talbott also blocked just one side on a case of double-sided frostbite on the hands and feet, obtained far better healing results and observed a more rapid healing process on this side than on the other side. The vast majority of surgeons and anaesthetists today undoubtedly confirm the value of a blockage of the sympathetic nervous system as a means of treating early cold damage. Unlike Isaacson and Harrel (1953) the author has never observed a deterioration either, rather more in nearly every case an improvement in the condition.

Neurovegetative Blocks

The disconnecting of neurovasal vegetative fibres to the arterial blood vessels can be carried out in two ways:
1) Via the medicinal administration of sympathicolytic and adrenolytic agents, which reduce the vascular tone by producing a paralysing effect on the vasoconstrictors.
2) By means of local anaesthetic and surgical measures:
a) Cross-section anaesthesia.
b) Periarterial blocking
c) Short-term blocking of the sympathetic trunk
d) Protracted blocking of the sympathetic trunk with long-term anaesthesia or definitive blocking with alcohol or phenol.
e) The resection of parts of the sympathetic trunk with its ganglia.
   The administration of vasoconstrictors together with local anaesthetic solutions should be avoided in the early treatment of cold damage.

1) Cross-section Anaesthesia. It appears that in 1931 Vischnevskij had already accomplished a temporary blocking of the nerves by means of local anaesthesia in cases of trophic disturbances. He referred to the procedure as „chemical neurotomy". His method – cross-section anaesthesia – has only been used by a few surgeons in the early treatment of frozen limbs, although the results of some animal experiments were positive. In 1937 Orloff (a, b) carried out comparative tests on rat tails, in which cold damage had been induced using an ethyl chloride spray. Without Novocaine cross-section anaesthesia mummification set in after 10 days and a shedding of the sections of the tail, which had been damaged by the cold, was observed. Of 20 animals with Novocaine blockages, carried out 6 h after exposure, 17 healed completely. Control injections with common salt were unsuccessful. Vischnevskij's method has been used by Osipovski (1935) and Kukin (1941) and was apparently successful. It is now, however, considered to be out-of-date.

2) Periarterial Blocking of the Sympathetic Nervous System, Blocking of the Ganglia and Sympathetic Trunk. After 1940, in accordance with the recommendations of Lériche, a periarterial blockage of the sympathetic nervous system with Novocaine was attempted. The method consists of an infiltration of the area around the vessels or of the periarterial sympathetic network with local anaesthetic solutions (at that time 5 − 10 ml of a 1 % procaine solution without adrenaline was mostly used), for example of the arteria femoralis for the treatment of cold injuries to the lower extremities, of the art. subclavia or axillaris for injuries to the hands and fingers (Starlinger 1942; Tantini and Raggio 1941a-c). If one is interested in reintroducing this method, the use of more effective Preparations than novocaine is to be recommended today, e.g. Xylocaine, Carbocaine, Citanest, Mepivacaine or the long-acting anaesthetic, Bupivacaine. The highest doses for injections recommended by the manufacturers must be observed according to the concentration.

The block of the stellate ganglion (D 1 and 2) is an appropriate means of treating cold injuries in the head region and to the upper extremities, for injuries to the lower extremities the blocking of the lumbar sympathetic chain on one or both sides. If it is necessary to treat both sides, one should leave an interval of 3 to 4 h after each blockage in order to prevent a circulatory breakdown.

Today it is also possible to block the sympathetic ganglia using the catheter method and to keep an extremity free of pain and with the blood vessels dilated for days.

Methods which are effective on both sides, like the *intradural spinal anaesthesia* in the lumbar region or an extradural lumbar blocking like *the higher caudal block* are not often used for the purposes mentioned and not to be recommended for early treatment since the patient's general condition after exposure is often poor.

An important condition for the use of ganglia and sympathetic trunk blocks is the ability to completely master the technique, to know all the danger factors and possible complications.

Within this monograph we cannot go into the details of the different methods and techniques and therefore refer to the following works for guidance:

H. Auberger: Praktische Lokalanästhesie, Thieme, Stuttgart.
H. Nolte: Die Technik der Lokalanästhesie, Springer Berlin, Heidelberg New York 1967.
J. Adriani: Labats Regional Anaesthesia, Saunders, Philadelphia London 1967.
D. C. Moore: Regional Block, 4th edn. Thomas, Oxford.
E. Erikson: Atlas der Lokalanästhesie, Thieme, Stuttgart 1970.
H. Killian: Lokalanästhesie und Lokalanästhetika, Textbook and Handbook. 1st edn. 1959, 2nd edn. 1973. Thieme, Stuttgart. spanish edn. 1979

Novocaine in 0.5%–1.0% solutions without adrenaline is no longer used for the early treatment of cold injuries (thawing out phase and initial treatment by means of blocking the ganglia), because of its short-term effectiveness, instead Citanest, Prilocaine, Scandicaine, Mepivacaine, Bupivacaine etc. are administered in equivalent amounts and concentrations, since they are effective for 2 to 4 h and more.

The blocking of the stellate ganglion can, of course, be carried out from the front, the side or from behind. For the treatment of cold damage in the facial area to the ears, the hands, the fingers and the lower arm, we recommend the frontal method according to Herget and Philippides, the unilateral method according to Lériche and Fontaine, or the posterior method according to White and Mendel. The success of the block is revealed by the appearance of Horner's syndrome after about 5—10 min on the same side.

For the lower extremity a block of the lumbar sympathetic chain is appropriate around L 2 — 4 by Kappis' posterior method, possibly even the lower block according to Reischauer to block L 4 — 5.

Alcohol or phenol blocks of the ganglions should not be attempted in early treatment.

3) Extradural Long-term Blocking for Early and Later Treatment of Cold Damage. Thanks to the introduction of long-acting anaesthetics of the Bupivacaine type, new possibilities have been opened to us for the permanent or one-time treatment of frostbite, freshly acquired or in its more advanced stages, and these should be made use of. Bupivacaine works on an average for a period of 6—8 h with about the same kind of anaesthetic conduction and toxicity as that of Pantocaine. Instead of a single application it is possible, according to Crul, to perform long-term treatment according to the continuous method of epidural anaesthesia for up to 10 days.

On the technique: The patient must lie on his side. Under strictly sterile conditions a skin weal is made 2 cm to the side of the interspinal area, beside the spinal processes, L 2 — 3 or 3 — 4. The special cannula (Salt) with an attachment for the penetration of the yellow ligament is used for the epidural puncture after contact with the fine stylet. This cannula is not introduced through the interspinal ligament on the median plane, but laterally via the soft dorsal muscles, as the interspinal ligament can often be very hard and ossified, which makes it difficult to insert the catheter. Crul (1970, 1971) introduced the cannula via the 2 cm lateral puncture point diagonally towards the median and upwards as far as the yellow ligament, and after penetrating it, injected the catheter 5—6 cm up into the epidural area. The Salt cannula is then carefully removed via the inserted catheter and the latter is locally sterilised and attached to the shoulder after the patient has been laid on his back. After breathing has been tested, a sample dose of 2 ml of a 5% Marcain solution (without adrenaline) is administered, its effects observed and then the main dose of 5—6 ml of the same solution injected. The anaesthetic usually reaches the segments 8—9. If this is not the case, another 4—5 ml of an 0.25% solution is injected. For treatment which is to last for some days doses of an average of three-quarters of the first dose of 0.5% Bupivacaine is used.

If Bupivacaine is only administered once 75 mg without adrenaline is considered to be a maximum dose. During long-term treatment the patients may take a few steps with the catheter still inserted after the myokinetic paralytic symptoms have disappeared, provided that the local condition allows this.

In the same way caudal anaesthesia may be used once or more often in the treatment of early and advanced stage cold injuries in the region of the buttocks, the perineum, the anus and the genitals. It is superior to the saddle-block anaesthesia in its old form, as it was used by Laewen (1942 a, b) Starlinger (1942) and Gally in the past.

In 1966 Martinez et al. pointed out that with severe cold injuries clot formation was not affected by the blocking of the sympathetic nervous system, nor by resection, but that it had been observed that oedemas around the demarcation line were absorbed more quickly.

Furthermore, in the case of fresh, 2nd or 3rd degree cold injuries, Spiegelberger et al. (1977) recently recommended not limiting treatment to the administration of vasodilators, but operating on the sympathetic nervous system itself, since this produces better results. (Experience with 67 cases.) Moreover, the endoscopic, endothoracal block has been used of late, i.e. the severing of the sympathetic trunk with a cauterising loop, according to Kux. The limbs subsequently become warm and dry, the prospects improve. For cold injuries to the upper extremities the severing of the sympathetic trunk between D2 and D6 is recommended as being without particular risk. The blocking of the stellate ganglion alone is only used in the case of slight cold damage to the fingers, hands and arms. For the lower extremities a block of the lumbar sympathetic trunk was used, a resection was avoided where at all possible, however, because of the danger of the disturbance of potency and was only then used when circulatory disturbance, trophic ulcers or causalgia were observed. The treatment is in accordance with our own opinion.

4) Operations on the Sympathetic Nervous System. In the years 1941–1945 many surgeons made use of the periarterial sympathectomy according to Lériche in the treatment of severe cold injuries. It was most frequently used in the area of the arteria femoralis in the case of cold damage to the lower extremities. On an average vasodilation was only achieved for 2 to 3 months. This ought to be enough in most cases to cure a cold injury, it is true, but unfortunately a lot of harm was done. Beside a number of successes, in particular those of Spanish surgeons, e.g. Pessmonid, Gill, achieved while the method was being tried out — also those of v. Schürer (1942), Starlinger (1942), Jung and Fell (1942a, b) Breitner (1944a, b), Philippides, Gerlach (1943), Demlainen and Philippowics (1942), there were also serious failures and incidents mostly concerning wound infections. The author discovered, for example, from Alius's report of his experiences that in 20 cases of periarterial sympathectomy five times in the region of the femoralis there were cases of purulence, phlegmonous processes in the vascular wall and heavy post-operative bleeding, which made it necessary to ligate the blood vessel. In one case the art. femoralis was found completely torn. As the author himself saw similar cases, he urgently warned against the use of the periarterial sympathectomy in field hospitals.

The surgical removal of the sympathetic trunk and its ganglia, the excision of the stellate ganglions or the resection of the lumbar sympathetic trunk may be used exclusively in the treatment of advanced stage damage, in particular of circulatory disturbances.

There are three different methods available of surgically blocking the peripheral, vegetative fibres of the sympathetic nervous system:
1) Periarterial sympathectomy according to Lériche.
2) The severing of the preganglionic cable.
3) Resection of the ganglia and sympathetic trunk.

Their use is only justified when other methods have failed or the effectiveness of blocking has been proved by means of anaesthetic tests.

Treatment of Manifest Cold Injuries According to Degrees

Treatment of 1st and 2nd Degree Cold Injuries and Related Conditions and Additional Treatment With Circulatory and Vasodilating Preparations

The aim of the treatment of a 1st degree cold injury is to improve the blood supply to the skin and to the hypodermis, to overcome the pain and the itching, to create an astringent, antiphlogistic influence and to quickly achieve an epithelialisation of open spots. Excessive sweating of the hands and feet must also occasionally be kept under control. Before treatment begins it must always be remembered that beneath a banal case of 1st degree frostbite there may be damage to the tissue substrata lower down, and this must be taken into consideration in the treatment.

The number of methods and preparations which exist for the treatment of superficial 1st degree frostbite is so great that our data must remain limited. Basically it is all the same whether one treats 1st degree frostbite by powdering it or uses a mild anti-frostbite ointment. Astringents have also often been brushed onto the affected areas and baths prescribed in such solutions (tannin). As with 1st degree frostbite it is only a case of frost erythema, the prognosis is favourable, the healing process takes place even without treatment.

In the past argentum nitricum, acidum nitricum or chromic acid, as well as acidum benzoicum and the tinctura cantharidal in different forms were often used for the treatment of 1st degree frostbite. These methods are old-fashioned and have been discarded (Ullmann 1932).

In 1918 Raymond and Parisot reported that camphor and alcoholic solutions produced favourable results. Of 2168 cases of cold injury, apparently over 95% were successfully treated, particularly those cases in which the top layer of skin was extremely wet. Camphor spirit dries the skin out and this much used preparation therefore seems appropriate.

Anti-Frostbite Ointments

The use of anti-frostbite ointments of various kinds has been and still is generally common. Three different substances have been reported as ointment admixtures: for dry frostbite: tar in one form or another (e.g.ichthyol), tanning agents (such as tannin, camphor and also iodine.) A coating of tincture of iodine on a frozen spot is disapproved of today because it makes the skin parched and chapped, causes intense pain and does more harm than good.

On the other hand many surgeons have used damp bandages with Dackin's solution and reported good healing results.

According to dermatological experience it seems to be of the utmost importance that the ointment bases do not irritate the skin. From the practical side Unguentulan, Desitin (a liver preparation), cod liver oil ointment, paraffin ointment etc. proved to be suitable. Different kinds of oils were also used as the bases of ointments, e.g. rosemary oil and similar substances with swelling properties.

For a long time it was common to treat mild frostbite and chilblains with a coating of ichthyol-resorcinol-tannin, (1 mg to 3 parts of water or 1% tannin solution with a glycerine admixture). Karwendel and Kadogel were also used.

In the less recent literature one of Hebra's prescriptions is to be found, diachylon ointment with the addition of tar, zinc and lead oxide, and a prescription of Lassar's for plumbi carbolisatum ointment. Ullmann (1932) mentions the following prescription: Unguentum plumbi vaselinum flavum anna 40 g, oleum olivarum 20 g, acidum carbolicum 2 g, olium lavendulae 30 g.

Furthermore we would like to refer to an old Russian prescription for anti-frostbite ointment: Sacidum hydrochloricum 30 g, extratum opii 2.5 g, camphor 10 g, oleum terebintinae 20 g, medul os 40 g, unguentum alteae 120 g. In 1941 Debrunner used 2%–5% acidum tannicum solution and in 1933 Grassmann used ichthyol glycerine. In 1942 Blanke reported having brushed on an ointment containing monochlorphenol, vaseline, glycerine and 2%–10% alcohol.

On the Russian side balsam oil in various compositions was preferred, namely almond oil, 10% Bromocolt, 10% Resorcinol in ointment form, gold creams, collodium elasticum and Tannobrom-collodium, 10% ichthyol-collodium etc.

Peruvian balsam is used a lot. The following prescription of Bruz (quoted according to Zicker-Sieber) is considered to be particularly effective against cold damage: ammonium sulph. ichthyolicum, balsam peruviani anna 6 g, camphor 3 g vaselinum flavum ad 30 g.

In 1928 Walsen recommended monochlor-benzol in a 10% alcohol solution against pruritis.

Anti-frostbite ointments can be mixed with local anaesthetics in small concentrations, e.g. Panthesin, Pantocaine, Xylocaine and others.

If one intends to heat the damaged limb in warm baths, it is strongly advisable to add small amounts of an astringent, oakbark extracts, tanning solutions, alum or potassium permanganate. Copper salts may also be used. In 1943 and 1944 Luetgens achieved good results by prescribing baths in a weak solution of copper sulphate (an old domestic remedy). A teaspoonful of copper sulphate was taken for a big tub of warm water. The limb was bathed in this solution for 20 to 40 min daily. In 1932 Takatsu used anti-frostbite ointments containing copper for the same purpose and in 1941 Simonetti used a mixture of copper salts and cholesterol with an addition of vitamins A and D. This apparently caused the purulent, serous secretions from the open spot to disappear remarkably quickly. The pain subsided rapidly, the regeneration process was considerably encouraged and accelerated.

Some authors like to treat 1st degree frostbite locally with a zinc bismuth paste or burn dressing, (bismuth with the addition of sulphonamides, e.g. Prontosil), also sulphonamide ointments, nowadays penicillin ointments (e.g. antibiotics), since they provide specific and very effective protection against infections, superficial erosions and rhagades, which is extremely important.

Histamine iontophoresis offers a particular kind of action to the peripheral vascular system in the region of the skin. In 1934 Cholnecky used solutions of 100,000 and $1-10$ μA. The pain-relieving effect was apparently excellent. Experimentally induced cold damage could apparently be alleviated in this way.

According to the reports of Saltner (1940) Acrothermal ointment, which contains histamine and acetylcholine to dilate the blood vessels, apparently proved to be good. Hopf carried out animal experiments in his day to determine the effects of Acrotherm and reported an increase in the defensive reaction of the tissue, a rapid improvement in the state of the oedema and an acceleration of the healing process. Acrothermal ointments were used by Lippert in 1936, Loos in 1941 (a, b), Saltner (1940), Hartwich (1940, 1941 a, b) and by others with good results in the treatment of 1st degree frostbite and chilblains. Some dermatologists have attempted to inject acetylcholine solutions under the affected area.

The introduction of ointments containing hormones has further improved the possibilities of the treatment of 1st degree frostbite. In 1940, for example, Wobker used the follicular hormone, Menoform or Progynon, on 45 cases of 1st and 2nd degree frostbite and apparently obtained good results.

Compare here also the reports made by Kloos in 1943. In 1941 Heyde used Cyren ointment on 24 cases of 1st and 2nd degree frostbite. He had his patients carefully massaged three times a day, on which occasion the Cyren ointment was rubbed into the skin. As early as 1939 Plath-Franke, Cobet (1926) and Ratschow (1953) had found that Cyren improves the blood circulation of the skin and produces a warm sensation. First degree frostbite disappeared after about 3 days when treated with Cyren ointment, as did the loss of sensation. In the case of 2nd degree frostbite with vesicles and ulceration the treatment took 12 days, with ammonium sulphide-ichthyol ointment, 24 days. Cyren ointment apparently affords a certain protection against frost, if applied as a prophylactic measure. (Plath-Franke 1939; Kühnau 1939). In 1939, working from an assumption of the same principles, Fiévez used granhormone ointment. It contains extracts from the thymus, the testis and the thyroid gland, plus admixtures of vitamins A and D. In literature, Peru skin ointment, Thiosept ointment, Forapin ointment and many others are mentioned. Dihydrocortisone ointment, as used for the treatment of burns, has recently gained importance in the treatment of frostbite. Apart from the use of such solutions and ointment, the treatment of 1st degree frostbite with talcum powder has proved to be good (Gomoyu and Vagliano 1948). It is advisable to add dehydrating powders, sulphonamides and penicillin (and other antibiotics) to avoid infection when cracks form.

If the cold damaged area is characterised by pronounced hyperhidrosis care must be taken that the perspiration does not mix too much with the powders and form an unpleasant greasy substance. In such cases, completely open air treatment, possibly with the use of a ventilator, can be of service.

Most surgeons and dermatologists did not restrict themselves to the local treatment of mild cold damage, especially not when there was a danger of tissue damage further down, but they made use of medication to activate the circulation and to dilate the blood vessels and of analeptic agents. Camphor, Cardiazol, and Coramine and also Glycoside may only be administered, however, if the patient is not suffering from loss of temperature. As far as the use of Efetonine, Sympatol and Veritol is concerned, great moderation is recommended, as these preparations cause peripheral vasoconstricition, which is not part of the aim of our treatment. An impressive experiment carried out by Lippross (see Fig. 76) shows the marked drop in the temperature of the finger tips due to the effect of adrenaline.

All vasodilative preparations, which were tried in the early treatment, may be used in this phase of treatment. These include, besides Euphylline, also acetylcholine, Ronicol, Dilatol, Doryl, Vasculat and many others, also hormone preparations such as Acrothermal pills, Dermotherm, Iamzol, Lacarnol, Myosten, Map. Progynon, Cyren, Lamuran. Prostigmin (Fig. 80), a dimethyl-carbamic acid-ester related to Eserin may also be used, (see the curve according to Lippross).

Brack (1940, 1941) observed favourable effects after the use of Priscol, a benzylimidazolin, on mild cases of frostbite. The peripheral warming effects are shown by 2 of Lippros's (1942) curves (Figs. 77–79). These good results were confirmed by Sneth, Singer (1940), Allendorf and Sarre, Buckreus (1941).

According to Brack (1940, 1941), Priscol works best on those persons, who tend to reveal abnormal, excessive reactions to the cold. The patients generally notice the effect of one to two Priscol tablets themselves and find it pleasant. The subjective reactions of the patients are an indication of the treatment technique and dose to be used: ($1-2$ cm^3 Priscol solution intramuscularly daily or at two to three day intervals or orally at the most three tablets daily (see Figs. 77 and 78).

According to Dogos et al. (1941), Celice et al. (1942) treatment with thiamine has been performed but we have no detailed information on this. Celice et al. (1942) tried nicotinic acid with the addition of vitamin B on 70 patients with chilblains and 1st degree frostbite. It had already been reccommended earlier by Courly and was apparently effective.

Furthermore, as early as 1941 it was found that the healing process could be favourably influenced if one tried to compensate vegetative disorders, *Bellergal, Neurovegetalin and tranquillizers,* i.e. preparations which calm the autonomous nervous system are most appropriate here.

Various kinds of calcium treatment have also been recommended to reduce the marked oedema and to seal the blood vessels in cases of 1st and 2nd degree frostbite and it was used particularly in recurrent cases as it is well known that with recidivation the oedema usually develops rapidly. Wright and Moffat (1934), Wright and Allen (1943) and Floerken (1914, 1915, 1920a, b) have praised calcium treatment. Barber (1926) saw no effect. It is claimed, however, that the administration of calcium salts combined with hormones and vitamins (cod liver oil) apparently reduces the tendency to chilblains, which boils down to a normalisation of the heat regulation. A diet rich in calories and vitamins is recommended. Vitamins A, C, D and E are of importance here.

Treatment of 2nd and 3rd Degree Frostbite

For the treatment of congelation bullosa and necroticans only treatment with powders may be considered today; the application of ointments or damp bandages with diseinfectant or astringent solutions is no longer used. Not until fresh granulation appears can ointments with appropriate admixtures be effective.

215

The main aim of the treatment of 2nd to 4th degree frostbite is not only to *improve the circulation* but also to *avoid infections,* since the latter not only cause ugly scars and keloids but in addition there is then danger to the limb or even to the patient's life, because of the possibility of superinfections (Pseudomonas etc.).

As soon as frostbite vesicles appear, an appropriate form of *tetanus prevention* should be sought and used. Passive protection is afforded by tetanus antitoxin, active protection by further doses of small amounts of tetanus anatoxin to raise the level of the titre, when active immunisation occurred too long before. The antitoxic tetanus serum only affords short-term protection for 10 to 12 days. Unlike the situation with burns, the germs in the upper layers of the skin are never killed due to the effects of the cold and thus every vesicle and every frostbite crack must be treated as being liable to becoming infected. Moreover, demarcation areas of every kind are always multi-infected, whereby types of germs belonging to the Di. group (pseudodiphteria) and anaerobes, putrid germs, proteus, pseudomonas etc. are often present in large numbers (see p. 171). Every cold injury, which involves vesicles and necrosis, hence requires an effective general form of *antibiotic protection,* which should affect more than just the commonplace pyogenic germs. This alone is not sufficient, however, one must combine general treatment with local infection treatment. This corresponds approximately today to the treatment which has proved of service in the handling of burns with vesicles and necrosis.

Open wound treatment under a current of cool air is preferred to all kinds of bandages. *Blisters,* which are not too big, should just be allowed to dry. The detached epithelium acts as a natural bandage. Large confluent vesicles can be punctured, but one should subsequently inject them with small amounts of antibiotic solutions. One can also open the vesicles and let the contents, which consists of histamine and is rich in protein (possibly pus or blood) drain off. One should not, however, remove the blister but use it again as a natural protection and let it dry up.

Open spots are best treated with jellies containing hydrocortisone, since these soothe the pain and increase the resistance of the tissue to infection. The necrosis is caused to dissolve tryptically with the help of collagenase. This does not affect the epithelialisation. In addition there is general treatment with vasodilators, possibly Pyrifers, and blocking of the sympathetic nervous system together with the administration of hormone and vitamin preparations.

Hydrotherapeutic Measures

Contrast baths are only of service if the blood vessels are still or once again capable of reaction. We have, however, stopped using them since the cold phase of this treatment encourages vasoconstriction and is found by the patient to be very uncomfortable (Goldhahn 1943a, b). If open spots are still present, astringents should be added to the bath water. Instead of contrast baths alternating douches and also mud packs and fango therapy can be used.

Vascular Training

In 1943 Mutschler (quoted according to von Brandis 1943a) and von Brandis tried rhythmic "throttling" for 3 minutes with 15 min intervals in order to activate the local circulation. The throttling phases can be gradually increased up to 10 min on 4 to 5 consecutive days. Subsequently there must be longer intervals of several days. Vascular training by means of active movements and resistance exercises making use of consensual reactions are the next step. Active myokinesis always has a favourable effect on the local circulatory condition.

Ray Treatment (Diathermy, X-rays and Short Waves)

Electrotherapy has been used in the most varied forms in the treatment of frostbite. In 1925 Hoffmann apparently achieved good results with galvanisation but diathermy proved to be a superior method. Chuiton treated frostbite areas for 20 min in a brine bath with a direct current of $5-20 \mu A$. In this way he was able to heal the last itching caused by chilblains and in the frostbitten areas of 1st degree cold injuries. They apparently healed quickly. In 1943 Jamin reported good results from short-wave treatment.

In the past the X-ray treatment of frostbitten areas was recommended by Revesz (1929) and Salzer (1930). Salzer (1930) used fairly hard X-rays with a 2–3 mm aluminium filter and a $3 \mu A$ current up to one-third until skin dose. He repeated the treatment once or twice with two-weekly intervals. If skin reactions due to ointments or rhagades are still present, X-ray treatment should not be undertaken. When they have healed it is necessary to lower the dose and to prolong the intervals.

Revesz (1922) used one-third to one-half unit skin doses with a 1 to 3 mm aluminium filter. If no effect was observed after the session he repeated the irradiation after an interval of 14 days. Obstinate cases he treated three to five times at three-weekly intervals. The pain-relieving effect of irradiation afforded considerable comfort. Its prophylactic use, on people who are susceptible to chilblains, was considered.

Short wave treatment is of greater significance for the therapy of frostbite (Weltz et al. 1943). It is referred to as an effective method of quickly rewarming a limb and improving the blood supply. It appears to have been mainly used by American surgeons and radiologists. In Germany, apart from Weltz et al. (1942a–c) and Moser (1942), Brückmann (1943), reported having been successful with short wave treatment on ten cases of cold damage.

Frostbite and chilblains on the hands, the fingers, the feet and the tip of the nose as well as some cases of erythrocyanosis crurum puellarum were chosen. Brückmann (1943) arranged six sessions of 15–20 min, placing a layer of felt between the electrodes and the skin. Buerlin and Matli (1940) used this method on 50 patients with cold damage and apparently the healing effects were very good. With 2nd degree frostbite considerable improvements were achieved with it and with 3rd degree frostbite the demarcation area benefited and healed more quickly. Stefanutti (1941a, b) confirmed these results. He did not use the electrodes in the affected area but around the base of the limbs. Evidently a spasmolytic effect takes place here because of the heat so that the main arteries are relaxed and dilated.

In comparative experiments, Moser (1942), found out that short wave treatment relieved the unpleasant pain in the frostbitten area.

General Principles and Practice Concerning the Surgical Treatment of 3rd and 4th Degree Frost Damage

When 3rd degree frostbite has developed, the question arises, whether it is possible to heal it completely in a purely conservative fashion or whether, and if so at what point, surgery is necessary. Simple treatment of the local cold damage with powders is definitely the most promising method. It has been shown, however, that its effects are limited. We have found that it is in fact possible to completely heal some cold damage with treatment with powders, but that in the majority of cases the scars which form are neither resistant to stress, nor durable and remain painful, so that later surgical corrections have after all to be made. As the sole method of healing treatment with powders can only be used for superficial localised necrosis, as it is sometimes found in the area of the soles of the feet, the edges of the feet and also around the knuckles, the ankles, and the patella, on the fingers and the tips of the toes. On the other hand, in necrotic stumps and forefoot stumps continued treatment with powders leads to scars, which show hyperkeratotic degeneration and deep cracks, grow together firmly with the bones beneath and remain very sensitive and painful. They can become a centre of vegetative stimulus, which not only causes vascular spasms, but also has an unfavourable influence on the patient's general condition. If one contents oneself with slow, spontaneous healing, the affected areas, the stumps, remain poorly supplied, and this very often leads to recurrent ulceration, which can be the cause of further damage.

Such old frostbitten areas open up again every winter. For this reason extremely conservative treatment administered until the local cold damage has healed, as was called for in the past by Gerulanos (1944), Mayer and Kohlschütter (1914), for reasons of the maximum saving of tissue, is today considered obsolete. Calls have been made, it is true, for surgical intervention to be restricted to an absolute minimum, taking into consideration the dangers of infection, but the development of a proper, adequately supplied stump must be achieved at all costs (Fig. 85).

A conservative approach is to be recommended in the 1st weeks, as one can never know in advance, how far into the tissue necrosis may reach and to what extent the cold damage has developed in the depths of the tissue. It is often found that skin which superficially looks completely black, can be peeled off in its lamellae to reveal beneath surprisingly intact, resistant tissue. If superficial necrosis of this kind is shed as a whole, further surgical treatment is sometimes not necessary. An over-hasty decision to operate could possibly lead to the amputation of larger sections of a limb. If, however, the tissue beneath the surface is also damaged necrosis may extent as far as the bone in some cases, in which case chronic ulcers develop, expecially on the edges of the scars and it is then necessary to operate, to remove osseous lamellae and to make a secondary closure, possibly by means of a grafting process. A skin graft to cover defects cannot be undertaken until all necrosis has been removed from the frostbitten area and the wound is forming good granulation.

Early Operations

In contrast to the above remarks we must mention that in the treatment of 3rd and 4th degree cold injuries one is sometimes forced to operate at an early stage, i.e. to intervene before the final demarcation line has formed. Such early operations require an exact indication, if dreadful mistakes are to be avoided. Over-hasty operations have frequently led to most severe infections, phlegmonous inflammations, venous suppuration, tendon sheath inflammations and even to the loss of the whole of an extremity. Systemic infections with a fatal outcome were not all that uncommon. These facts have prompted many surgeons to warn against rash decisions (Friedrich 1914; Hofheinz 1943, Floerken 1914, 1915, 1920a, b), Starlinger 1942; von Brandis 1943a, b; Killian 1942, 1946, 1959). Early operations should therefore be limited to extreme emergencies — in other words to cases with a rapidly progressing wet-type of gangrene accompanied by dangerous general symptoms, signs of the beginning of a systemic infection and intoxication of malignant gangrene or a new case of endocarditis when the extensive use of antibiotics with a wide range of action has failed.

A critical situation can be easily recognised by the patient's poor general state, the beginning of kraurosis, his rapid physical decline, deathly pallor and circulatory failure, which are all mostly accompanied by high septic temperatures. Rapidly progressing anaemia and hyperleucocytosis are observed and sometimes even haemolytic icterus, outbreaks of toxic sweating, vomiting, diarrhoea due to toxicity, states of agitation and drowsiness, all of which characterise an acute danger to life. Such a situation does not, however, mean today that one is absolutely forced to amputate. With phlegmonous areas which have developed from the frostbitten region one can often avert great danger and save the limb by opening wide the focus of inflammation and the abscesses, performing early resection of the vena saphena and by opening the tubular abscesses or suppurative joints, ensuring at the same time extensive antibiotic protection. Necrotic tissue must be removed on principle.

If there are signs of the beginning of tetanus this must be considered a special case. In such a case the initial focus of the tetanus, i.e. usually the deep demarcation region with its necrotic areas must be totally removed by surgery completely independently of other considerations. The amputation proximal to the demarcation area still does not guarantee that the patient can be saved. Amputation way up in the healthy part of the limb, as was recommended by the Sauerbruch school (Sauerbruch and Jung 1942a, b; Sauerbruch et al. 1944), is, on the other hand, no longer justifiable in our opinion, since it does not influence the course of the tetanus.

Treatment in One or Two Steps

Whereas agreement has been reached about the limits of the conservative treatment of fresh frost damage, there is more than one school of thought concerning the resumption of treatment after the demarcation area has fully developed and a state of mummification been reached. The one (Heller 1908) is namely in favour of encouraging complete cuticularisation of the granulating demarcation area until the stump heals, even using skin grafting according to Thiersch, Reverdin, if need be, before final surgical treatment.

Others, on the other hand, including Laewen (1944), Koehler (1916, 1921) Starlinger (1942), Michelson (1944), Killian (1942, 1946) and many Anglo-American surgeons recommend, on principle, *the one or two time* definitive treatment of the stump after the dry mummification stage has been reached or a demarcation furrow with good granulation has been formed, i.e. surgical correction at the earliest suitable time in order to shorten the duration of treatment.

If one waits for a cold injury stump which is not being properly supplied with blood to heal spontaneously this will usually take weeks or even months. This places a great strain on the patience of both physician and patient and prolongs the time of treatment considerably. As cold injuries are always accompanied by vascular damage many such stumps do not heal spontaneously, or superficially healed ulcers reopen again and again, which makes it necessary to perform various skin grafts to cover them. These are by no means always successful either, so that the moment of final treatment is sometimes postponed indefinitely. Such failures have led to an urgent need to force a complete cure by taking active steps. It must be admitted in the meantime, that the definitive surgical treatment of the stump can be carried out with the wound completely closed under safe, almost aseptic conditions. This is no longer of such importance today in the decision to operate, since antibiotic protection has proved to be extremely effective.

According to common observation the development of the demarcation area is generally completed in about 2 to 3 weeks, so that shortly after surgical treatment of the stump in one or two steps can be performed. According to the data provided by Laewen after the treatment of 58 cases of cold injury a decision to carry out corrective surgery could usually be made at the end of the 3rd week after exposure. This does not only apply to the removal of necrotic areas to enable the wound to granulate afterwards, which takes a further 6 to 7 weeks, but also final treatment. In accordance with the findings of Boehler (1942) and Michelson (1944), Starlinger (1942) and many other German and foreign surgeons, attempts are made to carry out final major treatment as early as the 3rd to 4th week after exposure.

The decision whether or not to amputate becomes difficult when *tendons, fasciae or osteonecrosis undergo lengthy suppuration,* further in those cases, in which relatively early attempts have been made with a circular cut to remove gangrenous areas, since this causes a retraction of the soft parts, which leads to a far greater loss of matter in the final treatment than would have been necessary without this previous intervention. Since, however, in particular in the area of the foot, every centimeter of tissue won is important, one can only warn urgently against the provisional use of a circular cut to remove the necrotic parts. Attempts must be made to make do with the simplest and most economical means.

Special Nature of Frostbite Amputation

Amputations in cases of cold damage have a special position compared with other amputations, since the limits of the tissue damage never coincide with the demarcation line. Changes to the tissue deeper down, to the blood vessels, the nerves, the muscles, the bones and the joints are always found above the demarcation area, although they are barely recognisable from the outside. Some of this damage is not discovered until much later, after months or even years. It is simply not possible to recognise the deeper damage from the external appearance (Killian 1942; Thorban 1962).

Kirschner (1917), Lorenz and many others have called for utmost economy in the amputation of feet after cold injuries, since it is important to create a stump, which will make walking possible.

Both feet placed together produce an elliptic-shaped longtitudinal arch, one foot represents half of this. In the case of an amputation in the region of the forefoot only half or a third of the foot is left. One would therefore expect it to be impossible to walk on a stump like this, but the patient can in fact still feel the ground with the stump and can move about without a prosthesis. Amputations higher up always make artificial limbs necessary. The patient becomes dependent on a prosthesis.

In the case of necrotising cold damage, an amputation must be carried out far enough away from the demarcation line in order to avoid mistakes and severe set-backs in the development of toe or forefoot stumps or stumps of the calcaneal part of the foot. Otherwise it will be found time and again that marginal necrosis or chronic, trophic ulcers form in the stump area, which cause delayed complications and make further amputations necessary.

Whereas Starlinger (1942) grafted his skin flaps very near the border between dead and healthy matter, we have, on principle, always left a space of at least 2 cm from the demarcation furrow in view of the blood supply situation. On arteriographs of frostbitten areas of this kind, one always sees that the afferent blood vessels never reach as far as the demarcation area itself but stop suddenly some way further up (Laewen 1944; Breitner 1944a, b). Kirschner's (1917) tenet of utmost economy would today run: *Amputate as seldom as possible but do so at all costs within the area where the blood supply is still good,* and in such a way that the soft tissue flaps can heal without any tension. This principle corresponds to Boehler's and our urgent advise not to be over-cautious in the final treatment of frostbite stumps.

From many sides the objection came that the strict call for dorsal and plantar flaps to close the stump without strain made the foot bones considerably shorter. That is undoubtedly correct. It is therefore necessary to decide in each individual case whether the final treatment of the stump should include flapping at all or whether it would not be better from the start to close a stump with a petiolated graft, so that the patient can walk on it. The excellent results of some surgeons make it right and even *essential to take into account all the possibilities of grafting.* If this method is unsuccessful, one still has the chance to operate again to produce satisfactory stump formation. However, grafting should only be carried out by those who have genuine experience in this field. Otherwise unfortunate mistakes may occur. Excessive economy, a graft which does not cover the affected area properly, have all too often led to the development of new marginal necrosis and ulcers, which make all efforts in vain. We often had to completely remove the remains of unsuccessful grafts and begin the treatment of the stump all over again.

The following-up of old cases of frostbite with necrotic areas which have healed spontaneously or unsatisfactory amputations has proved that in many cases chronic ulcers and *inflammatory processes of all kinds in time have a harmful effect on the afferent arteries.* Obliterative arterial vascular processes are the result and they can now in turn cause gangrene in the old affected areas due to the poor circulation. (Delayed damage which was usually considered to be the result of endangiitis obliterans and mistakenly referred to as constitutional.) This must be avoided all costs, as the author pointed out emphatically at the surgeons' conference in 1951 and the angiologists' conference in 1946 in Paris.

Amputation in Cases of Wet-type Gangrene

If it has not been possible to achieve a state of mummification, and *dangerous wet-type gangrene* has developed, accompanied by foul, purulent, putrid processes, early amputation will be necessary. In such cases simple circular amputations or amputations in the interarticular space are used in preference at first. It has been revealed namely that the opening of spongy areas, and the severing of the metaphyses in cases of wet-type gangrene can often lead to very lengthy osteomyelitic processes, which increase the damage. Sometimes it is still possible to dry up the rest of the tissue after a provisional amputation of this kind, so that later only the protruding parts of the bones will have to be resected in the definitive treatment. Even when the simple circular cut is used to amputate and treat open wounds foul progressive infections sometimes develop in the area of the tendons, the soft parts and the ends of the bones. The extensive use of appropriate antibiotics is necessary if even greater harm is to be avoided.

Comments on the Grafting of Ulcers and Stumps

Satisfactory results from the grafting of soft part defects after cold damage using the methods according to Thiersch and Reverdin are an exception. Since the blood supply to the affected areas usually is too poor the transplants are often shed. Split skin transplants can be used to advantage, however, for the provisional closure of an injury, before a resistant pedicle graft is applied (Hussel 1977). The red Lexer ointment containing Hg and also the Epigard gauze swabs used by Hussel have proved to be of service in the preparation of the transplantation. In all cases it has been difficult to find the convenient border between the area of dead or poorly supplied tissue and that of healthy or well supplied tissue. It can generally be recognised by the appearance of oozing blood.

Some authors recently tried to improve the methods of recognising the state of the blood supply to a limb before amputation or transplantation. Lisbona and Rosenthal (1976), for example, tried to determine the chances of survival of cold-damaged bones by using Szintigraphs (with 99m Te mythylendiphosphonate) because they are dependent on the volume of the circulation. Further, Erikson and Ponten (1974) tried the same using vasodilating preparations together with arteriography; and Kettelkamp et al. (1971) carried out experiments for the same purpose with labelled radioactive albumin, as did Sunner et al. (1971) and his colleagues, using Xenon-133. Such methods may only be used, however, when a great deal of time and the necessary equipment is available. In addition to compound flaps and split skin transplants, shift grafts or roll grafts may be used. Good results have recently been obtained with the free transfer of pedicle flaps, using the microtechnique. Whether or not it is particularly suitable for the treatment of cold damage has not yet been decided. In difficult cases we have made use of the technique of the round pedicle flap graft from the thigh, the upper or lower arm, or from the lower abdominal region, although this makes the time of treatment considerably longer.

For the upper extremity a graft is usually taken from the area of the abdomen and the thigh, for the foot and lower leg area, the flapped graft from the other leg, the thigh and lower leg or the different methods of jump and roll flap grafts with or without intermediary locations. Simple and time-saving procedures should be preferred. Shift grafts have not proved to be good when used in cold-damaged areas. The formation of bipedicled flaps, which have been recommended in many variations, is better. The jump flap should actually only be used if the joints have become stiff, so that it is difficult to get near to the extremities to transfer the tissue.

We abandoned the direct infolding of a petiolated skin flap in favour of implanting after preparation. The primary loosening of the flap required, and its infolding again for 8 days, as is recommended by nearly all experienced plastic surgeons, has the great advantage of considerably reducing the elasticity and the retraction of the transplant and of getting it accustomed to an inadequate blood supply via the base of the flap. This method has more or less guaranteed the success of our results. In the formation of roll and flaps too, we would strongly advise the surgeon first of all to peritonise the material to be transplanted once locally, to loosen it and infold it again, taking first the one side, before the decision is made, within a space of 8–10 days, to graft the transplant onto the surface to be closed. On an average the plastic flap should be about a third or a half larger than the area to be covered, a principle which is of particular significance for cases of frostbite with poor blood supply above the cold-damaged area. The blood supply to the edges of the transplant should always be satisfactory.

Special Information on the Region of the Hand and Fingers

Cold damage in the area of the hand and fingers is characterized by certain features which sometimes make treatment difficult. It has unfortunately been revealed that trophic disturbances after exposure in the region of the skin, the subcutaneous connective tissue, the bones, the joints and also the small muscles and the blood vessels of the hand can be considerable, which is evidently connected with the rapid loss of temperature to peripheral limbs resulting from their slight volume. The fingers usually remain reddish for a long time, they are extremely sensitive to the cold and easily injured. The skin is atrophic and tense and a marked wasting of the subcutaneous cell tissue can be observed. The fingers become thinner and sometimes stiffen, assuming and *open or extended position or forming a clawhand.* The joints lose their flexibility. These changes to the hand are far more unpleasant than those to the lower extremities in the area of the toe. *Shrinkage of the articular capsules, trophic disturbances of the joints of the fingers and disturbances of the articular surfaces, a deviation of the joint axes and an incongruence of the articular surfaces accompanied by osteophytosis* are the most unpleasant. Since parts of the limbs and skin suffer from acute atrophic disturbances it is sometimes difficult for a satisfactory stump to develop (see Figs. 52 and 53).

It has proved to be of great importance to encourage active movement of all the hand and finger joints during the early treatment so that the hands remain prehensile. Once the hand has stiffened into an open position or a clawhand has formed, experience has shown that it is very difficult to improve the situation (Starlinger 1942). Isolated necrosis of the digital pulp leads to painful trophic disturbances in the distal phalanges, hyperkeratotic scars, which grow together with the osseous distal phalanx. The nails are always lost. The regeneration products are brittle, deformed and tender, sometimes only a small piece of horn nail is left in swollen tissue. In cases like this the patient can only be helped by an amputation in the healthy area. It is important to form a skin flap from the volar side, which is still sensitive, in order to obtain a stump graft well supplied with blood and with a sense of touch. The tendons should not be allowed to simply be drawn back by the muscular traction, but should be given new points of attachment.

Furthermore it is advisable to be extremely cautious at first when amputating in the finger area until it is known to what extent the prehensile activity of the hand can be saved.

Attempts have also been made to graft skin to the tips or the stumps of the fingers, but this often proved not to be resistant enough. It has the disadvantage that the skin transferred is not sufficiently sensitive to ensure a proper sense of touch.

With the loss of the metacarpo-phalangeal joints of the second and fourth finger, it is still possible later, if the thumb is still partly or completely preserved, to ensure a prehensile hand by means of phalangisation of the metacarpal bone. The situation becomes particularly regrettable for the patient when the thumb is also lost, the loss of the first finger even as far as the proximal phalanx or as far as the region of the metacarpalia is extremely unpleasant. It is, however, possible in such cases to improve the prehensile activity of the hand considerably, not only with plastic substitutes, but also by means of a thumb prosthesis which fits well, as has been shown by Heller (1908).

Even with cold injuries which extend as far as the middle of the metacarpus or even as far as the wrist, the treatment should remain at first as economical as possible, so that it will still be possible to carry out an optimal skin graft later if necessary or to improve the prehensile activity of the hand with the use of suitable prostheses.

If the whole hand has been lost, which fairly seldom occurs, one is only left with the possibility of amputating in the area of the lower arm. One then has the opportunity of using Krukenberg's arm, Sauerbruch's method or other more modern methods, of which the former, inspite of its unattractive appearance, has proved to be of good service. Much can be achieved, however, just with a prosthesis, if the propinator and supinator muscles are made use of, without taking into account more recent electronic developments.

Special Findings Concerning 3rd and 4th Degree Cold Injuries in the Toe and Foot Area

The first, second and fifth toes are considered to be particularly susceptible to injury. Isolated frostbite on the big toe alone or on the fourth toe alone occur more frequently. Sometimes cold damage to the first and fifth toes spreads in both cases to the tips of the neighbouring toes or, on the other hand, to the area of the metacarpo-phalangeal joint and the metatarsal head. Since the skin covering these areas is tense, necrosis and chronic ulcers occur, so that, as reported by Starlinger (1942), in about half of the cases, further skin grafts or amputations become necessary. These necroses and chronic ulcers should not therefore be left unattended but should be treated as early as possible. If the necrosis has reached the bone, the stumps will always be painful and will form hyperkeratotic scars which will grow together with the bone. These must be attended to as well. One should not be over-economical, but should make the decision to exarticulate a toe in the area of the metacarpo-phalangeal joint rather than to be content to nip off an end-phalanx, which may be insufficient. With such cold injuries the joints and the small muscles of the feet are usually damaged as well, which can later cause unpleasant defective positions (Figs. 82 and 84).

If all the toes have been lost, it is not necessary to adopt too tragic a view of the situation. With skillfully formed flaps from the volar side excellent stumps, which it is possible to walk with, can be quickly obtained (Figs. 85a and b). In the past it was believed that one could not manage without support from the distal condyle head of the first metatarsal. This has fortunately been proved to be wrong. It is, of course, still important even today to preserve it, but it can be sacrificed if a plastic closure of the stumps makes it necessary.

Starlinger (1942) rightly drew attention to the fact that the hard diaphyses of the toe bones tend to splinter. Sharp pieces of bone which are left behind have often led to lengthy inflammations and fistulae and so considerably delayed the healing process.

In the formation of metatarsal stumps and stumps of the calcaneal part of the foot we have learnt not to stick exclusively to the classic rules of amputation any longer, but

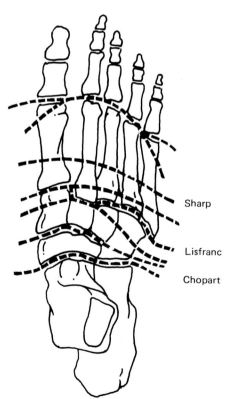

Sharp

Lisfranc

Chopart

Fig. 83. Established amputation lines for the preparation of forefoot and back of foot stumps after frostbite

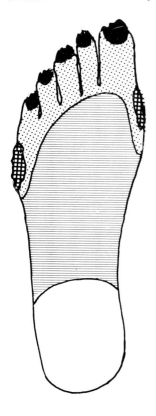

Fig. 84. Example of a poor stump. Shaded area: painful, frequently inflamed hyperkeratoses. Spontaneous stumpf after necroses of the distal phalanges (without operative correction). Hyperkeratoses, centres of irritation. Bad result after more than half a year of conservative treatment. The dead ossis (black) get free out of the open wounds. Early operative treatment could have reduced the time of treatment and healing to 1–2 months

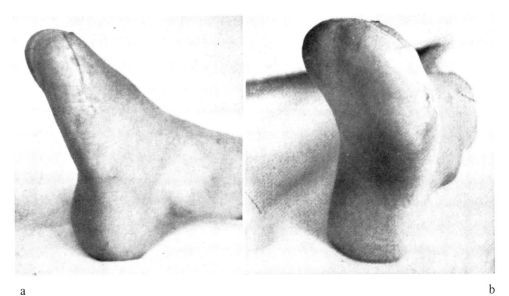

a   b

Fig. 85 a and b. Correctly prepared forefoot stump after frostbite (author's own case)

226

to act according to the needs of the situation. See our scheme of amputation rules which have proved good (Fig. 83). Before every amputation it must be remembered that the load capacity of the foot and the resistance of the stump can be considerably reduced by too close a resection and that this is therefore to be avoided (Boehler 1942; Killian 1942, 1946; Starlinger 1942; von Brandis 1943a, b and many others).

If the area which is becoming necrotic reaches as far as Lisfranc's joint the only possible solution then is usually to perform Chopart's amputation. Unfortunately it is then often no longer possible to close the end of the bone completely with a volar flap formation. The plantar soft parts which are left over are mostly too short. The decision must therefore be made in each individual case either to risk Chopart's amputation or to amputate straightaway above the ankle joint. In some cases we have risked Chopart's amputation and accepted the possibility from the start of having to graft to cover the stump, in order to be able to save part of the length of the foot. The resection was then made between the Lisfranc and Chopart joints. Here the anterior navicular articular surface is usually exposed, whereas the divisions are otherwise usually made in the spongy parts of the cuboid (Killian). This form of amputation is better than the Chopart stump, since the valuable os naviculare remains intact with all its tendon insertions (Fig. 86).

Judgement ot the Chopart stump has always been a controversial matter. Zurverth's rejection of it was met with heavy criticism as early as 1942, and attention was drawn to a series of excellent results. The reason for this rejection was the discovery that most Chopart stumps finish up in an equinovarus position, so that the patients are barely able

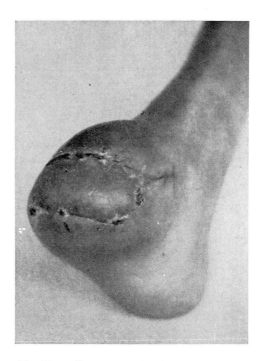

Fig. 86. Stump graft, which was performed to avoid a Pirogoff stump. Author's own case, shortly after completion of the graft after amputation close to the Chopart joint owing to frostbite necroses

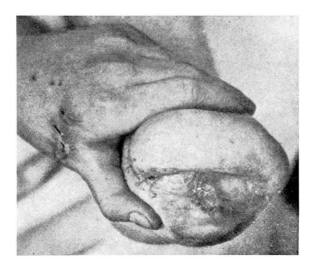

Fig. 87. Lower-leg roll-flap graft with intermediary siting on the left hand in order to cover a short lower-leg stump after frostbite with the aim of preserving the knee joint. Status after double implantation of the roll graft before unrolling. (Author's own case)

to walk on them. The cause of the shift to this taliped equinal position is the predominance of the gastrocnemius tibial group together with the total loss of the extensor traction and of the peroneal reins. The causes of most poor results are of a technical nature. The extensor tendons and the peroneal group must be given new points of attachment after amputation. Heller (1908), as the result of his vast experience, also strongly advised surgeons to sew on the tendons. According to statistical data, provided by Schüller (1915), Möllenhauer, Watermann and others, on-third of the Chopart stumps, which could not be used, and as many as about half of the Pirogoff stumps had to be amputated again in the area of the lower leg.

If the demarcation line reaches around the vicinity of Chopart's joint the decision must be made either to perform one of the many variations of Pirogoff's amputation or to amputate at once in the lower leg area. The bad experience of many surgeons with the original Pirogoff stump unfortunately resulted in the lower leg amputation being used far too often. The formation of any kind of Pirogoff stump is dependent on the state of the calcaneus. The method cannot be used if cold necrosis, extending as far as the bones, is present (Fig. 88 a, b).

The dissatisfaction with the original Pirogoff method found clear expression in the creation of a series of alternatives and variations of the technique, (see here our plan with the modifications according to Esmarch, Faure, Whiteman and Heller, Killian, Lorenz, Aberle and Spitzy). Today Aberle and Spitzy's methods are considered to be the best, since they never omit to amputate the protruding parts of the ankle joint.

In the opinion of orthopaedic specialists stumps according to Pirogoff, Syme, Chopart or Sharp are good. The original Pirogoff stump has been completely abandoned in favour of the modification according to Spitzy. If Chopart and Lisfranc stumps are to be at all usable, it is necessary to fix the tendons of the extensor digitorum to the lateral edge of the stump and to join the tendon of the tibialis ant, to the tendon of the peroneus longus subperiostal between the cuniforms 11 and 111 (Scagliotti and

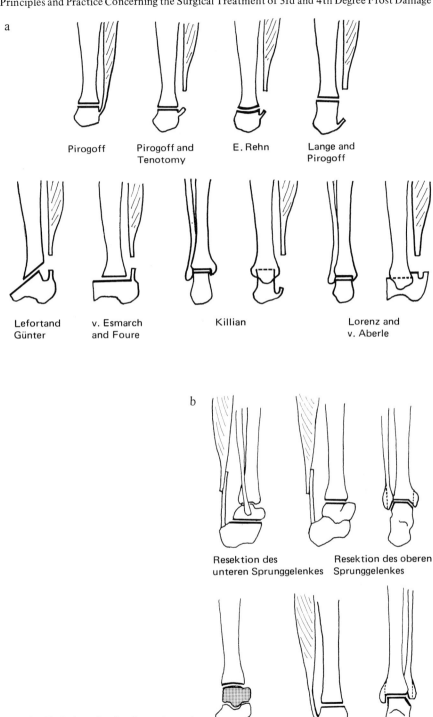

a

Pirogoff

Pirogoff and Tenotomy

E. Rehn

Lange and Pirogoff

Lefortand Günter

v. Esmarch and Foure

Killian

Lorenz and v. Aberle

b

Resektion des unteren Sprunggelenkes

Resektion des oberen Sprunggelenkes

Spitzy

Fig. 88 a and b. Variations in the formation of stumps for the calcaneal part of the foot according to Pirogoff

Todnitz). For more detailed data see Lange's monograph (1962). In the case of Chopart's stumps it is necessary to fix the extensor tendons to the Talus and to lenghten the Achilles tendon.

Isolated heel necrosis, which causes deep-seated, chronic ulcers and can penetrate far into the bones, is very unpleasant. The entire area which is poorly supplied with blood with adequate osseous lamellae from the calcaneus must be amputated. If the wound is healing well, a very simple, firm, petiolated skin graft from the calf or the thigh area according to Becker, or some other common graft can be made (Fig. 89).

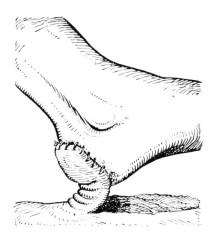

Fig. 89. Schemata of a simple heel graft for a localised necrosis of the heel (From Becker)

Remarks on the Follow-up Treatment and Orthopaedic Care of Local Cold Injuries

When the cold injury stump has healed the problems of follow-up treatment must be faced, so that the functioning of the limb can be maintained or encouraged as far as possible.

One cannot begin early enough with active movement of the fingers, the hands, the feet and the toes. It should already start during surgical treatment. These gymnastic exercises indirectly stimulate the circulation. Active movement during the critical period is of much more value than passive. In a warm bath the exercises are easier and better results ensured.

Almost all surgeons have made do with provisional plaster or felt boots of various kinds until an orthopaedic shoe has been fitted. These should be constructed in such a way that they first of all overcompensate the defective position to be expected for the stump in question, (e.g. Chopart stump).

Up as far as about the middle of the cuboid the treatment of the cold injury stump should be taken care of solely with orthopaedic shoes. Otherwise a proper prosthesis would have to be made.

Starlinger (1942), White and Scoville (1945) have stressed the fact that the *psychological aspect* of the post-operative treatment of such cold damage should not be neglected, since some patients exhibit an almost hysterical fear of using the sensitive limbs again. This can unfortunately become a habit and may conceal the desire for some sort of pension. Successful, suggestive treatment is, however, only possible if the stump and the tissue are well supplied with oxygen and free from ulceration. As long as the patient can still see the very smooth, bluish skin or ulcers, he will not believe that his condition is going to improve, his psychological attitude will change and he will consider himself unfit for work and expect to be pitied.

References

Abramson DJ (1944) Monograph. university of Chicago Press, Chicago
Adams RJ (1941) Acta Chir Scand 85:1
Adams RJ (1942a) Nord Med 915
Adams RJ (1942b) Bull Var Med 915
Adams RJ (1944) Acta Chir Scand 89:527
Adams RJ (1952) 2nd Conference on Cold Injuries. Josuah Macy Jr Foundation
Adams RJ (1956) Nord Med 56:1581
Adams RJ, Clemenson CJ (1944) Acta Chir Scand 89:527
Adams RJ, Falconer R (1951) Acta Chir Scand 101:269
Ariev TV (1937) Vestn Khir 52:63
Ariev TV (1939a) Vestn Khir 57:527
Ariev TV (1939b) Sov Krad Zhur 43:391
Ariev TV (1940) Kälteschäden, 2nd edn. Moscow
Ariev TV (1950) Klin Med (Mosc) 28:3,15
Barber (1926) Zentralbl Haut- und Geschlechtskrankh 23:57
Bellander G (1940a) Svensk Lag Tidn 37:487
Bellander G (1940b) Z Org Chir 107:488
Bernett P (1979) Med Forum 21:9
Bigelow GW (1942) Can Med Assoc J 47:523
Blain A (1951) Alexander Blain Hosp Bull 10:18
Blanke KV (1942) Dtsch Mil Arzt 7:735
Block W (1942) Arch Klin Chir 1:64,67
Block W (1943) Zentralbl Chir 70:1691
Boehler L (1942) Berichte der beratenden Ärzte
Bohnstedt RM (1932) Dermatol Wochenschr 2:1211
Bonika JJ (1953) Management of pain. Lea & Febiger, Philadelphia
Brack W (1940) Schweiz Med Wochenschr 40:948
Brack W (1941) Zentralbl Chir 107:848
Brambel CE, Locker FF (1944) Arch Surg 48:1
Brandis HJ von (1943a) Vorträge aus der praktischen Chirurgie, vol 27. Encke, Stuttgart
Brandis HJ von (1943b) Broschüre über Kälteschäden. Encke, Stuttgart
Breitner B (1944a) Dtsch Z Chir 259:273
Breitner B (1944b) Chirurg 16:8
Brooks B, Duncan GW (1940) Am Surg 112:130
Buckreus F (1941) Med Welt 15:347
Bundschuh E (1918) Munch Med Wochenschr 155
Campbell K, Lyon R, Berg R, Suttler M, Blain A (1946) Hosp Bull 5:108
Campbell R (1932) Schweiz Med Wochenschr 62:1153
Campbell R (1966) Vierteljahresschr Schweiz Sanitätsoffiz 43:20
Campbell R (1977) Report. V. Internationale Tagung der Bergrettungsärzte. Werk, p 73
Canty J, Sharf AG (1953) Ann Surg 138:65
Caputo B (1941) Med Contemp Tor 7:428
Celice, Duchessney, Pelizier (1942) Presse Med 50:627
Chalinot P, Benichon R, Guibal P (1954) Med Nancy 79:817
Chien S (1967) Physiol Rev 47:14
Crismon HJ, Fuhrmann FA (1946) Science 104:408
Crismon HJ, Fuhrmann FA (1947) J Clin Invest 259, 268, 286

Crul JF (1970) Symposium über Bupivacain, Bad Oeynhausen
Crul JF (1971) Brochure. Thieme, Stuttgart
Davis L, Scarff JE, Rogers N, Dickinson M (1943) Surg Gynecol Obstet 77:561
Debrunner H (1941) Report of the military surgeon on 26 cases of frostbite encountered while on ski maneuvres: In: Klinik und Behandlung der örtlichen Erfrierungen. Huber, Bern, p 128
Dogos, Gresset, Bonyguess (1941) Bull Soc Fr Dermatol 48:1246
Douglas WM (1952) Mil Surg 110:333
Edholm OG (1952) Practitioner 168:583
Entin MA, Baxter H (1952) Plast Reconstr. Surg 13:227
Entin MA, Schultz GA, Baxter H (1954) Anaesthesiology 5:486
Erikson U, Ponton B (1974) Injury 6:150
Fievez J (1939) Prog Med 67:1326
Finneran J, Shumaker HB (1950) Surg Gynecol Obstet 90:430
Fishman J (1951) US Armed Forces Med J 2:957
Floerken H (1914) Bruns Beitr Klin Chir 106:4
Floerken H (1915) Munch Med Wochenschr 7
Floerken H (1920a) Zentralbl Chir 47:1651
Floerken H (1920b) Die Kälteschäden im Krieg. Springer, Berlin (Ergebnisse der Chirurgie und Orthopädie)
Friedrich PH (1914) Munch Med Wochenschr 129
Frommel E, Piequet J (1946) Arch Int Pharmacodyn Ther 73:96
Fuhrmann FA, Crismon HJ (1947) J Clin Invest 26:229, 236, 245, 476
Gerlach F (1943) Zentralbl Chir 70:1337
Gerulanos M (1944) Bruns Beitr Klin Chir 93:487
Girgolaw SS (1943) Klin Naja 21:3
Glenn W, Maraist F, Braaten O (1952) N Engl J Med 247:191
Gödecke R (1971) Therapiewoche-Berichte 21:3632
Goldhahn R (1943a) Ther Gegenw 84:50
Goldhahn R (1943b) Med Welt 15:1173
Grassmann W (1933) Fortschr Ther 179
Greene R (1941) Lancet 689
Greene R (1942) Lancet 695
Greziller A (191) Medical dissertation, Paris
Guerasimenko NJ (1950) Klinika i letchneie otmorogeniy, vol 1. Moscow
Häussler H (1943) Munch Med Wochenschr 90:301
Harkins HH, Harmon PH (1937) J Clin Invest 14:213
Hartwich A (1940) Munch Med Wochenschr 603
Hartwich A (1941a) Med Klin 283
Hartwich A (1941b) Wien Med Wochenschr 2
Haydukievicz J (1977) Report. V. Internationale Tagung der Bergrettungsärzte. Werk, p 61
Heaton LD, Davis RM (1952) J Ky Med Assoc 50:206
Heller F (1908) Z Dermatol 630
Hempel (1930) Zentralbl Chir 51:3131
Hempel (1931) Zentralbl Chir 58:1467
Hempel (1933) Dtsch Z Chir 238:736
Heyde W (1941) Fortschr Ther 17:230
Hirsch WD, Phelbs W, Flora S (1977) Report. V. Internationale Tagung der Bergrettungsärzte. Werk, p 27
Höflin FG (1977) Report. V. Internationale Tagung der Bergrettungsärzte. Werk, p 25
Hofheinz S (1943) Berichte der beratende Chirurgen
Holmes TW Jr (1948) Alexander Blain Hosp Bull 7:12
Hurley LA, Roberts EJ, Buchanan AR (1951) Surg Gynecol Obstet 92:303
Hurley LA, Roberts EJ, Buchanan AR (1952) Surg Gynecol Obstet 95:423
Hussel H (1977) Report. V. Internationale Tagung der Bergrettungsärzte. Werk, p 61
Isaacson NH, Harrel JB (1953) Surgery 33:6,810
Jamin F (1943) Zentralbl Chir 70:54
Judmaier F (1952a) Munch Med Wochenschr 94:255
Judmaier F (1952b) Wien Klin Wochenschr 64:100
Jung A, Fell H (1942a) Dtsch Z Chir 285:244
Jung A, Fell H (1942b) Bull War Med 3:219
Kettelkamp DB, Walker M, Ramsay D (1971) Cryobiologie 8:79

Kettler D, Hellberg K, Kaess G, et al. (1976) Anaesthesist 25:132
Killian H (1942) Zentralbl Chir 1763
Killian H (1946) Dtsch Gesundheitswes 3:6
Killian H (1959) Wehrmed Mitt 3:11
Killian H (1966) Der Kälteunfall: Allgemeine Unterkühlung. Dustri
Killian H (1972) Lokalanästhesie, 2nd edn. Thieme, Stuttgart
Killian H, Vogt M, Hemmer, Koch (1946) Z Dtsch Gesundheitswes 3/6:129,176,206
Kirschner H (1917) In: Borchardt A, Schmieden (eds) Kriegschirurgie
Kiyaschev AP (1944) Klin Med (Mosc) 22:25
Klövekorn WP, Laks L, Pilon RN, Anderson WP, Maccalum J, Moore D (1973) Eur Surg Res (Suppl) 2:27
Klövekorn WP, Pichlmaier H, Ott E, Bauer H, Sunder-Plassmann L, Jesch F, Messmer K (1975) Bibl Haematol 41:248
Koehler H (1916) Virchows Jahresber Gesamte Med
Koehler H (1921) Veroeffentl Militaersanitaetswes 76
Kreyberg L (1949) Physiol Rev 29:156
Kronecker (1886) Korrespondenzblatt Schweiz Aerzte
Kühnau WW (1939) Arch Dermatol 179:322
Kukin NN (1941) Ark Biol Nauk 1:21
Kutschera-Aichen, Bergen (1943) Wien Klin Wochenschr 13:260
Kyösola K, Trasima J (1974) J Trauma 24:32
Laewen A (1942a) Dtsch Mil Arzt 7:479
Laewen A (1942b) Zentralbl Chir 69:1253
Laewen A (1944) Dtsch Med Wochenschr 70:141
Lake NC (1917) Lancet 2:557
Lange K, Loewe L (1946) Surg Gynecol Obstet 82:256
Lange K, Weiner D, Boyd L (1947) N Engl J Med 237:383
Lange K, Boyd L, Weiner D (1950) Proc Soc Exp Biol Med 74
Lange K, Davis D, Meyer WM (1955) J AM Physiol 181:675
Lange M (1962) Orthopädische Chirurgie. Bergmann, Munich
Larrey JD (1817) Meomoires du chirurgie militaire et de campagne, vol 4. Paris
Laufmann H (1951) JAMA 147:1201
Lee JA, et al. (1959) Synopsis of anaesthesia, 4th edn, chap 27
Leitner E, Kronberger E (1977) Aerztl Prax 29:983
Lempke HF, Shumaker HB (1949) Yale J Biol 21:321
Leriche R (1940) Presse Med 48:75
Leriche R (1945) In: Physiologie pathologique et traitement chirurgical des maladies artérielles de la vasomotricité. Masson, Paris, p 65
Leriche R, Kunlin J (1940) Mem Acad Chir 66:14,196
Lewis RB (1951) USA AFS AM-Report No 21-28016
Lewis RB (1952) Mil Surg 110:25
Lewis RB, Loewe L (1926) Heart 13:27
Lewis RB, Moen PW (1953) Surg Gynecol Obster 97:59
Lippert F (1936) Dermatol Wochenschr 102
Lisbona R, Rosenthal (1976) J Trauma 16:286
Lloyd E, et al. (1972) Scott Med J 17:73
Lippros (1942) Z Klin Med 3:140
Loos HO (1941a) Zentralbl Chir 10:449
Loos HO (1941b) Med Klin 37:54,84
Macht M, Bader M, Meat (1949) J Clin Invest 28:5646
Mallet-Guy P, Lieffring JJ (1940) Zentralbl Chir 98:491
Martinez A, Golding M, Surajer PN, Weslowski SA (1966) Cardiovasc Surg 7:495
Matais H (1942) Dtsch Mil Arzt 7:153
Mayer AW, Kohlschütter R (1914) Dtsch Z Chir 127:518
Meiding F, Kolsky M (1953) J Physiol (Lond) 45:182
Messmer K (1972) Anaesthesiol Wiederbeleb 60:149
Messmer K (1975) Surg Clin North Am 55/3:659
Messmer K (to be published) lecture held at the "Mittelrheinischer Chirurgenkongreß", Basel 29 Aug 1977
Messmer K, Sunder-Plassmann L (1973) Prog Surg 13:208
Messmer K, Sunder-Plassmann L, Klövekorn WP, Holper K (1971) Adv Microcirc 4:1

Michelson F (1944) Zentralbl Chir 71:997
Monseignon A (1940a) Presse Med 48:166
Monseignon A (1942b) Zentralbl Chir 18
Moser H (1942) Dtsch Med Wochenschr 68:549
Movrey FH, Farago PJ (1952) Mil Surg 110:249
Mundt EO, Long DM, Brown RB (1964) J Trauma 4:246
Nösske K (1910) Report. Chirurgenkongreß, Berlin
Nowack C (1942) Arch Med Chir 11:17
Orloff GO (1937a) Z Org Chir 89:353
Orloff GO (1937b) Z Org Chir 82:650
Orr KD, Fainer DC (1952) US Armed Forces Med J 3:95
Osipovski J (1935) Z Org Chir 76:318
Paunesco-Podeanu A, Tzurai I (1946) Kälteschäden. Masson, Paris
Pernato G (1941) Rif Med 57:177
Peter K, Lutz H (1975) Bibl Haematol 4:210
Philippowicz J (1942) Zentralbl Chir 69:1369
Pichotka J, Lewis RB, Freytag E (1949) Proc Soc Exp Biol Med 72:130
Pichotka J, Lewis RB, Freytag E (1951a) Texas Rep Biol Med 9:613
Pichotka J, Lewis RB, Ulrich HH (1951b) USA AFS AM-Report No 3
Pierau FK, Olesch K, Klüssmann FW (1965) Pflügers Arch 284:301
Plath-Franke F (1939) Dtsch Med Wochenschr 40
Pratt GH (1953) Gen Pract 7:34
Quintanilla R, Krusen FH, Essex HE (1947) Am J Physiol 149:149
Rahn BA, Höflin FG, Perras SH (1977) Aerztl Prax (Suppl) 41
Ratschow M (1953) Periphere Durchblutungsstörungen, 5th edn. Steinkopff, Berlin
Raymond V, Parisot J (1918) J Chir (Paris) 14:329
Reigber P (1945) Medical dissertation, Breslau
Revesz (1929) Zentralbl Chir 5
Ring J, Messmer K (1977) Anaesthesist 26:279
Rein H (1943) Lehrbuch der Physiologie. Springer, Berlin
Saltner L (1940) Dtsch Mil Arzt 5:123
Salzer O (1930) Z Org Chir 48:529
Sapin-Jaloustre J (1956) Enquêtes sur les gélures. Herman, Paris
Sauerbruch F, Jung H (1942a) Mil Arzt 477
Sauerbruch F, Jung H (1942b) Chirurg 267
Sauerbruch F, Jung H, Klapp R (1944) Dtsch Z Chir 258:319
Schaalf (1951) Aerztl Prax 3:5
Schleicher J, Gligore (1946) Zentralbl Kreislaufforsch 35:489
Schneider M (1949) Verh Dtsch Ges Kreislaufforsch 202
Schüller A (1915) Munch Med Wochenschr 62:1542
Schürer, F von (1942) Zentralbl Chir 69:486, 1797
Shanka CA (1975) Med J Aust 2/9:346
Shumaker HB, Lempke RE (1951) Surgery 30:873
Shumaker HB, Radigan LR, Zipermann HR (1951) Angiology 2:100
Siegmund H (1942a) Munch Med Wochenschr 827
Siegmund H (1942b) Arbeitstagung beratender Ärzte, Berlin
Siegmund H (1942c) Arch Dermatol 184:84
Simon R, Filhoulaud H (1940) Mem Acad Chir (Paris) 66:359
Simon R, Filhoulaud H (1941) Zentralbl Chir 103
Singer (1940) Wien Klin Wochenschr 53:462
Spiegelberger M, Flora G, Hölzl R, Margreiter R (1977) Report. V. Internationale Tagung der Berg-
    rettungsärzte. Werk, p 78
Starlinger F (1942) Zentralbl Chir 69:1179
Starlinger F, Frisch OW (1944) Die Erfrierungen. Steinkopff, Berlin
Stefanutti P (1941a) Zentralbl Chir 5
Stefanutti P (1941b) Policlinico 48:626
Sullivan B, Masterson W (1953) Am J Physiol 175:56
Sunder-Plassmann L, Klövekorn WP, Holper K, et al. (1971) Report. 6th European Conference on
    Microcirculation, Aalberg 1970. Karger, Basel, p 23
Sunner DS, Boswick JA, Cribley F (1971) Surgery 69:849
Talbott JH (1952) Trans Assoc Am Physicians 65:316

Tantini E, Baggio (1941a) Z Org Chir 107:294
Tantini E, Baggio (1941b) Clinica 7:549
Tantini E, Baggio (1941c) Ann Ital Chir 20:613
Telford ED (1943a) Br Med J 4315
Telford ED (1943b) Br Med J 2:360
Theiss F, O'Connor WB, Wahl FJ (1951) JAMA 146:992
Thorban W (1962) Bruns Beitr Klin Chir 207:87
Tonutti (1940) Z Mikrosk Anat Forsch 52:32
Ullmann (1932) In: Handbuch der Haut- und Geschlechtskrankheiten, vol 171, p 4
Vagliano M (1948) Erfrierungen. Masson, Paris
Vischnevskij AV (1931) Ark Biol Nauk 62:3
Wagner K (1915) Wien Klin Wochenschr 28:1385
Weatherley-White RCA, Knize DM, Geishofer DJ, Oatan BC (1969) Surgery 60:208
Webster DR, Woolhouse FH, Johnston JL (1942) J Bone Joint Surg 24:785
Weltz GA, Wendt HJ, Ruppin H, Werz R (1942a) Munch Med Wochenschr 25:1092
Weltz GA, Wendt HJ, Ruppin H, Werz R (1942b) Zentralbl Chir 1775
Weltz GA, Wendt HJ, Ruppin H, Werz R (1942c) Luftfahrtmedizin 25:12
Weltz GA, Wendt HJ, Ruppin H, Werz R (1943) Arch Exp Pathol 202:561
White JC, Scoville WB (1945) N Engl J Med 232:415
Whitelaw HJ, Woodman TJ (1950) J Clin Endocrinol 10:1171
Witteck A (1915) Munch Med Wochenschr 12
Wobker W (1940) Dtsch Med Wochenschr 66:1265
Wright JS, Allan EV (1943) Bull US Army Med Dept 65:136
Wright JS, Moffat D (1934) JAMA 103:318
Zicker-Sieber Therapie der Hautkrankheiten
Zink RA, Schaffer W, Lutz M, Bernett P, Messmer K (1977) Report. Angiologische Tagung,
    September 1977

Index of Names

Subject Index

247

Disaster Medicine

Editors: R. Frey, P. Safar
Sub-Editor: P. Baskett, K. Stosseck, P. Sands,
J. Nehnevajsa

Volume 1

Types and Events of Disasters Organization in Various Disaster Situations

Proceedings of the International Congress on Disaster
Medicine, Mainz 1977
Part I
Editors: R. Frey, P. Safar

1980. 97 figures, 33 tables. XX, 355 pages
ISBN 3-540-09043-6

Contents: Types and Events of Disasters. Definition of
Disasters. – Organization in Various Disaster Situations
(Local, Regional, National). – Workshops: Global
Disaster Situations. Local/Regional Disaster Situations.
Definite Care in Disaster Situations.

Volume 2

Resuscitation and Life Support in Disasters Relief of Pain and Suffering in Disaster Situations

Proceedings of the International Congress on Disaster
Medicine, Mainz 1977
Part II
Editors: R. Frey, P. Safar

1980. 81 figures, 52 tables. XIX, 280 pages
ISBN 3-540-09044-4

Contents: Resuscitation and Life Support in Disasters. –
Relief of Pain and Suffering in Disaster Situations. –
Workshops: Resuscitation. Intravenous Fluids. Relief of
Pain and Suffering. Free Topics.

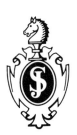

Springer-Verlag
Berlin
Heidelberg
New York

Acute Care

Based on the Proceedings of the Sixth International Symposium on Critical Care Medicine

Editors: B. M. Tavares, R. Frey
1979. 133 figures, 97 tables. XVI, 345 pages
(Anaesthesiology and Intensive Care Medicine, Volume 116)
ISBN 3-540-09210-2

Critical Care Medicine Manual

Editors: M. H. Weil, P. L. DaLuz
1978. 73 figures, 48 tables. XXIV, 371 pages
ISBN 3-540-90270-8

Endocrinology in Anaesthesia and Surgery

Editors: H. Stoeckel, T. Oyama
1980. 101 figures, 45 tables. XI, 203 pages
(Anaesthesiology and Intensive Care Medicine, Volume 132)
ISBN 3-540-10211-6

D. A. B. Hopkin

Hazards and Errors in Anaesthesia

1980. 5 figures, 2 tables. X, 298 pages
ISBN 3-540-10158-6

W. S. McDougal, C. L. Slade, B. A. Pruitt, Jr.

Manual of Burns

Medical Illustrators: M. Williams, C. H. Boyter, D. P. Russell
1978. 214 color figures, 4 tables. X, 165 pages
(Comprehensive Manuals of Surgical Specialties)
ISBN 3-540-90319-4

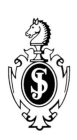
Springer-Verlag
Berlin
Heidelberg
New York